Pediatric Neuro-oncology

Katrin Scheinemann • Eric Bouffet

Editors

Pediatric
Neuro-oncology

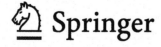 Springer

Editors
Katrin Scheinemann
Associate Professor of Pediatrics
Division of Hematology/Oncology
Department of Pediatrics
McMaster Children's Hospital
McMaster University
Hamilton, ON, Canada

Eric Bouffet
Garron Family Chair in Childhood
   Cancer Research
Department of Hematology/Oncology
The Hospital for Sick Children
University of Toronto
Toronto, ON, Canada

ISBN 978-1-4939-1540-8   ISBN 978-1-4939-1541-5 (eBook)
DOI 10.1007/978-1-4939-1541-5
Springer New York Heidelberg Dordrecht London

Library of Congress Control Number: 2014954085

Printed on acid-free paper

Springer is part of Springer Science+Business Media (www.springer.com)

To our patients and their families who teach
us the essence of life every day:
Do not look back in the past or plan for the future;
live life to the fullest today!

Foreword

Pediatric Neuro-Oncology is undergoing a rapid transformation within all of its key disciplines. Rapid advances in our understanding in the biology of medulloblastoma, pontine glioma, low-grade and high-grade glioma, ependymoma, embryonal tumors abundant neuropil and true rosettes (ETANER), and atypical rhabdoid teratoid tumor (ATRT) have ushered in a new era of clinical and molecular diagnostics. Modern treatment approaches are being introduced into the clinic based on this advanced understanding of tumor biology, and current treatment approaches are being modified to the clinical and biological risk so as to reduce the long-term toxicity for patients with good prognosis.

Newer imaging techniques along with availability of intraoperative MRI have facilitated surgical resections that one could only have wished for a few decades ago. Sophistication in radiation treatment planning and the gradual availability of proton beam radiation therapy hold the promise of decreased long-term morbidity in children treated with focal radiation therapy.

A better understanding of the pathophysiology of the damage to the developing brain caused by current therapies has allowed neuropsychologists to initiate intervention studies that seek to mitigate the damage and provide the children with coping mechanisms.

Emerging interest in studying the quality of life and symptom burden in this patient population has led to refined end-of-life care. The editors, Drs. Scheinemann and Bouffet, and their Canadian team of coauthors have done an outstanding job of presenting this complex information in a lucid manner—this book is a must-read for the global community of aspiring students and neuro-oncology practitioners.

Amar Gajjar, MD
Member, St. Jude Faculty, Scott and Tracie Hamilton
Endowed Chair in Brain Tumor Research Co-Chair,
Department of Oncology Interim Chair,
Department of Pediatric Medicine Director, Neuro-Oncology Division
Co-Leader, Neurobiology & Brain Tumor Program
St. Jude Children's Research Hospital
Memphis, TN, USA

Preface

Over the past decades the numbers of long-term survivors of pediatric brain tumors have increased. It was quickly recognized that this was influenced by modified multimodal treatment for which a multidisciplinary team was needed. In lots of large pediatric oncology units, specialized teams focused on pediatric neuro-oncology were created to take care of the complexity of these patients. Survivorship of this group also comes with significant long-term sequelae which have to be taken care of.

The purpose of this book is to provide a comprehensive practical, clinical, and research overview for pediatric neuro-oncology. It also emphasizes the role of national study groups as this book is authored by the members of the Canadian Pediatric Brain Tumor Consortium that involves many disciplines.

We would like to thank our chapter authors for their ideas, time, and knowledge devoted for this project.

We hope that this textbook will provide answers and guidance for healthcare professionals in this complex and challenging however fascinating field.

Hamilton, ON, Canada   Katrin Scheinemann
Toronto, ON, Canada   Eric Bouffet

Contents

Contributors

Samina Afzal, MBBS, FCPS, FRCPCH (UK) Department of Pediatrics, Division of Oncology, IWK Health Centre, Halifax, NS, Canada

Alaa Alkhotani, MD Department of Laboratory Medicine and Pathobiology, University of Toronto, Toronto, ON, Canada

Nisreen Amayiri, MD Department of Pediatrics, King Hussein Cancer Center, Amman, Jordan

Ali Amid, MD Department of Pediatrics, Division of Hematology/Oncology, Children's Hospital of Eastern Ontario, University of Ottawa, Ottawa, ON, Canada

Ute Bartels, MD Department of Hematology/Oncology, The Hospital for Sick Children, Toronto, ON, Canada

Kelsey C. Bertrand, MD Department of Developmental and Stem Cell Biology, The Hospital for Sick Children, Toronto, ON, Canada

Karina L. Black, BScN, MN, NP Pediatric Oncology Program, Stollery Children's Hospital, Edmonton, AB, Canada

Eric Bouffet, MD Department of Hematology/Oncology, The Hospital for Sick Children, University of Toronto, Toronto, ON, Canada

Anne-Sophie Carret, MD Department of Pediatrics, Division of Hematology/Oncology, CHU Sainte-Justine/Université de Montréal, Montréal, QC, Canada

Pierre-Olivier Champagne, MD Department of Neurosurgery, Hôpital Notre-Dame/Université de Montréal, Montréal, QC, Canada

Jennifer A. Chan, MD Department of Pathology & Laboratory Medicine, University of Calgary, Calgary, AB, Canada

Tiffany Sin Yu Chan, BSc Department of Cell Biology/Arthur and Sonia Labatt Brain Tumor Research Centre, The Hospital for Sick Children, Toronto, ON, Canada

Anne-Marie Charpentier, MD, FRCPC Department of Radiation Oncology, CHUM Notre-Dame Hospital, Montréal, QC, Canada

Louis Crevier, MD, MSc, FRCSC Department of Neurosurgery, Centre Hospitalier Universitaire de Sainte-Justine, Montréal, QC, Canada

Phedias Diamandis, MD, PhD Department of Laboratory Medicine and Pathobiology, University of Toronto, Toronto, ON, Canada

David D. Eisenstat, MD, MA, FRCPC Department of Pediatrics, Medical Genetics and Oncology, Stollery Children's Hospital, University of Alberta, Edmonton Clinic Health Academy, Edmonton, AB, Canada

Benjamin Ellezam, MD, PhD Department of Pathology, CHU Sainte-Justine, Université de Montréal, Montréal, QC, Canada

Adam J. Fleming, MASc, MD, FRCP(C) Division of Hematology/Oncology, The Montreal Children's Hospital (McGill University Health Center), Montréal, QC, Canada

Adriana Fonseca, MD Department of Pediatrics, McMaster Children's Hospital, Hamilton, ON, Canada

Carolyn Freeman, MBBS, FRCPC, FASTRO Department of Radiation Oncology, McGill University Health Centre, Montréal, QC, Canada

Sharon L. Guger, PhD Department of Psychology, The Hospital for Sick Children, Toronto, ON, Canada

Cynthia E. Hawkins, MD, PhD, FRCPC Department of Paediatric Laboratory Medicine, The Hospital for Sick Children, Toronto, ON, Canada

Annie Huang, MD, PhD Department of Cell Biology, The Hospital for Sick Children, Toronto, ON, Canada

Juliette Hukin, MBBS, FRCPC Division of Neurology and Oncology, British Columbia Children's Hospital, Vancouver, BC, Canada

Nada Jabado, MD, PhD Department of Pediatrics, McGill University Health Center/McGill University, Montréal, QC, Canada

Laura Janzen, PhD Department of Psychology, The Hospital for Sick Children, Toronto, ON, Canada

Donna L. Johnston, MD, FRCPC, FAAP Department of Pediatrics, Division of Hematology/Oncology, Children's Hospital of Eastern Ontario, University of Ottawa, Ottawa, ON, Canada

Daniel L. Keene, BSc (Med), MD, MA, FRCPC Department of Pediatrics, Children's Hospital of Eastern Ontario, Ottawa, ON, Canada

John-Paul Kilday, MBChB, MRCPCH, PhD Pediatric Brain Tumor Program, Department of Hematology/Oncology, Hospital for Sick Children, Toronto, ON, Canada

Anne-Marie Laberge, MD, PhD Medical Genetics Division, Department of Pediatrics, Université de Montréal, Montréal, QC, Canada

Lucie Lafay-Cousin, MD, MSc Department of Pediatrics, Division of Oncology, Alberta Children's Hospital, Calgary, AB, Canada

Joan Lee, BScPhm Department of Pediatrics, Division of Hematology/Oncology, McMaster Children's Hospital, Hamilton, ON, Canada

Victor Anthony Lewis, MD Department of Pediatrics, Alberta Children's Hospital, Calgary, AB, Canada

Donald Mabbott, BA, MA, PhD Department of Psychology, The Hospital for Sick Children, Toronto, ON, Canada

Stephen C. Mack, BSc Department of Developmental and Stem Cell Biology, The Hospital for Sick Children, Toronto, ON, Canada

Patrick J. McDonald, MD, MHSc, FRCSC Department of Neurosurgery and Pediatrics, Winnipeg Children's Hospital, University of Manitoba, Winnipeg, MB, Canada

Vivek Mehta, MD, MSc Division of Neurosurgery, Department of Surgery, Stollery Children's Hospital/University of Alberta, Edmonton, AB, Canada

Claude Mercier, MD, FRCSC Department of Neurosurgery, Centre Hospitalier Universitaire de Sainte-Justine, Montréal, QC, Canada

Diana Merino, BSc Department of Genetics and Genome Biology, The Hospital for Sick Children, Toronto, ON, Canada

Sami Obaid, MDCM Department of Neurosurgery, Centre Hospitalier Universitaire de Sainte-Justine, Montréal, QC, Canada

Lisa Pearlman, RN(EC) NP-P, BAMN, ACNP Department of Paediatric Symptom Management & Supportive Care, Children's Hospital London Health Sciences Centre, Victoria Hospital, London, ON, Canada

Annie-Jade Pépin, PhD Department of Hematology/Oncology, CHU Sainte-Justine, Université de Montréal, Montréal, QC, Canada

Sebastien Perreault, MD Division of Child Neurology, Lucile Packard Children's Hospital, Stanford University, Palo Alto, CA, USA

Department of Pediatrics, Division of Neurology, CHU Sainte-Justine/Université de Montréal, Montréal, QC, Canada

David Phillips, BASC (Eng), MScSS, MD, FRCSC Department of Neurosurgery, University of Manitoba, Winnipeg, MB, Canada

Vijay Ramaswamy, MD, FRCPC Division of Neurosurgery, Hospital for Sick Children, Toronto, ON, Canada

Shahrad Rod Rassekh, MD, MHSc Division of Pediatric Oncology, Department of Pediatrics, British Columbia's Children's Hospital, Vancouver, BC, Canada

Marc Remke, MD Department of Laboratory Medicine and Pathobiology, The Hospital for Sick Children, Toronto, ON, Canada

Luciana Torres Ribeiro, MD, MSc, PhD, FRCPC, ABR Department of Radiology, Hamilton General Hospital, McMaster's Children's Hospital, McMaster University, Hamilton, ON, Canada

David Roberge, MD, FRCPC Department of Radiation Oncology, CHUM Notre-Dame Hospital, Montréal, QC, Canada

Pierre Rousseau, MD Department of Radiation Oncology, CHUM Notre-Dame Hospital, Montréal, QC, Canada

Katrin Scheinemann, MD Division of Hematology/Oncology, Department of Pediatrics, McMaster Children's Hospital, McMaster University, Hamilton, ON, Canada

Patrick Sin-Chan, MSc Arthur and Sonia Labatt Brain Tumour Research Centre, The Hospital for Sick Children, Toronto, ON, Canada

Ash Singhal, MD, FRCS(C) Department of Pediatric Neurosurgery, University of British Columbia, BC Children's Hospital, Vancouver, BC, Canada

Tara Spence, MSc Department of Cell Biology, The Hospital for Sick Children, Toronto, ON, Canada

Nina Rodrigues Stein, MD, MSc Department of Diagnostic Imaging, McMaster University Hamilton Health Sciences, Hamilton, ON, Canada

Douglas R. Strother, MD Departments of Oncology and Pediatrics, Section of Oncology and Blood and Marrow Transplant, Cumming School of Medicine and Alberta Children's Hospital, Calgary, AB, Canada

Serge Sultan, PhD Department of Hematology/Oncology, CHU Sainte-Justine, Université de Montréal, Montréal, QC, Canada

Uri Tabori, MD Department of Hematology/Oncology, The Hospital for Sick Children/Institute of Medical Sciences, University of Toronto/The Arthur and Sonia Labatt Brain Tumour Research Centre, Toronto, ON, Canada

Michael D. Taylor, MD Department of Developmental and Stem Cell Biology, The Hospital for Sick Children, Toronto, ON, Canada

Jonathon Torchia, MSc Department of Lab Medicine and Pathobiology, Labatt's Brain Tumour Centre, SickKids, University of Toronto, Toronto, ON, Canada

Magimairajan Issai Vanan, MD, MPH, FAAP Departments of Pediatrics and Child Health, Oncology and Cell Biology, Cancer Care Manitoba, Manitoba Institute of Cell Biology, University of Manitoba, Winnipeg, MB, Canada

Xin Wang, BHSc (Hon) Department of Developmental and Stem Cell Biology, The Hospital for Sick Children, Toronto, ON, Canada

Beverly A. Wilson. BMSc, MD, FRCPSC Department of Pediatrics, Division of Hematology/Oncology, University of Alberta, Edmonton, AB, Canada

Kory Zayne, BSc Department of Developmental and Stem Cell Biology, The Hospital for Sick Children, Toronto, ON, Canada

Shayna Zelcer, BSc, MD Department of Pediatrics, Children's Hospital, London Health Sciences Center, London, ON, Canada

Introduction

Katrin Scheinemann and Eric Bouffet

Pediatric CNS tumors are the most common solid malignancy in childhood and the most common cause of cancer-related mortality and morbidity in this age group.

The diagnosis and treatment of these tumors have undergone significant improvement over the last decades, starting with the implementation of modern imaging techniques like computer tomography (CT) in 1972 and magnetic resonance imaging (MRI) in 1977. Since 1985 MRI has become widely available in tertiary care centers.

Given the significance of imaging, neurosurgeons are able to achieve more precise preoperative planning and they have progressively introduced new techniques such as stereotactic surgery, neuronavigation, neuroendoscopy, and more recently convention-enhanced delivery.

Neuropathology has moved from an essentially morphology-based approach to a sophisticated discipline using a battery of immunohistochemical markers. An increasing number of tumor subtypes have been identified, which has been reflected in updated

K. Scheinemann, M.D. (✉)
Division of Hematology/Oncology, Department of Pediatrics, McMaster Children's Hospital, McMaster University, Hamilton, ON, Canada
e-mail: kschein@mcmaster.ca

E. Bouffet, M.D.
Department of Hematology/Oncology, The Hospital for Sick Children, University of Toronto, Toronto, ON, Canada

versions of the World Health Organization (WHO) classification of tumors of the nervous system—the last version being published in 2007 and a new one is currently planned.

Adjuvant treatment options have been implemented started from stereotactic and conformal radiation to chemotherapy to high dose chemotherapy with stem cell rescue to targeted treatment.

Over the last three decades pediatric neurooncology has become a subspecialty within pediatric oncology. The treatment of pediatric CNS tumors requires an interdisciplinary approach with early and ongoing communication between all involved disciplines.

As the number of long-term survivors is growing, the issue of long-term sequelae has been clearly recognized. In return, this awareness increasingly influences up-front treatment decision depending on several factors such as tumor biology and age. Pediatric neurooncology program requires dedicated and specialized aftercare clinics that focus on prevention, early recognition, and management of long-term sequelae (see Table 1.1).

National and international working groups (in particular the CNS tumor committee of the Children's Oncology Group and the International Society of Paediatric Oncology) have collaborated to advance care of these patients and perform epidemiological as well as basic science and treatment research studies. The recent years have seen an explosion of knowledge thanks to collaborative research efforts by several groups

Table 1.1 Involved disciplines for a comprehensive pediatric neurooncology. Depending on the model, the neurooncologist, the neurosurgeons, or the radiation oncologist may be the team leader

Neurooncology (chair)	Case managers/nurses
Neurosurgery (chair)	Social work
Neuroradiology	Physiotherapy
Neuropathology	Occupational therapy
Radiation oncology (chair)	Dietician
Neuroophthalmology	Social work
Endocrinology	Child life
Neurology	Career counseling
Neuropsychology	Pharmacy
BMT oncologist	Research associate

around the world, including in Canada. Progress in molecular biology has provided new insight into this group of tumors and allowed identification of molecular target. Recent advances in genomics of pediatric CN tumors have transformed the research landscape in neurooncology and we can expect major changes in the management of these tumors in the coming years.

The aim of this comprehensive textbook is to highlight all aspects of the epidemiology, the diagnosis, the biology, the treatment, the follow-up as well as the long-term outcomes of the most common pediatric central nervous system tumors.

Presentation of Central Nervous System Tumors

2

Ali Amid, Daniel L. Keene, and Donna L. Johnston

Introduction

The clinical diagnosis of central nervous system (CNS) tumors can be challenging. There are no truly pathognomonic signs or symptoms of CNS tumors. This can lead to delay in diagnosis as often the initial signs and symptoms are mistaken for other childhood conditions such as migraine, behavioral problems, or gastroenteritis [1]. This is often further complicated by the inability of children to fully describe their symptoms early on in the disease process. The age of the child at the time of presentation complicates matters further. For this reason, physicians must have a high index of suspicion for CNS tumors in the appropriate clinical setting. A careful history of the presenting complaint, including growth and developmental milestones, and an age-appropriate neurologic examination are the key initial steps in making the diagnosis of tumors of the CNS.

A. Amid, M.D. • D.L. Johnston, M.D., F.R.C.P.C., F.A.A.P.
Department of Pediatrics, Division of Hematology/
Oncology, Children's Hospital of Eastern Ontario,
University of Ottawa, Ottawa, ON, Canada

D.L. Keene, B.Sc. (Med), M.D., M.A., F.R.C.P.C. (✉)
Department of Pediatrics, Children's Hospital of
Eastern Ontario, Ottawa, ON, Canada
e-mail: DKeene@cheo.on.ca

The clinical presentation of CNS tumors is variable. In some situations, when invasion of the brain is involved, the symptoms are localized. In this situation the symptoms depend on the region of the brain involved. In other situations, the clinical presentation will be nonspecific or diffuse secondary to increased intracranial pressure or pressure on adjacent brain structures. It also varies with the age of the child. Symptoms can vary from acute, subacute, or chronic in nature [2].

The evaluation of the patient with a suspected tumor of the CNS begins with a focused history and physical examination. Based on the information obtained, a clinical localization of the most probable location of the tumor can be made and appropriate confirmatory investigations considered.

The CNS is divided into three main compartments: the spinal cord, the infratentorial region, and the supratentorial region. The infratentorial region includes the brainstem and the cerebellum, while the supratentorial region included the cerebral hemispheres, thalami, basal ganglion, diencephalon, optic tracts/chiasmatic region, and the pituitary fossa. The presentation varies with the region involved.

Infratentorial Tumors

Tumors involving the infratentorial region are more common than those involving the supratentorial region in children. They can arise either in

K. Scheinemann and E. Bouffet (eds.), *Pediatric Neuro-oncology*,
DOI 10.1007/978-1-4939-1541-5_2, © Springer Science+Business Media New York 2015

3

the brainstem or the cerebellum. The clinical presentation differs based on the region in which the tumor arises.

Tumors involving the cerebellum often present in a subtle manner. As the tumor grows, it blocks the flow of cerebral spinal fluid (CSF) through the fourth ventricle. As the brain parenchyma, CSF, and blood are enclosed by a rigid skull and the skull cannot expand to accompany the increase in CSF, increased intracranial pressure (ICP) occurs. The initial presentation of raised ICP often consists of morning headaches occurring upon awakening [3]. The headache may or may not initially be associated with effortless, projectile vomiting. When the child has been standing or sitting for a few minutes, the symptoms can significantly decrease as a result of reestablishment of CSF flow due to the effect of gravity and change in position of the tumor mass. Though headaches are common in children, early morning headache with vomiting, an intense headache or one that awakens the child from sleep, a headache that worsens with cough, defecation or Valsalva maneuver, and the presence of papilledema on fundoscopy should alert the physician of possibility of a cerebellar tumor [1, 4, 5].

Increased ICP can also be associated with non-localizing palsy of the sixth (abducens) cranial nerve, impaired light reflex, and a head tilt. The abducens nerve innervates the ipsilateral lateral rectus muscle which abducts the eye. It has the longest intracranial course of all the cranial nerves and is usually the first nerve affected by elevated ICP. Symptoms include binocular horizontal diplopia which is worst at distance and esotropia. In order to minimize diplopia, children may tilt their head to reduce double vision. A more extreme presentation of rapidly rising ICP consisting of a decreased level of consciousness or Cushing's triad (elevated blood pressure, bradycardia, and irregular respiration) is uncommon. In these situations, a rapidly growing tumor of the midline brainstem or posterior fossa should be suspected and immediate intervention is critical [3].

Cerebellar signs such as clumsiness in movements, speech, dysmetria, and nystagmus often occur late and are more common in tumors that involve the cerebellar hemispheres. Truncal ataxia, when present, suggests that the cerebellar vermis is involved.

Brainstem tumors present in a different manner. Increased intracranial pressure, if it occurs at all, occurs late. As the brainstem contains the cranial nerve nuclei and the motor long tracts, cranial nerve palsies with or without motor difficulties are common at presentation. The motor difficulties can be hemiparesis, monoparesis, tetraparesis, or quadriparesis.

Cranial neuropathies are another common presentation of brainstem tumors. Abnormalities of extraocular movements are common findings. Diplopia and head tilt suggest impairment of cranial nerve IV or cranial nerve VI. Involvement of other cranial nerves may cause facial weakness, hearing loss, abnormal corneal or gag reflex, or difficulties with swallowing [1].

Supratentorial Tumors

Supratentorial tumors include tumors of the cerebellar hemispheres, basal ganglia, and thalamus and hypothalamus regions (gliomas); ventricular neoplasms (choroid plexus papillomas and ependymomas); parasellar tumors (craniopharyngiomas, optic pathway gliomas, germinomas); and other less common tumors such as pinealomas. In addition to raised intracranial pressure, supratentorial tumors often present with localizing symptoms and signs. These symptoms are generally related to the location of the tumor and can vary from indolent progression to an acute presentation based on the tumor growth rate.

A focal seizure can be a common presenting symptom of a tumor involving the cerebral hemisphere. As a rule, seizures do not occur in patients with infratentorial tumors [3]. Depending on the site of the tumor, the pattern of seizure may be different and occasionally identification of patient's symptoms based on seizure is challenging, especially in infants and toddlers. The seizures are often resistant to standard antiepileptic drug therapy.

Supratentorial tumors may involve any part of the optic pathway and cause visual complaints.

The pattern of visual symptoms and signs secondary to these tumors is different from those of infratentorial and brainstem tumors. Tumors of the optic nerve anterior to the optic chiasm (e.g., optic gliomas) produce a unilateral monocular visual deficit. *Marcus Gunn pupil* or relative afferent pupillary defect is a finding associated with tumors of the optic nerve or optic chiasm and indicates a relative afferent pupillary defect. During the swinging-flashlight test, the patient's pupils dilate when the light source is moved from the unaffected eye to the affected eye. The test may also indicate retinal disease. These patients may also have proptosis and strabismus. Patients with a diagnosis of optic pathway gliomas should be screened for signs of neurofibromatosis type I as they are commonly associated with this syndrome [6].

Suprasellar tumors may also cause various forms of visual field defects as well as decreased visual acuity commonly referred as chiasmal syndrome. Anterior lesions may cause *junctional scotoma*. *Bitemporal hemianopsia* (visual loss of temporal half of both left and right visual fields) represents lesions of the body of chiasm while paracentral bitemporal field loss and contralateral *homonymous hemianopsia* (visual field loss on the same side of both eyes) can be signs of posterior chiasmal lesions. Other symptoms of posterior chiasmal tumors include nystagmus in a younger child or pituitary endocrinopathies more commonly in patients older than 4 years of age [7]. Hemianopsia can also be observed in more dorsal tumors that affect the optic tract, lateral geniculate nucleus, optic radiations, or occipital cortex.

Depending on the site of brain lesion, patients may present with other symptoms such as hemiparesis, hemisensory loss, or aphasia. Thalamic *Dejerine–Roussy syndrome* (a pain syndrome with poor localization of stimuli) may be seen in patients with thalamic tumors, but sensory-motor deficits are more frequent findings [8]. Children with frontal lobe tumors may have behavioral problems. *Parinaud's syndrome* (also known as dorsal midbrain syndrome) is characterized by upward gaze palsy, abnormal pupillary responses, retraction of eyelids (Collier's sign), and retraction nystagmus. This is a pathognomonic feature of pineal region tumors and is usually associated with endocrinopathies. Patients may exhibit more than one type of dysfunction and up to one third of these patients will also have visual symptoms associated with involvement of the optic chiasm, due to proximity of the optic chiasm to the hypothalamic region [9].

Hormonal abnormalities can also occur, the most common of which is growth hormone deficiency, resulting in short stature, followed by sex hormone dysfunction manifested as precocious or delayed puberty. However, almost every pituitary hormone system can be affected by a tumor. These abnormalities may precede the diagnosis of a brain tumor by months to years. It is imperative that patients with chiasmal lesions have a complete endocrinology evaluation and their baseline hormone levels should be checked and followed by an endocrinologist [7].

Behavioral and sleep disturbances also can occur in hypothalamic tumors. *Diencephalic syndrome* is a rare but potentially lethal finding which includes failure to thrive and emaciation but a normal linear growth and an increased appetite, a euphoric mood, hyperkinesis, and occasionally macrocephaly, nystagmus, and visual deficits. This syndrome predominantly affects younger children who have hypothalamic or optic pathway gliomas [10].

Spinal Tumors

Primary tumors of the spine in children are uncommon. They account for only 2 % of childhood malignancies. As in intracranial tumors, the timing and pattern of clinical presentation vary based on the child's age and children are frequently symptomatic for long time before diagnosis. In children older than 4 years of age, the most common symptom is *back pain* which can be the presenting symptom in up to two thirds of patients. Realizing that back pain is always abnormal in children is paramount in the diagnosis of primary spinal tumors or other solid tumors with intraspinal invasion (e.g., neuroblastoma) as well as other spinal pathologies such as infections.

Any child with continued back pain unresponsive to analgesics should be investigated with appropriate imaging. The pain may fluctuate in intensity and is commonly worse when lying down and at night. The absence of abnormal neurologic findings does not exclude tumors of the spine. In contrast, in adolescents, paraspinal pathologies (mostly musculoskeletal) may be the cause of the back pain; however, associated neurological findings make paraspinal processes more likely. Other symptoms of spinal tumors may include *scoliosis* or *kyphosis* or in the cervical region, *torticollis*. Suspicion for spinal tumors should be high if spinal deformity is associated with pain or if there is a rapid increase in spinal curvature.

The most common neurologic symptoms of spinal tumors are gait disturbances, loss of fine motor skills, or regression in motor milestones. Gait abnormality can be difficult to differentiate from more common and normal developmental variations such as in-toeing or transient tip-toeing. The progressive nature of changes in spinal tumors can be a helpful hint to the underlying diagnosis. Other deficits include sensorimotor (weakness, numbness, pain) or bowel and bladder dysfunctions (like incontinence, dysuria, or constipation). Muscle atrophy and abnormal muscle reflexes are also commonly seen. As a general rule, these manifestations should be interpreted based on the complete knowledge of neuroanatomy and neurophysiology. Horner syndrome may also be observed in spinal tumors in the cervico-thoracic region [3, 11, 12].

CNS Tumors in Infants

The presentation of CNS tumors in the neonatal group is varied and differs from those of children. Infants are unable to articulate their symptoms, so the presenting features are generally vague and include irritability, poor feeding, emesis, failure to thrive, hypotonia, regression of acquired milestones, apneic episodes, and other nonspecific symptoms. Most infants will have symptoms with indolent progression for a long duration prior to diagnosis. As well, in infants the fontanels are not closed and any enlargement of an intracranial mass or development of hydrocephalus will be compensated with increased head circumference. As a result, symptoms of increased ICP and papilledema or headache are not common presenting features of intracranial tumors in infants. Macrocrania (a head circumference in excess of that appropriate for patient's height and weight, or crossing growth percentiles), full and budging fontanels, splayed sutures, prominent veins on the scalp, and sunset eyes are the most common presenting signs, observed in up to two thirds of infants with CNS tumors. Cranial nerve deficits or other focal motor deficits as well as seizures are uncommon presenting signs, although seizures can occur. *Spasmus nutans* characterized by the triad of pendular nystagmus, head nodding, and head tilt suggests chiasmatic tumors [1, 3, 13].

Syndromes Associated with Brain Tumors

Several genetic syndromes are associated with an increased risk of development of brain tumors in children. Physicians should be familiar with the clinical signs of these syndromes. If a child is diagnosed with one of these syndromes, regular surveillance for a tumor of the CNS is warranted.

The presence of *café au lait spots*, axillary freckling, *Lisch nodules* of the iris, neurofibromas, and bony abnormalities suggests *neurofibromatosis type 1* (NF-1). Optic pathway glioma is commonly seen in these patients and regular monitoring with physical exam including assessment of visual fields and acuity is warranted [6]. The role of regular imaging in these patients is controversial as the majority of optic pathway gliomas in these patients are asymptomatic and they may regress without any interventions.

Tuberous sclerosis is another autosomal dominant genetic disorder resulting in hamartomatous lesions in different organs. Seizures, developmental delay, and adenoma sebaceum are among its clinical symptoms. These patients are at increased risk of subependymal giant cell astrocytoma and malignant gliomas [2, 14].

Cancer predisposing syndromes such as *Li–Fraumeni syndrome* may be initially diagnosed with non-CNS malignancies, and brain tumors may occur later [2].

Patients with *bilateral retinoblastoma* are at risk of developing tumors of the pineal region. Close follow-up of these patients and special attention to a detailed history and neurological exam help in the timely diagnosis of associated CNS tumors [2].

Conclusion

While CNS tumors are rare in children and adolescents, their diagnosis poses difficulties and the majority of the patients are symptomatic for a long period of time prior to their diagnosis. Presentation of a child with any potential symptoms or signs of brain tumors should lead to a careful assessment including a systematic enquiry for associated symptoms, complete physical examination, including detailed neurologic exam. Knowledge of neuroanatomy and the clinical course of CNS tumors are essential for timely diagnosis. Once a CNS tumor is within the differential diagnosis, appropriate diagnostic imaging must be undertaken to confirm or exclude its presence.

References

1. Blaney SM, Haas-Kogan D, Young Poussaint T, et al. Gliomas, ependymomas, and other nonembryonal tumors of the central nervous system. In: Pizzo P, Poplack DG, editors. Principles and practice of pediatric oncology, vol. 26A. 5th ed. Philadelphia: Lippincott Williams & Wilkins; 2011. p. 717–71.
2. Fleming AJ, Chi SN. Brain tumors in children. Curr Probl Pediatr Adolesc Health Care. 2012;42:80–103.
3. Wilne S, Collier J, Kennedy C, et al. Presentation of childhood CNS tumours: a systematic review and meta-analysis. Lancet Oncol. 2007;8:685–95.
4. Newton RW. Childhood headache. Arch Dis Child Educ Pract Ed. 2009;93:105–11.
5. Lewis DW, Qureshi F. Acute headache in children and adolescents presenting to the emergency department. Headache. 2000;40:200–3.
6. Listernick R, Charrow J, Greenwald M, Mets M. Natural history of optic pathway tumors in children with neurofibromatosis type 1: a longitudinal study. J Pediatr. 1994;125:63–6.
7. O'Kelly DJ, Rutka JT. Optic pathway gliomas. In: Berger MS, Prados MD, editors. Textbook of neuro-oncology. St Louis: Elsevier Saunders; 2005. p. 579–86.
8. Souweidane MM. Thalamic gliomas. In: Berger MS, Prados MD, editors. Textbook of neuro-oncology. St Louis: Elsevier Saunders; 2005. p. 579–86.
9. Packer RJ, Rorke-Adams LB, Lau CC, et al. Embryonal and pineal region tumors. In: Pizzo P, Poplack DG, editors. Principles and practice of pediatric oncology, vol. 26B. 5th ed. Philadelphia: Lippincott Williams & Wilkins; 2011. p. 772–808.
10. Fleischman A, Brue C, Poissant TY, et al. Diencephalic syndrome: a cause of failure to thrive and model of partial growth hormone resistance. Pediatrics. 2005;111:e742.
11. Wilne S, Walker D. Spine and spinal cord tumours in children: a diagnostic and therapeutic challenge to healthcare systems. Arch Dis Child Educ Pract Ed. 2010;95:47–54.
12. Walton KA, Buono LM. Horner syndrome. Curr Opin Ophthalmol. 2003;14:357.
13. Hwang SW, Su JM, Jea A. Diagnosis and management of brain and spinal cord tumors in the neonate. Semin Fetal Neonatal Med. 2012;17:202–6.
14. Krueger DA, Care MM, Holland K, et al. Everolimus for subependymal giant-cell astrocytomas in tuberous sclerosis. N Engl J Med. 2010;363:1801–11.

Epidemiology of Central Nervous System Tumors

3

Daniel L. Keene and Donna L. Johnston

Introduction

When a child is diagnosed with a tumor of the central nervous system, parents often search for answers as to why this has happened to their child; how it could have been prevented; how long their child will survive; are other members of the family at risk; is treatment available and if available, does it work; and what are the side effects. Epidemiology provides the scientific framework to start to answer these questions. This is done by providing information about the occurrence of a condition in relation to the factors about the individual, their environment, and their lifestyle.

Epidemiological studies begin by describing the condition/disease (i.e., number of persons, their sex, their age at the time of onset, where they had lived, their lifestyle, the duration of the disorder in question, any interventions done). Studies examining a causal relationship between the condition/disease and the personal characteristics or prior exposures follow the description of the condition/disease. Based on the information gained from these studies, interventions to control, treat, or prevent the condition/disease are developed and tested.

This chapter provides the basic information to answer the above questions. It includes the global descriptive epidemiology of tumors of the central nervous system (CNS), changes in the reported survival rates, and possible environmental factors. As interventional studies will be covered in other chapters of this book, they are not covered in this chapter.

Descriptive Epidemiology

Overall, tumors of the CNS in children are more prevalent amongst males (1.29:1 male to female ratio). They tend to be slightly more frequent in the infratentorial region than supratentorial region [1]. However, for children under three years of age, tumors more frequently occur in the supratentorial region (59 %) [2]. It has been reported that the most common histological diagnoses are astrocytoma (37.6 %), medulloblastoma (17.7 %), ependymoma (9.9 %), craniopharyngioma (7.3 %), and germ cell tumors (4.4 %) [1]. This distribution, however, varies with age. The distribution of cases with a histological diagnosis of ependymoma or medulloblastoma decreases with age. Both account for a greater percentage of diagnoses in patients under

D.L. Keene, B.Sc. (Med), M.D., M.A., F.R.C.P.C.
Department of Pediatrics, Children's Hospital of Eastern Ontario, Ottawa, ON, Canada

D.L. Johnston, M.D., F.R.C.P.C., F.A.A.P. (✉)
Department of Pediatrics, Division of Hematology/ Oncology, Children's Hospital of Eastern Ontario, University of Ottawa, Ottawa, ON, Canada
e-mail: djohnston@cheo.on.ca

K. Scheinemann and E. Bouffet (eds.), *Pediatric Neuro-oncology*,
DOI 10.1007/978-1-4939-1541-5_3, © Springer Science+Business Media New York 2015

4 years of age than in older age groups. In contrast, the percentage of cases of astrocytoma is fairly constant across the pediatric age groups.

Incidence Rate

Determining an exact incidence figure for the occurrence of tumors of the CNS can be confusing. Varying estimates have been reported depending on the source of the data, the age in question, and the time period used. What is known about the incidence of childhood tumors of the CNS has been obtained using information from regional or national databases. Caution must be taken in the interpretation of these figures. Much of the data that has been reported regarding primary brain and CNS tumors has been limited to primary malignant tumors. Less often have nonmalignant tumors been included. Often only summary estimates of tumor location and histology are provided. The histological classifications can be different between geographic locations and have also changed over time. A lack of agreement on diagnostic criteria and the small size of available tissue mean that the histological diagnoses are infrequently confirmed by a second review. As well, the ages used often have varied between reported studies. The populations from which the cases are drawn have varied, with varied degrees of completeness. This has resulted in a variation of the reported incidence rates of tumors of the CNS between the populations under study and the time period of interest.

Despite these limitations, the reported incidence rates have been similar. For example, in the United States, there are principally three large, centralized databases: the National Cancer Data Base (NCDB), the Central Brain Tumor Registry of the United States (CBRTRUS), and the Surveillance, Epidemiology, and End Results (SEER) database [3]. Each covers a different population base. The NCDB is sponsored by the American College of Surgeons and the American Cancer Society. The case ascertainment is derived from hospital-based follow-up of all primary tumors from institutions accredited by the American College of Surgeons. The collection of

data on malignant tumors is mandatory for each participating hospital as part of its accreditation; however, data collection for benign tumors is voluntary. Though it can provide valuable information on diagnosis and outcome, it was not designed to provide estimates of incidence rates. However, annually the American Cancer Society, Centers for Disease Control and Prevention, the National Cancer Institute, and the North American Association of Central Cancer Registries collaborate to provide incidence rates in the United States. For the period 1992, the reported overall incidence was 4.8 per 100,000 children [4]. For the same period, CBTRUS, a population-based registry which draws data from several regional registries in the United States reported an incidence rate of 3.76 per 100,000 persons [5]. In comparison, SEER, a population-based national cancer registry program funded by the National Cancer Institute, reported an incidence rate of 3.5 per 100,000 [6]. For the same time period, the European incidence rate for persons 14 years or less was reported to be 2.9 per 100,000 [7]. However, within Europe, the incidence figures have varied. Denmark, based on the Danish Cancer Registry, Danish Hospital Discharge diagnosis, and clinical databases from major Danish centers, had an incidence rate of 3.95 per 100,000 population years [8]. In Germany, a rate of 2.6 per 100,000 children under age of 15 years was reported. This figure was based on data obtained from a tumor registry involving130 pediatric hospitals and centers for pediatric oncology in Germany [9]. For the same time period, the Japanese incidence was reported as 3.43 per 100,000 children [10].

The incidence of tumors changes with age; however, this has differed between registries. Kaatsch et al. [9] noted that the incidence rate in German children less than 1 year of age was 2.7 per 100,000 compared to 3.1 per 100,000 for children between the ages of 1–4 years, 2.7 per 100,000 children between the ages of 5–9 years, and 2 per 100,000 children between the ages of 10–14 years. For a similar time period, Kuratsu et al. [10] reported the age-specific Japanese annual incidence rates to be 2.43 per 100,000 for the 0–4-year age group, 4.67 per 100,000 for the

4–9-year age group, and 3.08 per 100,000 for 10–14-year age group. This difference is most likely due to the different mix of tumors between the two populations of children; specifically the number of cases of germ cell tumors was different (0.1 per 100,000 incidence rate in the German cohort compared to 0.6 per 100,000 in the Japanese cohort). In both cohorts, germ cell tumors were not reported in patients under 4 years of age; however, germ cell tumors accounted for approximately one third of the tumors in the older children.

The question has been raised as to whether incidence figures have increased over time. In 1973 SEER reported an annual incidence rate of 2.4 per 100,000 children; however, in 1994, as previously mentioned, SEER reported the annual incidence rate to be 3.5 per 100,000 children, which was a significant difference. The change was reported not to have occurred at a constant rate, but rather "jumped" from a relatively constant rate prior to 1985 to a higher rate [11]. It was felt that this jump in incidence rate was a reflection of better diagnostic imaging technology (i.e., the introduction of magnetic resonance imaging). Raaschou-Nielsen et al. [8] also reported an increase in the incidence rate for the period 1980–2006 in Denmark (3–5 per 100,000 population years); however, the increase occurred at a constant rate rather than in jump fashion. This increase was present across all the age groups. However, another Nordic country study using the national tumor registries in Denmark, Norway, Sweden, and Finland along with the Nordic Society of Pediatric Hematology and Oncology database for the period 1984–2005 did not find a time trend [12].

Survival Rates

The survival rates are dependent on the tumor type, location of the tumor, and age at the time of diagnosis. For example, patients with supratentorial low-grade astrocytomas which are completely resected do well, having an expected 5-year survival of greater than 90 %, whereas patients with diffuse brain stem tumors and ana-

plastic astrocytomas do poorly with an expected 5-year survival of less than 20 %. Children under one year of age do not do as well as older children (i.e., ~45 % 5-year survival for children less than 1 year of age compared to greater than 70 % for children over 10 years of age). The 5-year survival rates for childhood CNS tumors, however, have improved over time (59 % in 1984 compared to 67 % in 1994). This improvement has been driven mostly by improved patient risk stratification and treatment protocols [11].

Possible Risk Factors

The etiology of tumors of the CNS is not fully understood. A small number of children will have a strong genetic predisposition for tumor development. For example, the risk of cancer in children with neurofibromatosis, tuberous sclerosis, nevoid basal cell cancer, Turcot syndrome, and Li–Fraumeni syndromes has been known for some time. The risk of cancer in these syndromes is associated with mutations in known developmental biological pathways resulting in deregulation of the natural cell life cycle. For example, in neurofibromatosis type 1, this is related to the NF1 gene, a tumor repressor gene. Mutations in this gene result in changes to the gene product, neurofibromin, which plays a role in the down-regulation of p21-ras which is an essential signal transduction molecule for several tyrosine growth factor receptors [13]. Yet, not every person with neurofibromatosis will develop the same type of tumor at the same age.

For most children, the cause of a CNS tumor is not clear. It is likely to be the result of a complex interaction between the child's genetic background and specific environmental exposure(s). Gene copy number aberrations, structural arrangements, and/or deregulation of the number transcriptome have been found to contribute to tumors occurring in children in the absence of underlying genetic syndromes [14]. For example, in tumor tissue from children with medulloblastoma, deregulation of the Shh, Wnt, NOTCH, MYC family, PDGF/MAPK, and p53 signalling pathways has been reported. Similarly in tumor tissue from children with ependymoma, NOTCH, EGFR signalling pathway, and MYC family have been found [14]. What causes these changes in normal tissue to occur is not completely understood. Epidemiological studies have been used to attempt to identify possible causal relationships that might play a role in tumor genesis [15]. Risk factors that have been suggested to be associated with a greater risk of development of a CNS tumor include race, a family history of prior fetal loss/birth defects/brain tumors/cancer/mental retardation, father's occupation/exposures to N-nitroso compounds, maternal dietary history particularly as related to cured meat consumption, maternal age at the time of conception of the child, birth order, increased head circumference at birth, increased birth weight, exposure to infectious disease in the first year of life, exposure to pesticides/irradiation, history of prior head injuries, and more recently prolonged use of mobile telephones [11]. However, the rarity of tumor occurrence, variability of age of onset, and the retrospective nature of the cohort case study designs have made the finding of a definite etiological agent difficult.

References

1. Rickert C, Paulus W. Epidemiology of central nervous system tumors in childhood and adolescence bases on the new WHO classification. Childs Nerv Syst. 2001;17:503–11.
2. Balestrini MR, Micheli R, Giordano L, et al. Brain tumors with symptomatic onset in the first two years of life. Childs Nerv Syst. 1994;10:104–10.
3. Davis FG, McCarthy BJ, Berger MS. Centralized databases available for describing primary brain tumor incidence, survival and treatment: Central Brain Tumor Registry of the United States; Surveillance, Epidemiology and End Results; and National Cancer Data Base. Neuro Oncol. 1999;1:205–11.
4. Kohler B, Ward E, Mc Carthy B, et al. Annual report of the nation on the status of cancer, 1975–2007, featuring tumors of the brain and other nervous system. J Natl Cancer Inst. 2011;103:714–36.
5. Suarwicz T, McCarthy B, Kupelian V, et al. Descriptive epidemiology of primary brain and CNS tumors: results from the Central Brain Tumor Registry of the United States 1990–1994. Neuro Oncol. 1999;1:14–25.
6. Bishop A, McDonald M, Chang A, et al. Infant brain tumours: incidence, survival and the role of radiation based on surveillance, epidemiology, and end results (SEER) data. Int J Radiat Oncol Biol Phys. 2012;82:347.
7. Peris-Bonet R, Martinez-Garcia C, Lacour B, et al. Childhood central nervous system tumours- incidence and survival in Europe (1978–1997): report from automated childhood cancer information system project. Eur J Cancer. 2006;42:2064–80.
8. Raaschou-Nielsen O, Sorensen M, Cartensen H, et al. Increasing incidence of childhood tumours of the central nervous system in Denmark, 1980–1996. Br J Cancer. 2006;95:416–22.
9. Kaatsch P, Rickert C, Kuhl J, et al. Population-based epidemiological data on brain tumors in German children. Cancer. 2001;92:3155–64.
10. Kuratsu J, Ushio U. Epidemiological study of primary intracranial tumors in childhood. Pediatr Neurosurg. 1996;25:240–7.
11. Bleyer W. Epidemiologic impact of children with brain tumors. Childs Nerv Syst. 1999;15:758–63.
12. Schmidt L, Schmiegelow K, Lahteenmake P, et al. Incidence of childhood central nervous system tumors in Nordic countries. Pediatr Blood Cancer. 2011;56:65–9.
13. Spyk S, Thomas N, Cooper D, et al. Neurofibromatosis type 1 tumours: their somatic mutational spectrum and pathogenesis. Hum Genomics. 2011;5:623–90.
14. Dubuc A, Northcott P, Mack S, et al. The genetics of pediatric brain tumors. Curr Neurol Neurosci Rep. 2010;10:215–23.
15. Baldwin R, Preston-Martin S. Epidemiology of brain tumors in childhood—a review. Toxicol Appl Pharmacol. 2004;199:118–31.

Pediatric Neuroimaging

Nina Rodrigues Stein and Luciana Torres Ribeiro

Introduction

Neuroimaging is a key tool in the diagnosis and follow-up of neuro-oncologic patients. Magnetic resonance imaging (MRI) and computerized tomography (CT) are the main imaging modalities involved in neuroimaging diagnosis of these patients. However, MRI is the main imaging tool in the daily practice of pediatric neuro-oncology. The main reason is that CT involves radiation exposure risks and MRI has the ability to show significant more details about the brain parenchyma.

PET (positron emission tomography) and molecular imaging are rapidly developing as new techniques to evaluate brain tumor. The results provided by PET and molecular imaging appear to corroborate the findings of MRI studies and may contribute to decision-making in the treatment and follow-up of patients. Therefore understanding general principles of different imaging modalities can help the clinician to improve patient care.

N.R. Stein, M.D., M.Sc. (✉)
Department of Diagnostic Imaging, McMaster University Hamilton Health Sciences,
Hamilton, ON, Canada
e-mail: steinnina@hhsc.ca

L.T. Ribeiro, M.D., M.Sc., Ph.D., F.R.C.P.C., A.B.R.
Department of Radiology, Hamilton General Hospital, McMaster's Children's Hospital, McMaster University, Hamilton, ON, Canada

CT Principles

Neuroimaging is essential for diagnosis of both primary and secondary central nervous system (CNS) neoplasms, and magnetic resonance imaging (MRI) remains the main imaging modality for characterization of these lesions. However, computerized tomography (CT) is often used in patients with acute presentations. The two main reasons that CT may be preferred over MRI in cases presenting acutely are: faster image acquisition than MRI, within few seconds, and diagnostic images are accrued more rapidly, which is important if the patient's clinical status is unstable. In addition, there is rarely a need for sedation [1] and CT may often be more instantly available than MRI [2]. However, a downside of CT is the ionizing radiation exposure, of particular importance in children who are more sensitive to its effects than adults (Fig. 4.1) [3].

Radiation Safety

Biological radiation effects can be divided into two categories: stochastic and deterministic effects. Deterministic effects are set by exposure threshold, and doses above the cutoff cause damage (e.g., cataract occurs if the crystalline lenses are exposed above 5 Gy (gray is the radiation unit for absorbed dose of radiation)) [3]. Stochastic effects are the result of cumulative doses of radiation and are related to genetic abnormalities and

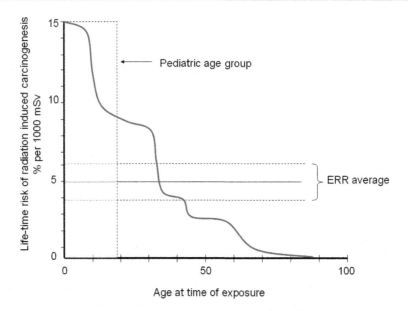

Fig. 4.1 The graphic demonstrates the increased carcinogenic risk related to radiation exposure for the pediatric population compared to the adult population. Reprinted from Peck DJ, Samei E. How to Understand and Communicate Radiation Risk. Image Wisely. Available at: http://www.imagewisely.org/Imaging-Professionals/ Medical-Physicists/Articles/How-to-Understand-and-Communicate-Radiation-Risk. Reprinted with permission of the American College of Radiology, Reston, Virginia. No other representation of this material is authorized without express, written permission of the American College of Radiology

carcinogenic effects. There are no safe levels of radiation exposure related to stochastic effects, and the cancer risk increases as cumulative doses increase [3].

Recently, Pearce et al. (2012) demonstrated the association of low doses of radiation administrated on CT with occurrence of brain tumors and leukemia in a pediatric population (Fig. 4.2). This was the first time that this association was proven, although previous publications based on information gathered from the survivors following atomic explosions had raised the concern about the use of low dose radiation in medical imaging modalities [4]. Therefore, extra care should be taken when requesting a CT scan in the pediatric population, weighing the risks and benefits for each case.

There are three principles of radiation safety that should be kept in mind when requesting and performing a CT examination: justification, optimization, and dose limitation (Table 4.1) [5].

The North American radiological societies have mounted campaigns in an effort to educate doctors and the general population regarding radiation effects and radiation safety. The most important radiation safety campaigns (Image Gently® for pediatric population (http://www. pedrad.org/associations/5364/ig/) and Image Wisely® for the adult population (http://www. imagewisely.org/)) have made optimization ("as low as reasonably achievable" (ALARA)) a very popular principle. However, justification is also very important, not only because it justifies the investigation, but also because it helps to decide which adjustments are necessary in the imaging technique in order to make the diagnosis.

There are several techniques that can be applied in CT imaging acquisition. For example, a patient who needs to have only the size of the cerebral ventricles assessed can have a study performed with low radiation exposure. In contrast, for brain parenchyma assessment, a scan with a regular radiation dose exposure is required to prevent artifacts related to low doses [6] (Fig. 4.3).

The clinical information provided in the request form also helps the radiologist to decide if the study requires contrast. For

Fig. 4.2 Relative risk of leukemia and brain tumors in relation to estimated radiation doses to the red bone marrow and brain from CT scans: (**a**) Leukemia and (**b**) brain tumors. *Dotted line* is the fitted linear dose–response model (excess relative risk per mGy). *Bars* show 95 % CIs. Reprinted Pearce MS, Salotti JA, Little MP, McHugh K, Lee C, Kim KP, et al. Radiation exposure from CT scans in childhood and subsequent risk of leukaemia and brain tumours: a retrospective cohort study. Lancet. 2012 Aug 4;380(9840):499-505. With permission from Elsevier

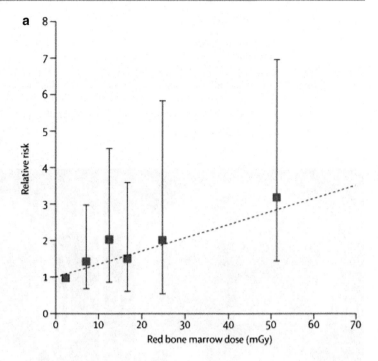

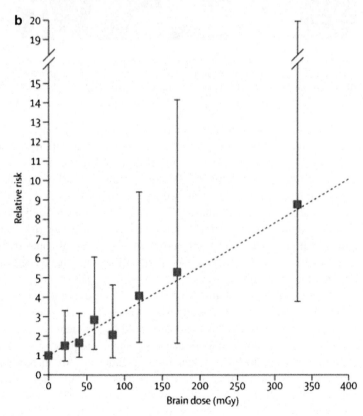

Table 4.1 Radiation safety principles

Justification	Any radiation exposure should be justified and judge. It only should be adopted if the benefit outweighs the harm it may cause
Optimization	Radiation doses and risks should be kept as low as reasonably achievable (ALARA). Technical aspects should be respected to achieve minimal radiation exposure and maximize benefits
Dose limitation	Exposure of individuals should not exceed specified dose limits above which the dose or risk would be deemed unacceptable. The limits are usually set by ICRP[a]

[a]International Commission on Radiation Protection

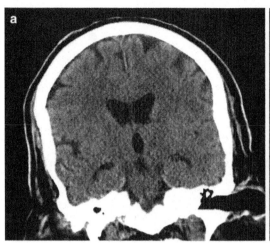

Fig. 4.3 (a) CT head regular dose is acquired showing detailed imaging of the brain parenchyma and ventricles. (b) Low-dose CT of the head does not have the same parenchymal imaging details but is enough to demonstrate presence of hydrocephalus

example, melanoma metastases are easier to depict after intravenous contrast injection. However, if the radiologist is not informed about a clinical suspicion of melanoma, intravenous contrast might not be used, thereby increasing the chance of missing lesions. The same problem applies for leptomeningeal disease in patients with history of malignancy as this can be difficult to visualize without the administration of intravenous contrast media as illustrated in Figs. 4.4 and 4.5.

The contrast used in CT scans is an iodine-based media. The use of this contrast should be cautious since it is not innocuous and contraindications to its use must be taken into account (Table 4.2) [7]. In addition, if a pre- and post-contrast study is needed, the patient will need to be scanned twice, receiving two doses of radiation.

In conclusion, every time a physician fills out a requisition with adequate clinical information, the radiologist is being helped to decide if the image modality chosen by the clinician is the most appropriate for the diagnosis and what is the best technical approach to perform it. The clinician must also flag any risk factors or contraindications for the use of contrast media. The chosen diagnostic test will have adequate sensitivity and specificity and patients will be saved from unnecessary radiation exposure if all these principles are followed.

Here are some questions that might help physicians to evaluate the appropriateness of a CT request:

– Are there publications or protocols to support the choice of a CT study for the condition?

The American College of Radiology website (http://www.acr.org/Quality-Safety/Appropriateness-Criteria) has published a list of

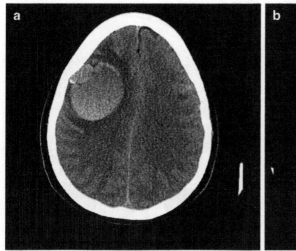

Fig. 4.4 (a) CT without contrast demonstrates a hyperdense hemorrhagic metastasis from melanoma on the right hemisphere. (b) Enhanced CT showing a second metastatic lesion on the left frontal lobe (*black arrow*). This was poorly visualized without contrast

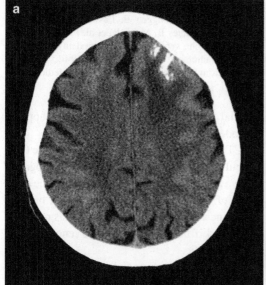
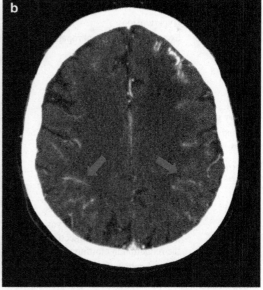

Fig. 4.5 (a) CT without contrast shows multiple hyperdense sulci in the cerebral convexity bilaterally with focal calcification on the left frontal lobe. (b) Enhanced CT of the same patient showing extensive leptomeningeal disease (*red arrows*)

appropriateness criteria for different clinical scenarios. The use of this website may be helpful when questions about appropriateness are raised.

- In the knowledge that the younger the patient, the greatest the risk for tumors related to radiation exposure, does the benefit of a CT diagnosis outweigh the risk of cancer?

- Is there any contraindication to iodine contrast media if this is needed for the imaging study?
- What is the history of previous radiation exposure? Is this patient pregnant or at risk of pregnancy?
- Are there alternative tests available for the diagnosis?

Table 4.2 Adverse effects from the administration of iodine-based contrast agents

Adrenal glands	Hypertension (in patients with pheochromocytoma after intra-arterial injection)
Brain	Headache
	Confusion
	Dizziness
	Seizure
	Rigors
	Lost or diminished consciousness
	Lost or diminished vision
Gastrointestinal tract	Nausea
	Vomiting
	Diarrhea
	Intestinal cramping
Heart	Hypotension
	Dysrhythmia (asystole, ventricular fibrillation/ventricular tachycardia)
	Pulseless electrical activity (PEA)
	Acute congestive heart failure
Kidney	Oliguria
	Hypertension
	Contrast-induced nephropathy (CIN)
Pancreas	Swelling/pancreatitis
Respiratory system	Laryngeal edema
	Bronchospasm
	Pulmonary edema
Salivary glands	Swelling/parotitis
Skin and soft tissues	Erythema
	Urticaria
	Pruritus
	Compartment syndrome (from extravasation)
Thyroid	Exacerbation of thyrotoxicosis
Vascular system	Hemorrhage (due to direct vascular trauma from contrast injection or from the reduction in clotting ability)
	Thrombophlebitis

Based on data from [7]

Basic Principles of CT Interpretation

CT image formation is based on a gray scale of tissue X-ray attenuation. Tissues that can attenuate more X-rays appear whiter or hyperdense (e.g., bone) and tissues that allow the passage of X-rays appear blacker or hypodense (e.g., cerebrospinal fluid spaces). Fat tissue, for example, attenuates less X-rays than the

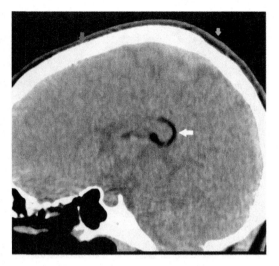

Fig. 4.6 Examples of different CT densities. A hypodense structure is seen in the posterior aspect of the corpus callosum (*white arrow*), in keeping with a lipoma. The *red arrow* is showing the parietal bone (hyperdense structure) and the *blue arrow* is pointing to the subcutaneous tissues of the scalp, which is also hypodense due to the presence of fat. Reprinted Senggen E, Laswed T, Meuwly JY, Maestre LA, Jaques B, Meuli R, et al. First and second branchial arch syndromes: multimodality approach. Pediatric radiology. 2011 May;41(5):549-61. With permission from Springer Science + Business Media

normal brain tissue and therefore appears hypodense (Fig. 4.6) [8].

CT is a very good technique to assess the CNS vasculature. CT arteriograms and venograms have a high sensitivity and specificity in the diagnosis of vascular disease. Nevertheless, because of the increased radiation exposure, it is normally only used if the MR arteriogram/venogram was not diagnostic.

Interpretation of pediatric imaging has its own peculiarities as compared to adult imaging, as the different stages of development result in different appearances of the normal brain. The lack of myelin in the early stages of development and increased water content in the white matter is one example. This characteristic results in differences between the gray and white matter contrast that does not resemble what is seen in an older child, when the myelination process is complete (Fig. 4.7). Therefore, when looking at a pediatric study, it is very important to know the patient's age before coming to any conclusions.

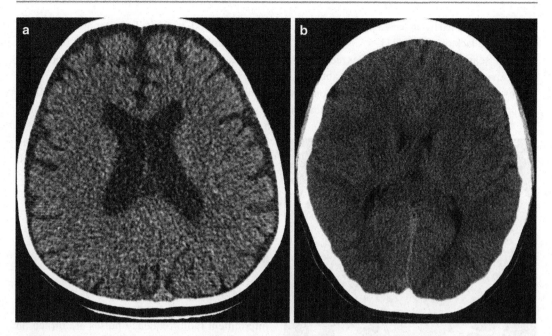

Fig. 4.7 (**a**) Axial CT image of an 11-month-old patient showing fairly homogeneous brain density with decreased gray white matter differentiation due to the small amount of myelin in the white matter. This is a normal finding in this age group due to the myelination process. (**b**) CT image of a fully myelinated brain of a 14-year-old showing the well-demarcated gray/white matter differentiation. The relative hypodensity of the white matter is due to the presence of myelin

Table 4.3 Imaging characteristics of hemoglobin degradation in intraparenchymal hemorrhages

| Phase | Time | Hemoglobin | Appearance | | |
			CT	T1-weighted MRI	T2-weighted MRI
Hyperacute	< 12 h	Oxyhemoglobin	Hyperdense	Isointense or hypointense	Hyperintense
Acute	Hours to days	Deoxyhemoglobin	Hyperdense	Isointense or hypointense	Hypointense
Early subacute	Few days	Methemoglobin	Isodense	Hyperintense	Hypointense
Late subacute	4–7 days to 1 month	Methemoglobin + cell lysis	Hypodense	Hyperintense	Hyperintense
Chronic	Weeks to years	Ferritin and hemosiderin	Hypodense	Isointense or hypointense	Hypointense

Adapted from Parizel P, Makkat S, Van Miert E, et al. Intracranial hemorrhage: principles of CT and MRI interpretation. Eur Radiol 2001; 11: 1770-1783. & Osborn AG (ed). Osborn's Brain, Pathology and Anatomy. Salt Lake City, UT: Lippincott Williams & Wilkins; 2012

The same principles apply for the interpretation of MRI images [9].

The assessment of a CNS bleed also has some pitfalls. There are different stages of hemoglobin degradation (Table 4.3) [10, 11]. In acute stages a bleed will be hyperdense compared with the rest of the brain parenchyma. However, if the patient is anemic, the attenuation of the signal from an acute bleed can be similar to that of the brain parenchyma. Therefore, a small bleed can be easily missed.

Another problem is the lack of myelin in young children, which produces a relative diffuse hypodensity of the parenchyma and makes the blood vessels (in particular the venous sinuses) appear more hyperdense than usual (Fig. 4.8). This should not be confused with acute thrombosis of the venous sinuses. A similar effect can be seen in patients with cyanotic conditions such as cardiac shunts or chronic lung disease, if they are polycythemic. However, in these cases the relative hyperdensity of the vessels is caused by an increased hematocrit and is not due to lack of myelin [11].

A CT scan can determine the degree of mass effect over the parenchyma when evaluating a space-occupying lesion. It can also demonstrate the presence of intralesional cysts, calcification,

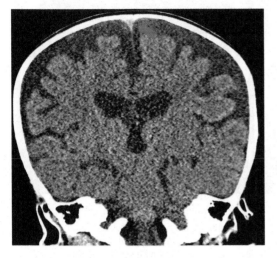

Fig. 4.8 Coronal CT image of an 11-month-old infant showing the relative hyperdensity of the superior sagittal sinus (*red arrow*) in the background of non-myelinated brain parenchyma. This should not be interpreted as venous sinus thrombosis

necrosis, blood, or fat. CT almost always defines the anatomical location of the lesion, except in some cases of infiltrative lesions and posterior fossa lesions. However, MRI allows a more detailed assessment of brain anatomy and its associated pathology (Fig. 4.9). Therefore, once a space-occupying lesion is identified on CT, an MRI is carried out as the next step in the imaging investigation to further characterize the mass and its relationship to the rest of the parenchyma.

Magnetic Resonance Imaging

MRI Image Formation

The principle of MRI imaging acquisition is based on the spin movement of hydrogen atoms. Intermittent radiofrequency pulses are turned on to cause resonance of these atoms. The atomic resonance is extinguished when the radiofrequency pulse is turned off. At this moment, there is a relaxation period while the atoms are losing resonance in which a radiofrequency pulse is emitted by the atoms and then captured by the MRI coils (a device placed around the patient

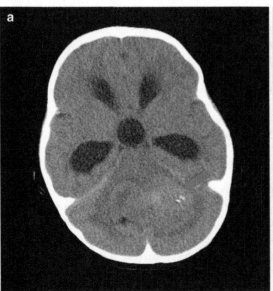
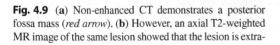
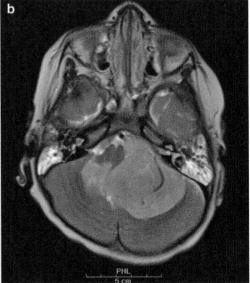

Fig. 4.9 (**a**) Non-enhanced CT demonstrates a posterior fossa mass (*red arrow*). (**b**) However, an axial T2-weighted MR image of the same lesion showed that the lesion is extra-axial in location involving the 4th ventricle and foramen of Luschka on the left side. This demonstrates the superior tissue characterization obtained with MR technique

Table 4.4 Characteristics of frequently used MRI sequences

Sequence	Characteristic	Main importance for CNS tumor imaging
Turbo spin echo (TSE) and spin echo (SE)	High-resolution and detailed anatomy	Helps in determining:
		– Anatomy of the lesion and its effect over the parenchyma
		– Evaluation of cystic/solid components
		– T1 and T2 signal characteristic of the lesion for differential diagnosis
FLAIR (T2 weighted)	Highlights with high signal abnormal water content and presence of gliosis in the brain parenchyma	– Helps in delineating infiltrative lesion's extension
		– Shows the presence of perilesional edema
Diffusion-weighted imaging (DWI)	Demonstrates presence of diffusion restriction of water molecules in the tissues	– Increased cellularity, decreased extracellular space, and a high nuclear to cytoplasm ratio are responsible for water diffusion restriction in high-grade tumors
		– If water restriction is present, it also may indicate the presence of necrosis, pus, acute blood products within the lesion
		– ADC map[a] measurements have an inverse relationship with tumor grading (the higher the measurement, the lower the grade)
Susceptibility-weighted imaging (SWI)	Highlights with low signal, the presence of gas, calcifications, and blood products	– Helps to establish the presence of intralesional calcifications and blood, adding information for the differential
		– Helps in demonstrating postsurgical changes or formation of post-radiation cavernomas

[a]Apparent diffusion coefficient (ADC) map is a mathematical subtraction of the true diffusion acquisition necessary to show the true diffusion of water throughout the tissues

which acts as a receptor), giving the necessary information for the image formation. The set of images obtained with a specific combination of radiofrequencies is called a sequence.

Depending on how the radiofrequency pulse is applied, the sequences can highlight the signal of water (T2-weighted images) or the signal of fat tissue (T1-weighted images). Other radiofrequency combinations result in different sequences and other contrasts (e.g., proton density-weighted imaging). The study protocol details are the combination of sequences. There are several types of MRI sequences (e.g., spin echo (SE), turbo spin echo (TSE), FLAIR (fluid-attenuated inversion recovery), and susceptibility-weighted image (SWI)).

The clinical history provided by the physician will help the radiologist to set up the MRI protocol and to make the decision regarding the need for intravenous contrast administration. Standard MRI protocols of the brain and spine vary among institutions. In our institution, the standard brain tumor imaging protocols are volumetric sagittal T1 with reconstructions, coronal T2 TSE, axial FLAIR, axial diffusion-weighted image (DWI), and axial SWI (Table 4.4). A volumetric gradient

T1 with reconstructions is applied after intravenous gadolinium contrast media administration.

Accurate anatomical localization of a space-occupying lesion is the key for the differential diagnosis of a brain tumor in the pediatric population. Nevertheless, signal intensity, presence of restricted diffusion, calcifications, fat, hemorrhage, and enhancement pattern of the lesion are additional features that help to narrow down the differential diagnosis [12].

The routine MRI sequences are usually enough for an accurate differential diagnosis (Fig. 4.10). Nevertheless, newer sequences and techniques provide additional information to help in the diagnosis and treatment management of difficult and atypical cases.

Commonly, neuro-oncology MRI studies will need post-contrast imaging for the characterization of a space-occupying lesion. Particular attention should be paid to studies post-surgery. Ideally, these should be performed within the first 24 h after a surgical procedure in order to avoid misinterpretations of residual tumor enhancement with leakage across the blood–brain barrier. Enhancement of the surgical bed due to such leakage starts within

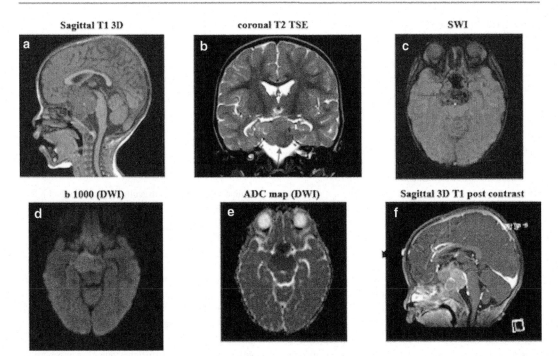

Fig. 4.10 (**a**) Sagittal T1 3D MPRAGE showing large heterogeneous slightly hypointense lesion centered in the suprasellar/hypothalamic region. Small punctate areas of high T1 signal within the lesion may represent small areas of hemorrhage or calcification. Mass effect is seen over the pons but the lesion also appears invading adjacent structures like sella turcica and anterior aspect of third ventricle. (**b**) Coronal T2 turbo spin-echo showing that the same lesion has areas of slightly high and low T2 signal. (**c**) sequence is showing abnormal susceptibility. The DWI (**d**, **e**) is showing restricted diffusion within the lesion. The post-contrast sagittal T1 (**f**) shows heterogeneous enhancement of the lesion. FLAIR images were not acquired as this was an 18-month-old child. The characteristics of this lesion are aggressive and the main differential was primitive neuroectodermal tumor which was confirmed after biopsy

72 h after surgery and is maintained clearly for up to 6–8 weeks, decreasing progressively for up to 12 months after surgery. A further aspect post-intervention is the enhancement of lesions 4–6 months after radiotherapy, which may be related to radiation necrosis [13]. In these cases frequent follow-up is necessary, and other MRI techniques can be used in an attempt to differentiate radiation necrosis from tumor recurrence.

MRI Special Considerations

MRI contrast media are gadolinium-based agents, and its use in the pediatric population is off-label for individuals younger than 2 years. Gadolinium-based contrast media is not nephrotoxic in the approved dosages for MRI studies [7]. However, patients with previous renal failure can develop nephrogenic systemic fibrosis (NSF) if gadolinium-based contrast is administered. NSF is a rare irreversible disease. The hypothesis is that it is caused by deposition of gadolinium in the tissues. To date, there are approximately 370 cases reported in the literature associating this pathology to the use of gadolinium contrast. The age range of reported cases is from 8 to 87 years [14]. The majority of NSF cases are described in patients with previous chronic renal failure. Patients with acute renal failure can also develop NSF especially if superimposed to chronic renal failure. Due to the risk of NSF, the procedure of administering gadolinium-based contrast "just in case" has been removed from the daily practice. The American College of Radiology also advocates cautious use of gadolinium-based agents in newborn and infants due to renal immaturity, even though no case has been reported in patients younger than 8 years [7].

Enhanced CT is the alternative for patients at increased risk of NSF that need an enhanced study,

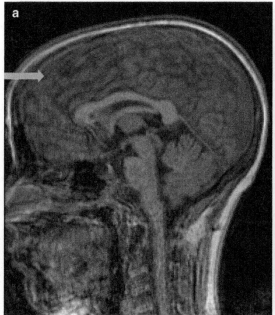
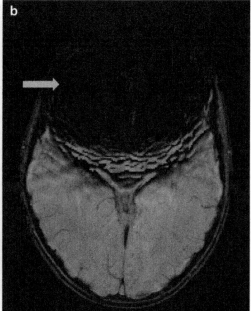

Fig. 4.11 (a) Sagittal T1 3D of the brain showing imaging quality degradation secondary to motion artifact. The multiple curved lines overlying the midline gyri correspond to artifacts. (b) Nondiagnostic axial SWI showing marked imaging degradation secondary to metallic artifacts produced by dental braces (*arrow*)

but iodine contrast media can potentially worsen the renal function. In addition, the risk of ionizing radiation needs to be weighed up in the risk-benefit analysis when a CT study with contrast is carried out instead of an MRI especially in the pediatric population. However, CT iodine contrast can be removed from the blood stream through hemodialysis. It is unknown if hemodialysis performed soon after an enhanced MRI scan to remove gadolinium from the blood stream can prevent NSF. Nevertheless, this practice is advised if the enhanced MRI study is indeed performed [7].

Imaging Artifacts

MRI is a technique that is highly susceptible to imaging artifacts. In brain imaging, artifacts related to dental hardware are very common and it may be impossible to diagnose any pathology. Motion artifact is another common artifact in pediatric studies, and this can also degrade the quality of images significantly (Fig. 4.11). For this reason some pediatric MRI studies need to be performed under sedation.

MRI Safety

Another important consideration is the MRI safety area and procedures. When approaching the area of an MRI scanner, safety zone alerts should be evident. Metallic objects can fly towards the magnet due to the magnetic field strength and this can be deadly. Patients with metallic implants can have the implant damaged or displaced. Injury can also occur by heat of a metallic foreign body or implant. Anyone that approaches an MRI scanner should be initially screened for the presence of metallic hardware and other contraindications (Table 4.5) [15].

Pediatric Sedation

Imaging pediatric patients can be challenging. Motion artifact can ruin an MRI or CT study. Therefore, sedation may be needed to perform an imaging examination.

The age group most likely to require sedation is for children younger than 8 years.

Table 4.5 Important screening information for an MRI study

Problems in previous MRI scan (e.g., claustrophobia)
Previous surgery and dates
Injury by metallic object or presence of foreign body?
History of kidney disease, asthma, or allergies?
History of previous allergy of MRI or CT dye? Which kind of reaction?
Pregnancy? Lactation?
Any type of electronic, mechanical, or magnetic implant or device?
Cardiac pacemaker/implanted cardiac defibrillator/artificial heart valve
Aneurysm clip
Neurostimulator/biostimulator
Internal electrodes or wires/any type of surgical clip or staple
Any type of coil, filter, or stent
Cochlear implant/hearing aid/any type of ear implant
Implanted drug pump
Halo vest/spinal fixation device/artificial limb or joint
Penile implant
Artificial eye/eyelid spring
Any type of implant held in place by a magnet
Any IV access port/shunt
Medication patch
Tissue expander
Removable dentures, false teeth, or partial plate
Diaphragm, IUD, pessary
Surgical mesh
Body piercing
Wig/hair implants
Tattoos or tattooed eyeliner
Radiation seeds (e.g., cancer treatment)
Any implanted items (e.g., pins, rods, screws, nails, plates, wires)
Any hair accessories (e.g., bobby pins, barrettes, clips)
Jewelry
Any other type of implanted item

Adapted from Expert Panel on MRS, Kanal E, Barkovich AJ, Bell C, Borgstede JP, Bradley WG, Jr., et al. ACR guidance document on MR safe practices: 2013. Journal of magnetic resonance imaging : JMRI. 2013 Mar;37(3):501-30. With permission from John Wiley & Sons, Inc.

Overall, the failure rate of sedation varies in the literature from 1 to 20 % [16]. In addition, major cardiovascular and respiratory events can occur in approximately 0.4–1 % [17]. Alternative techniques are safer for the patients and can avoid a significant number of sedations. Audiovisual systems in the MRI suits, for example, can reduce the number of sedations in children between 3 and 10 years old by 25 % and by 50 % in children older than 10 years [18]. Other examples of alternative techniques are feed and sleep (which works very well in neonates and young infants), sleep deprivation, melatonin administration, and MRI simulation training. Alternative techniques should be applied whenever is possible [19].

Advanced Imaging Techniques

Functional MRI (fMRI)

Imaging acquisition in fMRI is based in the principle that oxygen consumption increases in the brain area used for a particular activity. The sequence used for this technique is known as blood-oxygen-level-dependent (BOLD) contrast. In neuro-oncology this technique can add information about involvement of eloquent areas of the brain by a space-occupying lesion (Fig. 4.12) [20].

Functional studies are carried out with the patient awake and able to collaborate [20]. Standard MRI scanners might have the BOLD sequence available; however, special software is necessary to perform the functional examinations.

Diffusion Tensor Imaging (DTI)

DTI imaging principle is based in the three directional movements of water molecules throughout the tissues. Isotropy is the term used when the water molecules diffuse equally in all directions. However, in the brain, due to the parallel micro movement of water molecules within the axons, there is anisotropy of water molecule movement, which is measured by the fractional anisotropy (FA) index. DTI also allows determination of fiber bundle directionality, also known as tractography study [21].

Nowadays, tractography studies have been used alone or in association with fMRI to determine the degree of white matter tract involvement by a CNS tumor (Fig. 4.13). This information is extremely helpful for surgical and radiotherapy treatment planning, especially if the tumor is located in an eloquent region of the brain [21].

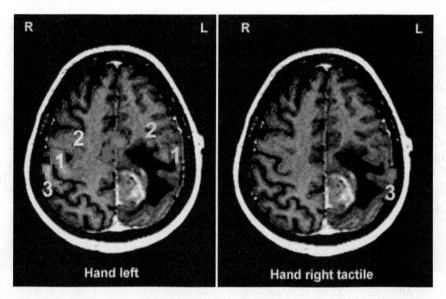

Fig. 4.12 Presurgical fMRI in a hemiparetic patient (grade 3/5) with a left malignant glioma only weak BOLD activation was available from contralateral (*right*) hand movements precluding reliable localization of the motor hand area (not shown). By using complex finger opposition of the unimpaired hand ipsilateral to the tumor (*left*) and fully automated tactile stimulation of the right digits BOLD activation is achievable in the motor hand area (1), premotor cortex (2), and primary somatosensory cortex (3) on the tumor side. Note the corresponding activations in the unimpaired hemisphere (*right*) associated with the left finger movements (*white numbers*). Bilateral supplementary motor activation is in the midline. Reprinted from Stippich C. Preoperative Blood Oxygen Level Dependent (BOLD) functional Magnetic Resonance Imaging (fMRI) of Motor and Somatosensory Function. In: Ulmer S, Jansen O (eds). fMRI: Basics and Clinical Applications: Heidelberg, Germany: Springer-Verlag; 2013. p. 91-110. With permission from Springer Science + Business Media

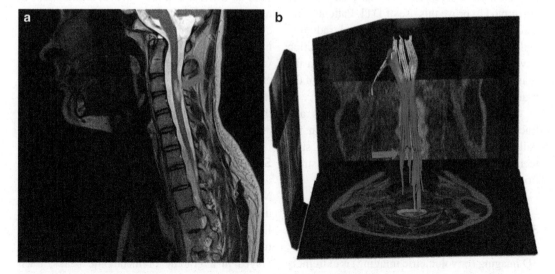

Fig. 4.13 (a) Spinal cord tumor (pilocytic astrocytoma) is demonstrated on a sagittal T2-weighted image (*red arrow*). (b) The same lesion is demonstrated causing disruption of tract direction by using a 3D tractography imaging reconstruction technique (*red arrow*)

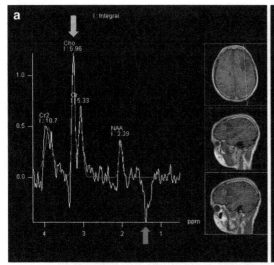 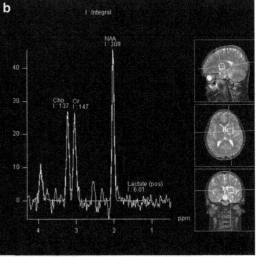

Fig. 4.14 (**a**) MRS study (PRESS technique—single voxel—TE 135 ms) showing a malignant signature with high choline (Cho) (*orange arrow*), low NAA peaks in relation to creatine (Cr), and the presence of a lactate peak (*red arrow*) in the surgical margin of a left frontal lobe lesion. (**b**) Normal MRS study acquired with the same technique for comparison in left basal ganglia

A promising application of DTI technique in neuro-oncology is the FA index measurement in high-grade gliomas. This measurement may help to detect infiltrative portions of the tumor and differentiate it from perilesional edema [22]. It also could potentially help to depict tumor recurrence. However, further research in this area is being performed to prove this use of DTI. Patients with medulloblastoma who have received radiation and present with decreased cognitive function have shown low FA index measurements in the brainstem, even though the overall imaging of the brainstem may be normal [23].

Unfortunately, FA index measurements and tractography studies are not carried out in the daily practice of most institutions since such techniques demand special software reconstructions that are not always available.

3D Imaging and Stereotaxy

3D imaging (or volumetric imaging) is extremely helpful for anatomical reconstructions. There are several different MRI sequences that can be acquired as volumetric images. Several different kinds of reconstructions also can be performed from it if adequate software is available.

In neuro-oncology, 3D imaging is especially used for stereotaxy. Stereotaxy is a technique that makes use of 3D imaging to create a coordinate system that will guide the localization of a lesion in a surgical procedure or radiotherapy treatment. Nowadays it is associated with other techniques, such as fMRI and direct cortical stimulation, to reduce morbidity in CNS tumor resection especially if the lesion is located in eloquent areas of the brain [24]. Association of 3D MRI imaging with other imaging modalities such as positron emission tomography (PET) scan is possible and it has been studied to improve surgical and radiotherapy planning.

Spectroscopy

MR spectroscopy (MRS) is a technique widely used in brain imaging. It is used to assess metabolites in the brain parenchyma and lesions. The results of an MRS acquisition are typically displayed in a graphic of metabolite peaks. Each metabolite has its own location in the MRS graphic and the height of the peak indicates its concentration in the parenchyma (Fig. 4.14). The most commonly assessed metabolites are choline, creatine, N-acetylaspartate (NAA), and lactate.

Choline is a substance related to the cell membrane and it is elevated therefore in situations in which there is increased cell density and high cellular turnover. Creatine is related to the cell's metabolic rate. NAA is a protein present in the cells, which reflects the neuronal density. The most common spectral signature of a brain tumor is increased choline and decreased NAA compared to creatine peaks. If present, lactate peak usually reflects areas of ischemia and necrosis within the tumor, suggesting a higher grade tumor. The lipids peak is related to cell proliferation. Therefore this peak is usually present in high-grade CNS tumors [13].

Attempts have been made in the use of MRS to determine the type and grading of CNS tumors. However, there is a significant overlap of metabolite peaks pattern that exists between low- and high-grade CNS tumors as well as between neoplastic and nonneoplastic lesions. For example, pilocytic astrocytoma and oligodendrogliomas are low-grade tumors that may have a similar MRS spectrum to that of a high-grade tumor [13].

In general, MRS does not add much information to the differential diagnosis of an initial investigation. Nevertheless, it has been shown to be useful in some atypical cases differentiating brain tumor from brain abscess. It can also potentially help to differentiate areas of radiation necrosis or postsurgical changes from recurrent or residual tumor. Ratios between choline peak and other peaks such as creatine and NAA peaks can also be helpful in assessing response of therapy.

Perfusion Techniques

Perfusion technique can be applied with both MRI and CT. However, CT perfusion is usually not performed in the pediatric population due to the risks involved in radiation exposure.

The standard perfusion technique uses intravenous contrast. Nevertheless, there is a new MRI sequence called arterial spin labeling (ASL) that can be used to study brain perfusion without the use of contrast media. This technique does not require IV access and avoids the off-label use

of gadolinium contrast media in patients younger than 2 years [13].

The perfusion images are frequently interpreted in a color map. The red zones usually demonstrate increased perfusion and the blue zones decreased perfusion. More detailed analysis can also be made with numerical estimations of cerebral blood volume using post-processing techniques.

Research studies suggest that perfusion technique may help to differentiate between low- and high-grade tumors. It also has been described to help in the differentiation of radiation necrosis (decreased perfusion) from tumor recurrence (normal to elevated perfusion) (Fig. 4.15) [25]. Another application of this technique is to help in defining an ideal area for surgical biopsy, avoiding areas of necrosis. It can be used in association with MRS for this purpose. Future applications of this technique are related to evaluation of tumor angiogenesis and treatment response in patients using antiangiogenic drugs [13].

Unfortunately, MRI perfusion technique is not available in all institutions since it is not a standard MRI sequence.

PET Scan and Future Molecular Imaging

PET scan is considered to be a conventional molecular technique. Its principle is based on the injection of a radiopharmaceutical containing a positron-emitting radionuclide (tracer) into the body. This tracer emits two gamma rays in opposite directions to the imaging receptor located in the PET scanner forming the image. The highlighted areas in the images usually demonstrate higher concentration of the radiopharmaceutical in the tissues. The main difference between PET and single-photon emission computed tomography (SPECT) is that the gamma-emitting radionuclide used in SPECT produces a random emission of gamma rays, while in PET the emission of gamma rays is always in opposite directions (180°) giving better resolution. Use of a PET scan is often carried out together with low dose CT images or MRI to improve the anatomical

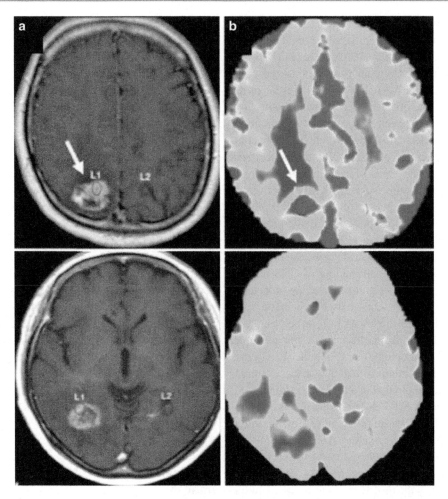

Fig. 4.15 Contrast-enhanced T1-weighted (**a**) and perfusion-weighted (**b**) MRI in cases of tumor recurrence (upper) and radiation-induced necrosis (lower) after radiosurgery of metastatic brain tumors. Note the clear difference in the cerebral blood volume of lesions. Reprinted from Mitsuya K, Nakasu Y, Horiguchi S, et al. Perfusion weighted magnetic resonance imaging to distinguish the recurrence of metastatic brain tumors from radiation necrosis after stereotactic radiosurgery. Journal of Neuro-Oncology 2010; 99(1): 81-88. With permission from Springer Science + Business Media

analysis. The difference between PET/SPECT scan from CT scan is that the radiation source is within the patient while in CT the source is external.

Radiopharmaceuticals are radionuclides bonded to specific biological markers. Numerous radiopharmaceuticals are available and each one has a special diagnostic or treatment target. Common radiopharmaceuticals applied in brain imaging are fludeoxyglucose (FDG), L-[methyl-^{11}C]methionine ([^{11}C]MET), and 3′-deoxy-3′-[^{18}F]fluorothymidine ([^{18}F]FLT).

Neoplastic lesions demonstrate increase uptake of FDG in PET studies due to increased glucose metabolism (Fig. 4.16). Thus an FDG scan can be used in the evaluation of tumor grading, localization for biopsy, differentiation of radiation necrosis from tumor recurrence, therapeutic monitoring, and assessment for malignant transformation of what were originally low-grade gliomas [26]. However, its applicability in clinical practice is low because normal gray matter also demonstrates increased glucose metabolism, effacing lesions.

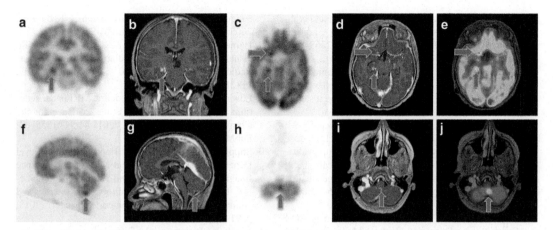

Fig. 4.16 An 11-year-old patient with metastatic pineo-blastoma. 18F-FDG PET (**a, c, f, h**) brain images with correspondent MRI images (**b, d, g, i**) and PET-MRI fusion images (**e, j**). 18F-FDG PET study demonstrated lesions with focal increase in activity corresponding to abnormal leptomeningeal enhancement in the MRI images. Courtesy of Dr. Amer Shammas (Hospital for Sick Children—Toronto, Canada)

L-[methyl-^{11}C]methionine ([^{11}C]MET) is an amino acid-based agent. The advantage of this radiopharmaceutical over FDG is that it does not have a high uptake by the normal brain parenchyma. It has been used to differentiate neoplastic from nonneoplastic lesions and to differentiate recurrence from radionecrosis [26].

3′-deoxy-3′-[^{18}F]fluorothymidine ([^{18}F]FLT) is a marker for cell proliferation since it is trapped by thymidine kinase, an intracellular proliferation pathway enzyme. It is useful to differentiate recurrence from radionecrosis and in differentiation of low- and high-grade tumors [26].

MR-based molecular imaging is another example of molecular imaging technique. MR molecular imaging can be based on physical principles of imaging acquisition or on the use of special combinations of gadolinium with specific macromolecules or nanoparticles.

MRS is an example of MR-based molecular imaging since it demonstrates presence and quantities of different metabolites. Its applicability in neuro-oncology was described previously in this chapter. Nowadays, a significant amount of research has been carried out using a new MRI technique called chemical exchange saturation transfer (CEST) imaging. This technique is able to image specific molecules. Amide proton transfer (APT) imaging is a type of CEST imaging that has been used in studies of brain tumor. This technique is able to depict endogenous mobile proteins and peptides in the tissues. Potentially it may be able to assess tumor boundary and detect tumor recurrence [27].

A large number of special combinations of gadolinium and nanoparticles have been investigated in preclinical research projects. The hypothesis is to explore the possibility of this type of gadolinium contrast acting in a similar way as a radiopharmaceutical. This is another promising research field in MRI techniques, which could revolutionize brain tumor imaging in the near future.

References

1. Kaste SC, Young CW, Holmes TP, Baker DK. Effect of helical CT on the frequency of sedation in pediatric patients. AJR Am J Roentgenol. 1997;168(4):1001–3. PubMed PMID: 9124104.
2. Ginde AA, Foianini A, Renner DM, Valley M, Camargo Jr CA. Availability and quality of computed tomography and magnetic resonance imaging equipment in U.S. emergency departments. Acad Emerg Med. 2008;15(8):780–3.
3. Peck DJ, Samei E. How to understand and communicate radiation risk. Image Wisely; American College of Radiology; 2010. http://www.imagewisely.org/Imaging-Professionals/Medical-Physicists/Articles/How-to-Understand-and-Communicate-Radiation-Risk?referrer=search. Accessed 24 Apr 2013.
4. Pearce MS, Salotti JA, Little MP, McHugh K, Lee C, Kim KP, et al. Radiation exposure from CT scans in

childhood and subsequent risk of leukaemia and brain tumours: a retrospective cohort study. Lancet. 2012;380(9840):499–505. PubMed PMID: 22681860. Pubmed Central PMCID: 3418594.

5. IAEA. Radiation, people and the environment: a broad overview of ionizing radiation, its effects and uses, as well as the measures in place to use it safely. Vienna: IAEA; 2004. p. 23–8.

6. Udayasankar UK, Braithwaite K, Arvaniti M, Tudorascu D, Small WC, Little S, et al. Low-dose nonenhanced head CT protocol for follow-up evaluation of children with ventriculoperitoneal shunt: reduction of radiation and effect on image quality. AJNR Am J Neuroradiol. 2008;29(4):802–6. PubMed PMID: 18397968.

7. ACR Manual on Contrast Media - version 8. ACR Committee on Drugs and Contrast Media. American College of Radiology; 2012.

8. Senggen E, Laswed T, Meuwly JY, Maestre LA, Jaques B, Meuli R, et al. First and second branchial arch syndromes: multimodality approach. Pediatr Radiol. 2011;41(5):549–61. PubMed PMID: 20924574.

9. Barkovich AJRC. Pediatric neuroimaging. Philadelphia: Lippincott Williams & Wilkins; 2012. p. 20–80.

10. Parizel PM, Makkat S, Van Miert E, Van Goethem JW, van den Hauwe L, De Schepper AM. Intracranial hemorrhage: principles of CT and MRI interpretation. Eur Radiol. 2001;11(9):1770–83. PubMed PMID: 11511901.

11. Osborn AG. Osborn's brain: imaging, pathology and anatomy. 1st ed. Philadelphia: Amirsys and Lippincott Williams & Wilkins; 2012. p. 215–43.

12. Barkovich AJ, Raybaud C. Pediatric neuroimaging. 5th ed. Philadelphia: Lippincott Williams & Wilkins; 2012. p. 637–807.

13. Rao P. Role of MRI in paediatric neurooncology. Eur J Radiol. 2008;68(2):259–70. PubMed PMID: 18775616.

14. Zou Z, Zhang HL, Roditi GH, Leiner T, Kucharczyk W, Prince MR. Nephrogenic systemic fibrosis: review of 370 biopsy-confirmed cases. JACC Cardiovasc Imaging. 2011;4(11):1206–16. PubMed PMID: 22093272.

15. Expert Panel on MRS, Kanal E, Barkovich AJ, Bell C, Borgstede JP, Bradley Jr WG, et al. ACR guidance document on MR safe practices: 2013. J Magn Reson Imaging. 2013;37(3):501–30. PubMed PMID: 23345200.

16. Cravero JP, Blike GT. Review of pediatric sedation. Anesth Analg. 2004;99(5):1355–64. PubMed PMID: 15502031.

17. Sanborn PA, Michna E, Zurakowski D, Burrows PE, Fontaine PJ, Connor L, et al. Adverse cardiovascular and respiratory events during sedation of pediatric patients for imaging examinations. Radiology. 2005;237(1):288–94. PubMed PMID: 16183936.

18. Harned 2nd RK, Strain JD. MRI-compatible audio/visual system: impact on pediatric sedation. Pediatr Radiol. 2001;31(4):247–50. PubMed PMID: 11321741.

19. Edwards AD, Arthurs OJ. Paediatric MRI under sedation: is it necessary? What is the evidence for the alternatives? Pediatr Radiol. 2011;41(11):1353–64. PubMed PMID: 21678113.

20. Stippich C. Preoperative Blood Oxygen Level Dependent (BOLD) functional Magnetic Resonance Imaging (fMRI) of motor and somatosensory function. In: Ulmer S, Jansen O, editors. FMRI: basics and clinical applications. Heidelberg: Springer; 2013. p. 91–110.

21. Assaf Y, Pasternak O. Diffusion tensor imaging (DTI)-based white matter mapping in brain research: a review. J Mol Neurosci. 2008;34(1):51–61. PubMed PMID: 18157658.

22. De Belder FE, Oot AR, Van Hecke W, Venstermans C, Menovsky T, Van Marck V, et al. Diffusion tensor imaging provides an insight into the microstructure of meningiomas, high-grade gliomas, and peritumoral edema. J Comput Assist Tomogr. 2012;36(5):577–82. PubMed PMID: 22992609.

23. Palmer SL, Glass JO, Li Y, Ogg R, Qaddoumi I, Armstrong GT, et al. White matter integrity is associated with cognitive processing in patients treated for a posterior fossa brain tumor. Neuro Oncol. 2012;14(9):1185–93. PubMed PMID: 22898373. Pubmed Central PMCID: 3424215.

24. Stapleton SR, Kiriakopoulos E, Mikulis D, Drake JM, Hoffman HJ, Humphreys R, et al. Combined utility of functional MRI, cortical mapping, and frameless stereotaxy in the resection of lesions in eloquent areas of brain in children. Pediatr Neurosurg. 1997;26(2):68–82. PubMed PMID: 9419036.

25. Chernov MF, Ono Y, Abe K, Usukura M, Hayashi M, Izawa M, Diment SV, Ivanov PI. Differentiation of tumor progression and induced effects after intracranial radiosurgery. Acta Neurochir Suppl. 2013;116:193–210.

26. Petrirena GJ, Goldman S, Delattre JY. Advances in PET imaging of brain tumors: a referring physician's perspective. Curr Opin Oncol. 2011;23(6):617–23. PubMed PMID: 21825989.

27. Zhou J, Tryggestad E, Wen Z, Lal B, Zhou T, Grossman R, et al. Differentiation between glioma and radiation necrosis using molecular magnetic resonance imaging of endogenous proteins and peptides. Nat Med. 2011;17(1):130–4. PubMed PMID: 21170048. Pubmed Central PMCID: 3058561.

Sami Obaid, Pierre-Olivier Champagne,
Claude Mercier, and Louis Crevier

Introduction: The Role and Timing of Pediatric Neurosurgery Involvement as Part of the Multidisciplinary Neuro-oncology Team

The diagnosis of brain tumors in children bears heavy psychological involvement for both the children and their family. Accordingly, families expect a detailed discussion including the precise diagnosis and treatment options for the condition. In addition, the question of long-term morbidity and survival if treatment is initiated is a common concern. The role of the multidisciplinary neuro-oncology team is thus to offer the optimal management while respecting the patient and his family's wishes.

S. Obaid, M.D.C.M. • C. Mercier, M.D., F.R.C.S.C.
• L. Crevier, M.D., M.Sc., F.R.C.S.C. (✉)
Department of Neurosurgery, Centre Hospitalier
Universitaire de Sainte-Justine, Montréal,
QC, Canada
e-mail: louis.crevier.hsj@ssss.gouv.qc.ca

P.-O. Champagne, M.D.
Department of Neurosurgery, Hôpital Notre-Dame/
Université de Montréal, Montréal, QC, Canada

The pediatric neurosurgeons are essential to that neuro-oncology team and should be involved early in the diagnostic phase. Indeed, a multidisciplinary team composed of both medical and surgical specialists with their respective expertise is essential in elaborating a treatment plan for the management of CNS pediatric brain tumors. Discussion within the multidisciplinary team allows for decision on whether observation, radiation, chemotherapy, surgical intervention, or a combination of these should be the best treatment. Of course, the best option varies depending on the tumor type, location, invasiveness as well as the patient's age and overall medical condition. As a general rule and apart from a few specific lesions, if a tumor is accessible and risk of morbidity is acceptable, resection should be considered. Neurosurgeons should also actively follow patients even if a nonsurgical approach is preferred since their services might be required for treating unsuccessful cases or complications of the chosen method.

The following chapter will discuss the role of the pediatric neurosurgery team in the management of CNS neoplasms in children. More specifically, multiple surgical modalities for the treatment of such tumors including indications, technique description, associated complications, and outcome will be detailed.

K. Scheinemann and E. Bouffet (eds.), *Pediatric Neuro-oncology*,
DOI 10.1007/978-1-4939-1541-5_5, © Springer Science+Business Media New York 2015

Goals of Pediatric Neurosurgery in the Context of CNS Tumors

Pediatric neurosurgeons are usually involved in the early stages of management of pediatric CNS tumors. Before a precise neurosurgical opinion can be emitted, thorough evaluation of the patient should be performed, including the clinical condition, neuroimaging studies, and case-specific pertinent investigations (e.g., serum hormone levels, tumor markers, genetic syndrome features, etc.). Imaging of the entire neuraxis should be done for most cases, especially for tumors with a tendency for CNS dissemination such as medulloblastomas, germ cell tumors, ependymomas, and primitive neuroectodermal tumors (PNETs).

Following proper evaluation of the tumor, neurosurgeons should have three main objectives in mind:

- Maximal safe tumor resection when possible
- Histopathological diagnosis
- Treatment of associated conditions (e.g., hydrocephalus)

Tumor Resection

As a general rule, tumors that can be safely resected are considered for surgical excision. What is considered a safe resection can be arguable but usually involves a lesion for which significant neurological impairments can be avoided after its surgical removal, keeping in mind that the prognosis often correlates with the extent of resection [1, 2]. Nowadays, the mainstay of treatment of many pediatric CNS tumors including gliomas, medulloblastomas, and ependymomas is maximal surgical resection followed by adjuvant therapy in selected cases [1, 3]. There are a few exceptions to this rule: germ cell tumors of the pineal or sellar region, tumors located in eloquent areas, and low-grade tumors for which observation might be an option.

The diagnosis of germ cell tumor of the pineal or sellar region may indeed be obtained via serum and/or CSF markers. When this is the case, initial surgery can be avoided and treatment with chemotherapy initiated [4]. Second-look surgery may then be considered for residual tumor before radiation therapy is started. However, for marker-negative germ cell tumors (e.g., pure germinomas), surgery followed if needed by chemotherapy and/or radiation remains the treatment of choice. Germinomas respond very well to chemotherapy and thus surgery should be limited to a biopsy. Biopsy of a pineal region tumor can be done during endoscopic third ventriculostomy (ETV) performed in the context of hydrocephalus, as discussed below.

When a tumor is located in a zone of the brain responsible for important functions (eloquent), resection may be deemed too dangerous and nonsurgical management may be preferred. In such cases, if imaging features and/or other paraclinical investigations are sufficient to establish the specific diagnosis including the nature of the tumor, treatment can be initiated. However, if uncertainty persists, a biopsy is performed and histopathological analysis will then guide subsequent nonsurgical treatment [4]. The risks and benefits of both the surgical and nonsurgical approach should be weighted when conservative management of tumors in eloquent areas is considered.

Histopathological Diagnosis

As mentioned earlier, most pediatric CNS tumors will be amenable to surgical resection. When this is not the case and if a doubt persists on neuroimaging studies regarding the likely histopathological diagnosis, a biopsy of the lesion may be required. Various biopsy techniques have been described and choice of the appropriate method is largely influenced by tumor location.

Stereotactic Biopsy

This method uses stereotactic coordinates to precisely guide a needle inside the tumor. It is the method of choice for deeply located tumors. The neurosurgeon may proceed with a frame-based system using a metallic head frame or use a more modern frameless neuronavigation device. Based on preoperative acquired images, the neurosurgeon can determine the coordinates for adequate placement of the burr hole and angulation and depth of the needle.

Open Biopsy

An open biopsy can be performed through a small craniotomy and allows for direct access to the tumor. This method is traditionally used for superficial tumors near or within the cerebral cortex or when leptomeninges also need to be biopsied. Imaging adjuvant such as neuronavigation can be used to allow for precise localization of the tumor in relation to the skull surface.

Endoscopic Endonasal Biopsy

Tumors such as those of the anterior skull base, sellar region, and those invading sinuses can sometimes be accessed through an endoscopic endonasal approach. Done under general anesthesia, the endoscope is passed through the nostril and the sinuses until the lesion is reached. The assistance of an ENT surgeon is usually required.

Endoscopic Intraventricular Biopsy

Tumors located within the ventricular system or adjacent to it may be amenable to an endoscopic transventricular approach. This procedure has the advantage to allow for CSF sampling as well as treatment of associated hydrocephalus via an endoscopic third ventriculostomy (ETV).

Treatment of Associated Conditions

In addition to the mass effect and infiltrative effect of the tumor itself, secondary brain insults (SBIs) can result from conditions such as hydrocephalus. Other causes of SBIs such as vasogenic edema and seizures which require medical rather than surgical treatment will not be discussed in this section.

The main mechanism of hydrocephalus in the context of CNS tumors is obstruction of the ventricular system by tumors of the posterior fossa and tumor located around the third ventricle. Signs and symptoms of hydrocephalus result from elevated intracranial pressure (ICP). These include nausea, vomiting (often in the morning),

irritability, sixth nerve palsy, headaches, and a decline in mental status [1, 3]. An upward gaze deficit and other associated signs of the Parinaud syndrome can be seen with compression of the midbrain tectum by the enlarged third ventricle at the level of its suprapineal recess or via direct tumor compression. Bulging fontanelles, splayed sutures, and an increase in skull circumference are additional manifestations of elevated ICP seen in infants with open sutures.

In the presence of hydrocephalus from tumor compression, the patient's clinical state should dictate initial management. In a stable patient with little clinical evidence of significant hydrocephalus and normal neuro-ophthalmologic examination, conservative management is recommended until tumor surgery. Contribution of vasogenic edema to the compression should warrant glucocorticoid administration acting as a temporizing measure until surgical resection. On the other hand, an unstable patient with clinical evidence of elevated ICP should undergo emergent surgery consisting of the insertion of an external ventricular drain (EVD). A catheter is inserted through a burr hole in the skull until the anterior horn of the lateral ventricle is accessed and CSF flow is observed. The EVD is connected to an external collecting device and allows the excess CSF to drain [4]. Endoscopic third ventriculostomy (ETV) is another treatment option in the face of triventricular hydrocephalus from posterior fossa or pineal region tumors.

Hydrocephalus can persist despite resection of the obstructing tumor. This is especially true for posterior fossa lesions in which persistent hydrocephalus is observed in up to 30–40 % of cases following surgical resection [4, 5]. Such patients will need permanent diversion of CSF. The two main methods for permanent diversion of CSF are the ventriculoperitoneal shunt (VPS) and endoscopic third ventriculostomy (ETV). The VPS consists of a three-part device. A proximal catheter is inserted inside the lateral ventricle. The device is then connected to a distal catheter tunnelized subcutaneously ultimately reaching the peritoneum where CSF will be freely reabsorbed. A valve is commonly inserted between the proximal and distal catheter and allows for drainage control. One of the disadvantages of VPSs includes the theoretical risk of dissemination of neoplastic cells. An ETV consists in the creation of a communication between the third ventricle and the interpeduncular cistern under endoscopic guidance within the ventricular system. This technique allows diversion of CSF flow and obviates the need of extrinsic devices such as VPSs.

Considering the risk of postoperative hydrocephalus, neurosurgeons should answer the two following questions: (1) should a shunt be inserted prior or after surgical resection and (2) which CSF diversion procedure should be performed? We recommend the following management. If validated risk factors associated with postoperative hydrocephalus such as young age (<2 years), transependymal edema, type of tumor, and moderate to severe hydrocephalus are present, a preoperative ETV can be performed to avoid long-term shunt dependency [6]. If not, the risk of developing hydrocephalus is lower and tumor resection ± the insertion of an EVD during surgical removal of the tumor should be sufficient. If an EVD has been placed, the ICP is then monitored over the following days to determine the need for permanent CSF diversion such as a VPS.

Spinal Cord Neoplasms

Intramedullary spinal cord tumors are rare in the pediatric population, representing 4.2 % of all CNS tumors [7]. The general approach for such tumors consists of surgical excision. Tumor debulking often leads to favorable outcome and is thus the preferred surgical option. In fact, removal of 80 % of the lesion has been associated with good survival rate in low-grade tumors (70 % at 5 years for nonmalignant lesions, which represent 80 % of these tumors) [8]. In addition to tumor removal, debulking provides specimens for histopathological analysis. Another option in the initial management of these tumors consists of a more conservative surgical resection followed by radiation therapy, which has revealed an overall comparable survival rate [9–13].

In this context, the choice between the two treatments should be guided by the risk of morbidity. Since the introduction of intraoperative physiological monitoring, morbidity rate from spinal cord surgeries has considerably decreased [14]. In addition, irradiation of the spine in children has been associated with significant side effects, including myelopathy [15], alteration of bone growth [16], and potential induction of other malignancies [17]. However, these secondary effects were mostly described with radiotherapy techniques used in the 1980s and are thus less likely to occur nowadays with modern radiation therapy.

Treatment of Complications

The refinement of neurosurgical procedures in the recent years has led to improvement of outcome following both cranial and spinal procedures. Nevertheless, postoperative complications remain an important component to which the involved medical specialists are faced on a daily basis. For that reason, prevention, early recognition, and treatment of such complications by a multidisciplinary team is an essential aspect of postoperative management.

Overall the rate of postoperative complications following pediatric brain tumor surgery varies from 10 to 70 % [18–26] whereas mortality rates range from 0 to 20 % [18–23, 27]. Several factors justify the wide range in these values. These include the type of surgery performed, patient's age and condition, tumor characteristics such as location, size, and nature of tumor as well as the surgeon's experience [22].

All patients undergoing brain tumor resection should be closely monitored in an intensive care unit postoperatively. Neurologic deterioration should prompt immediate imaging in order to guide subsequent management. Furthermore, we recommend postoperative MRI for all cases in the first 24–48 h following surgery to document the degree of tumor resection and to screen for postoperative complications.

The goal of the following section is to give a brief overview of the major complications that may occur and should be identified following surgery for pediatric CNS tumor.

Neurological Complications

Following intracranial brain tumor resection in a pediatric population, the most common complication is a new-onset neurological deficit (12–54 % of cases) [22, 23, 26, 28, 29]. Although no clear consensus for defining "neurological complications" has been established, most authors encompass deficits including mutism, muscle weakness, ataxia, speech disturbances, diminished consciousness, epilepsy, eye movement disturbances, and visual field deficits [22, 28–30].

Tumor location seems to influence the rate and severity of postoperative neurological complications: infratentorial surgeries are associated with a higher rate of deficits, in particular the occurrence of cerebellar mutism [28]. This syndrome is characterized by muteness, ataxia, irritability, and hypotonia. Muteness is probably the component that tends to resolve spontaneously, while other features of the syndrome tend to persist [28]. Supratentorial surgeries tend to produce visual deterioration and focal deficits [28].

The main concern following the occurrence of such deficits is whether long-term consequences will ensue. According to a study by Lassen et al., a large proportion of postoperative neurological deficit remained permanent despite improvement of the patient's condition [28]. In this study, 12.8 % of children that underwent craniotomy and tumor excision were found to exhibit some evidence of neurological deficit in the postoperative period. Most of these patients were found to have permanent deficits. In another study by Cochrane et al., the rate of permanent neurological morbidity attributable to surgery was 24 % [28, 31]. Despite that risk, it is the severity rather than the frequency of these deficits that should be taken into account. The plasticity of the brain in children allows for remarkable improvements of surgically related deficits, allowing good recovery and long-term outcome. For that reason, pediatric patients meeting surgical criteria should not be withheld from an intervention if benefits and improvement of quality of life are expected.

Although no surgical treatment is effective to restore new-onset neurological deficits, affected patients should be referred to a multidisciplinary team of health care professionals including speech, occupational, and physiotherapist in order to optimize rehabilitation.

Endocrinological Disturbances

Any single hormone secreted by the pituitary gland can be altered following tumor resection—mainly in (supra)sellar lesions—sometimes resulting in the necessity of long-term hormonal replacement. The most significant ones are vasopressin (diabetes insipidus) and cortisol (hypocortisolism) disturbances since alteration of secretion of these hormones can lead to life-threatening consequences. Syndrome of inappropriate antidiuretic hormone secretion can also be challenging and should be looked for in the face of hyponatremia. In addition, hypothalamic injuries with concomitant increase risk of morbid obesity and personality changes are of great concern.

The rate of various endocrinological disturbances following tumor resection varies greatly according to the tumor location. Neervoort et al. reported a rate of 22 % following resection of tumors from various locations [22]. However, this number increases greatly for (supra)sellar lesions. For example, new-onset hypopituitarism (excluding transient diabetes insipidus) following resection of craniopharyngiomas was observed in 38.4 % in a series by Caldarelli et al. [32].

CSF Disturbances

Common complications include pathologies related to an obstructed or a divergent flow of CSF. CSF fistulas and hydrocephalus are both complications for which surgical intervention might be needed and should be addressed appropriately.

Other Complications

These include epilepsy/seizures, hemorrhage/
hematomas, deep and superficial infections, and
metabolic and hematologic disturbances. Specific
complications related to neuroendoscopic procedures include intraventricular hematomas, third
nerve palsy, basilar artery injury, short-term
memory deficit, and CSF fistulas.

Mortality

Mortality following resection of pediatric
brain tumors ranges between 0 and 20 % [22].
The incidence varies greatly according to the
location and type of tumor, patient's characteristics (age, performance status) as well as
the volume of cases annually treated in each
center [22]. Such heterogeneity suggests that
no general guideline can be formulated and
the decision to operate should be taken on a
case-by-case basis after a careful evaluation of
risks and benefits.

Spinal Procedures

Spinal cord tumors represent only 4–8 % of pediatric central nervous system tumors and are
mostly benign [33]. Nevertheless, screening for
complications following tumor resection remains
essential to avoid long-term sequelae. Patil et al.
revealed that 17.5 % of the 19 017 admissions
identified from the US National Inpatient Sample
for spinal cord tumor resection developed an in-
hospital complication [14]. Hemorrhagic, neurological, and infectious complications were
observed in 2.5 %, 1.7 %, and 0.5 % of patients,
respectively [14]. Other complications include
CSF leak and spinal deformity. In-hospital mortality following intramedullary tumor resection is
low (approximately 0.5 %) and often results from
complication of the surgery. This low rate of
mortality is reassuring and allows the surgeon to
emphasize on the risk of morbidity in order to
decide if a surgical procedure should be
performed.

Management of Tumoral Cysts

Various pediatric CNS tumors are composed of a
cystic component. The potential space of the cystic portion creates an isolated microenvironment
into which local treatment in the form of chemotherapy or radiotherapy can be administered
when resection of the cyst is associated with a
risk of significant morbidity. The main advantage
of such method is the administration of intracystic therapy while avoiding the undesired damage
to the surrounding normal parenchyma. In addition, the fluid that composes the cyst allows for
simple aspiration which can sometimes be a sufficient treatment.

Although surgical resection can be considered
for most cystic tumors, local treatment may be
considered and includes the insertion of a device
in which medical therapy will be administered.
More specifically, the use of intracystic radiotherapy and intracavitary chemotherapy may be used
in selected cases. Furthermore, fluid aspiration
alone through a subcutaneous reservoir may be
sufficient to control a cystic tumoral component.
Examples of such cases include cystic craniopharyngiomas and cystic pilocytic astrocytomas
when complete resection is not possible.

Intracavitary brachytherapy commonly uses
phosphorus 32 [34] or iodine-125 (^{125}I) seeds
inside the cystic cavity and allows for administration of continuous low-dose irradiation rather
than intermittent high-dose irradiation of external
beam therapy. The main advantage of low-dose
treatment is the low rate of normal brain parenchyma radiation necrosis. Long-term sequelae,
which are of particular concern in children, are
thus minimized.

Intracystic chemotherapy has been advocated
by some authors to delay aggressive treatment
such as radical resection or irradiation. This
method of delivery allows for administration of a
high dose of effective therapy and dampens the
systemic toxicity associated with intravenous
chemotherapy and the severe morbidity that can
result from surgical resection. Insertion of an
Ommaya reservoir and instillations of single or
multiple doses of active drugs have been the

method of choice for intracystic chemotherapy. Bleomycin and interferon alpha (INFα) are the most commonly used therapeutic agents.

Management of Tumor Recurrence

Screening for tumor recurrence in the postoperative period is essential as it will influence subsequent management. Differentiating between postoperative changes, radionecrosis, and tumor recurrence can be challenging. In this context, opinions from neuroradiologists and the use of nuclear imaging such as single-photon emission computed tomography (SPECT) and positron emission tomography (PET) can be beneficial.

The decision to re-operate a tumor that has recurred must be taken in the light of the patient's life expectancy and quality of life, tumor histology, the time length between initial resection and recurrence, the risks and benefits of a second surgery, and the potential for adjuvant therapy such as radiotherapy and chemotherapy. Each case should be individually evaluated and discussed with the involved specialists and the patient's family.

In general, surgical treatment of recurrent tumors should be considered since re-operation has improved survival for choroid plexus tumors [35], localized recurrent ependymomas [36], and cerebellar astrocytomas [37]. As for other tumors such as supratentorial high grade gliomas, there are insufficient data to support that a reoperation might improve outcome.

Nonsurgical Management of Potentially Surgical Lesions

Not all tumors found on neuroimaging require surgical management. For example, low-grade tumors such as DNET or gangliogliomas presenting with epilepsy may be followed with serial MRIs if the patient is clinically well and seizures are well controlled with medical treatment. Surgical resection may become necessary if the tumor grows or epilepsy becomes refractory to medical treatment. Other examples include some hypothalamo-

chiasmatic gliomas for which conservative management may be considered, especially in the context of neurofibromatosis. The role of surgical biopsies in diffuse pontine gliomas is currently a matter for debate, but most centers nowadays will consider irradiation without a biopsy if the clinical presentation and the radiological findings are typical. Tumors known to respond well to chemotherapy and/or radiotherapy, such as germinomas, should not undergo aggressive surgical resection as the first modality. Similarly in the context of non-germinomatous germ cell tumors, serum or CSF markers are often sufficient to achieve the correct diagnosis. The management of tumors located in eloquent region is the subject of extensive discussions. The pros and cons of such surgery should be well discussed within the medical team and with the family before excluding conservative follow-up as a potential option.

In conclusion, surgical management of children with CNS tumors should be done within a specialized multidisciplinary team by experienced pediatric neurosurgeons. Each case is unique and multifactorial and the many different treatment options should be individualized for each patient.

References

1. Ullrich NJ, Pomeroy SL. Pediatric brain tumors. Neurol Clin. 2003;21:897–913.
2. Wilne S, Collier J, Kennedy C, Koller K, Grundy R, Walker D. Presentation of childhood CNS tumours: a systemic review and meta-analysis. Lancet Oncol. 2007;8:685–95.
3. Duffner PK, Cohen ME, Freeman AI. Pediatric brain tumors: an overview. CA Cancer J Clin. 1985;35:287–301.
4. Maher CO, Raffel C. Neurosurgical treatment of brain tumors in children. Pediatr Clin North Am. 2004;51:327–57.
5. Crawford JR, MacDonald TJ, Packer RJ. Medulloblastoma in childhood: new biological advances. Lancet Neurol. 2007;6:1073–85.
6. Foreman P, McClugage III S, Naftel R, Griessenauer CJ, Ditty BJ, Agee BS, et al. Validation and modification of a predictive model of postresection hydrocephalus in pediatric patients with posterior fossa tumors. J Neurosurg. 2013;12:220–6.
7. Central Brain Tumor Registry of the United States. 2009–2010 CBTRUS statistical report: primary brain

and central nervous system tumors diagnosed in eighteen states in 2002–2006. Hinsdale: CBTRUS; 2009.

8. Constantini S, Miller DC, Allen JC, Rorke LB, Freed D, Epstein FJ. Radical excision of intramedullary spinal cord tumors: surgical morbidity and long-term follow-up evaluation in 164 children and young adults. J Neurosurg Spine. 2000;93:183–93.

9. Abdel-Wahab M, Corn B, Wolfson A, Raub W, Gaspar LE, Curran Jr W, et al. Prognostic factors and survival in patients with spinal glioma after radiation therapy. Am J Clin Oncol. 1999;22:344–51.

10. Jyothirmayi R, Madhavan J, Nair MK, Rajan B. Conservative surgery and radiotherapy in the treatment of spinal cord astrocytoma. J Neurooncol. 1997;33:205–11.

11. Mansur DB, Hekmatpanah J, Wollman R, Macdonald L, Nicholas K, Beckmann E, Mundt AJ. Low grade gliomas treated with adjuvant radiation therapy in the modern imaging era. Am J Clin Oncol. 2000;23:222–6.

12. Rodrigues G, Waldron J, Wong CS, Laperrierre NJ. A retrospective analysis of 52 cases of spinal cord gliomas managed with radiation therapy. Int J Radiat Oncol Biol Phys. 2000;48:837–42.

13. Sandler H, Papadopoulos S, Thorton Jr AJ, Ross DA. Spinal cord astrocytomas: results of therapy. Neurosurgery. 1992;30:490–3.

14. Patil CG, Patil TS, Lad SP, Boakye M. Complications and outcomes after spinal cord tumor resection in the United States from 1993 to 2002. Spinal Cord. 2007;46:1–5.

15. Sundaresan N, Gutierrez F, Larsen M. Radiation myelopathy in children. Ann Neurol. 1978;4:47–50.

16. Mitchell M, Logan P. Radiation-induced changes in bone. Radiographics. 1998;18:1125–36.

17. O'Sullivan C, Jenkin RD, Doherty MA, Hoffman HJ, Greenberg ML. Spinal cord tumors in children: long-term results of combined surgical and radiation treatment. J Neurosurg. 1994;81:507–12.

18. Albright AL, Pollack IF, Adelson PD, Solot JJ. Outcome data and analysis in pediatric neurosurgery. Neurosurgery. 1999;45:101–6.

19. Dirven CMF, Mooij JJA, Molenaar WM. Cerebellar pilocytic astrocytoma: a treatment protocol based upon analysis of 73 cases and a review of the literature. Childs Nerv Syst. 1997;13:17–23.

20. Due-Tonnessen B, Helseth E, Scheibe D, Skullerud K, Aamondt G, Lundar T. Long-term outcome after resection of benign cerebellar astrocytomas in children and young adults (0–19 years): report of 110 consecutive cases. Pediatr Neurosurg. 2002;37:71–80.

21. Gonc EN, Yordam N, Ozon A, Alikasifoglu A, Kandemir N. Endocrinological outcome of different treatment options in children with craniopharyngioma: a retrospective analysis of 66 cases. Pediatr Neurosurg. 2004;40:112–9.

22. Neervoort FW, Van Ouwerkerk WJ, Folkersma H, Kaspers GJ, Vandertop WP. Surgical morbidity and mortality of pediatric brain tumors: a single center audit. Childs Nerv Syst. 2010;26:1583–92.

23. Sandri A, Sardi N, Genitori L, Giordano F, Peretta P, Basso ME, Bertin D, Mastrodicasa L, Todisco L, Mussa F, Forni M, Ricardi U, Sandri A, Sardi N, Genitori L, Giordano F, Peretta P, Basso ME, Bertin D, Mastrodicasa L, Todisco L, Mussa F, Forni M, Ricardi U, Cordero di Montezemolo L, Madon E. Diffuse and focal brain stem tumors in childhood: prognostic factors and surgical outcome. Childs Nerv Syst. 2006;22:1127–35.

24. Sinson G, Sutton L, Yachnis A, Duhaime A, Schut L. Subependymal giant cell astrocytomas in children. Pediatr Neurosurg. 1994;20:233–9.

25. Wisoff JH, Boyett JM, Berger M, Brandt C, Li H, Yates AJ, McGuire-Cullen P, Turski PA, Sutton LN, Allen JC, Packer RJ, Finlay JL. Current neurosurgical management and the impact of the extent of resection in the treatment of malignant gliomas of childhood: a report of the Children's Cancer Group Trial No CCG-945. J Neurosurg. 1998;89:52–9.

26. Young HK, Johnston H. Intracranial tumors in infants. J Child Neurol. 2003;19:424–30.

27. Akay KM, Izci Y, Baysefer A, Atabey C, Kismet E, Timurkaynak E. Surgical outcomes of cerebellar tumors in children. Pediatr Neurosurg. 2004;40:220–5.

28. Lassen B, Helseth E, Rønning P, Scheie D, Johanneses TB, Maehlen J, Langmoen IA, Meiling TR. Surgical mortality at 30 days and complications leading to recraniotomy in 2630 consecutive craniotomies for intracranial tumors. Neurosurgery. 2011;68(5):1259–68.

29. Drake JM, Riva-Cambrin J, Jea A, Auguste K, Tamber M, Lambert-Pasculli RN, Drake JM, Riva-Cambrin J, Jea A, Auguste K, Tamber M, Lambert-Pasculli RN, Drake JM, Riva-Cambrin J, Jea A, Auguste K, Tamber M, Lambert-Pasculli RN. Prospective surveillance of complications in a pediatric neurosurgery unit. J Neurosurg Pediatr. 2010;5(6):544–8.

30. Drake JM, Singhal A, Kulkami AV, DeVeber G, Cochrane DD, Canadian Pediatric Neurosurgery Study Group. Consensus definitions of complications for accurate recording and comparisons of surgical outcomes in pediatric neurosurgery. J Neurosurg Pediatr. 2012;10(2):89–95.

31. Cochrane DD, Gustavsson B, Poskitt KP, Steinbok P, Kestle JR. The surgical and natural morbidity of aggressive resection for posterior fossa tumors in childhood. Pediatr Neurosurg. 1994;20(1):19–29.

32. Caldarelli M, Massimi L, Tamburrini G, Cappa M, Di Rocco C. Long-term results of the surgical treatment Of craniopharyngioma: the experience at the Policlinico Gemelli, Catholic University, Rome. Childs Nerv Syst. 2005;21(8–9):747–57.

33. Bansal S, Suri A, Borkar SA, Kale SS, Singh M, Mahapatra AK. Management of intramedullary tumors in children: analysis of 82 operated cases. Childs Nerv Syst. 2012;28(12):2063–9.

34. Kobayashi T, Kageyama N, Ohara K. Internal irradiation for cystic craniopharyngioma. J Neurosurg. 1981;55(6):896–903.

35. Kaufman BA. Choroid plexus tumors. In: Winn HR, editor. Youman's neurological surgery. Philadelphia: Elsevier; 2011. p. 2062–8.

36. Duntsch CD, Taylor MD, Boop FA. Ependymoma. In: Winn HR, editor. Youman's neurological surgery. Philadelphia: Elsevier; 2011. p. 2086–94.

37. Lapras C, Patet J, Mottolese C, Vitale G. Cerebellar astrocytomas in children. Prog Exp Tumor Res. 1987;30:128.

Histopathological Features of Common Pediatric Brain Tumors

Phedias Diamandis, Alaa Alkhotani,
Jennifer A. Chan, and Cynthia E. Hawkins

Introduction

Collectively, central nervous system (CNS) tumors are the most common solid tumors in the pediatric population and are the leading cause of cancer-related death in this age group. These tumors display diversity in their cellular origin, biology, management options, and long-term outcomes. Microscopic examination combined with molecular signatures of these tumors continues to identify and define features specific to CNS tumor subtypes. Intra- or postoperative histological analysis of biopsies and resections thus continues to play an important role in providing a specific diagnosis that helps guide the appropriate subtype-specific management and care for each patient.

In this chapter, we provide a brief overview of the main diagnostic histopathological features of

the common pediatric CNS tumors to aid in the appreciation of how brain tumors are subclassified by neuropathologists. Some diagnoses can be made immediately on standard hematoxylin and eosin stains based on classic architectural features alone, while more challenging cases often require ancillary studies including immunohistochemistry, electron microscopy, cytogenetics, and/or molecular studies. For the interested readers, texts dedicated to the neuropathology of brain tumors may be consulted for a more detailed review [1, 2].

Neuroepithelial Tumors

Astrocytic Tumors

Pilocytic Astrocytoma

Pilocytic astrocytomas (WHO grade I) are the most common group of pediatric gliomas, and typically present in the cerebellum or midline along the hypothalamic/optic pathways [3]. Grossly, pilocytic astrocytomas are well-circumscribed, soft, and often cystic lesions. Microscopic examination of classic pilocytic astrocytomas characteristically shows a biphasic histologic pattern comprised of a compact fibrillary component that neighbors a spongy microcystic element (Fig. 6.1a). The compact component is formed by parallel fascicles of bipolar hair-like (piloid) astrocytic cells with

P. Diamandis, M.D., Ph.D. • A. Alkhotani, M.D.
Department of Laboratory Medicine and
Pathobiology, University of Toronto, Toronto,
ON, Canada

J.A. Chan, M.D.
Department of Pathology & Laboratory Medicine,
University of Calgary, Calgary, AB, Canada

C.E. Hawkins, M.D., Ph.D., F.R.C.P.C. (✉)
Department of Paediatric Laboratory Medicine,
The Hospital for Sick Children, Toronto, ON, Canada
e-mail: Cynthia.hawkins@sickkids.ca

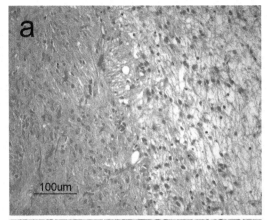

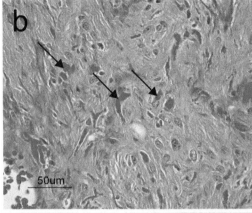

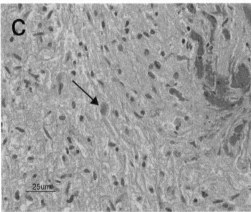

Fig. 6.1 (**a**) Pilocytic astrocytoma showing biphasic architecture, with both a loose, hypocellular pattern (right half) and a compact cellular pattern (left half). H&E, original magnification ×100. (**b**) Rosenthal fibers (*arrows*) scattered within the compact piloid component of a pilocytic astrocytoma. H&E, original magnification ×200. (**c**) Eosinophilic granular body (*arrow*) within a loose area in a pilocytic astrocytoma. H&E, original magnification ×200

bland nuclei and long, narrow cytoplasmic processes in a fibrillary background rich in Rosenthal fibers (Fig. 6.1b, c). These fibers are brightly eosinophilic, proteinaceous, intracytoplasmic, glial fibrillary acidic protein (GFAP)-positive masses that are characteristic of, but not specific for, pilocytic astrocytoma. The less cellular component consists of loose, hypocellular, microcystic areas made up of cells with small round nuclei and fine processes and with scattered cells containing another type of globular, brightly eosinophilic, aggregate known as eosinophilic granular bodies (EGBs) (Fig. 6.1c). Although prognosis is generally good, incomplete resection of the lesion is associated with recurrence of the cystic component [4].

The presence of microscopic foci of brain or subarachnoid space infiltration, occasional mitotic figures, isolated foci of necrosis, or microvascular proliferation does not necessarily indicate malignancy or poor survival [5]. Innocent degenerative changes such as nuclear atypia and pleomorphism associated with smudgy chromatin and nuclear pseudo-inclusions can occur and may lead to misdiagnosis of a malignant glioma. Other degenerative changes that can be seen include the presence of multinucleated giant cells (often referred to as "pennies on a plate"). Malignant transformation is rare and typically results following radiation therapy of this low-grade lesion [5].

Immunohistochemically, pilocytic astrocytomas have a low Ki67/MIB-1 proliferative index of 1–4 % (but sometimes higher) and stain for GFAP. When the location of these tumors limits adequate biopsies, it is often difficult histologically to differentiate them from other low-grade lesions such as diffuse astrocytomas (WHO grade II). Molecular testing in these cases may provide some aid, as the majority (70 %) of cerebellar pilocytic astrocytomas exhibit activation of the RAS/BRAF/MAPK pathway commonly due to BRAF duplication/fusion with the KIAA1549 gene, something less commonly seen in diffuse astrocytomas [6].

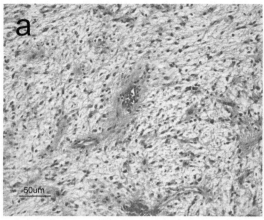 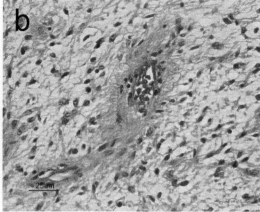

Fig. 6.2 (**a**) Pilomyxoid astrocytoma showing a monophasic architecture in a myxoid background. There is an impression of the angiocentric pattern at this low power that is better seen at higher power. H&E, original magnification ×200. (**b**), Angiocentric pattern of pilomyxoid astrocytoma. H&E, original magnification ×400

A potential diagnostic mimic of pilocytic astrocytoma is nonneoplastic reactive gliosis which can resemble a pilocytic astrocytoma due to increased numbers of astrocytes and the presence of Rosenthal fibers. Such so-called piloid gliosis classically occurs at the rim of a craniopharyngioma or a hemangioma where the surrounding brain tissue creates a dense gliotic background filled with Rosenthal fibers, but can occur around any long-standing or slowly expanding lesion. Biopsies from these areas may be misinterpreted as findings consistent with a pilocytic astrocytoma, underscoring the need for adequate surgical sampling.

Pilomyxoid Astrocytoma

This pediatric tumor entity shares many of the gross and microscopic features of pilocytic astrocytomas. Like pilocytic astrocytomas, these tumors tend to occur in midline structures, with a predominance for the suprasellar/hypothalamic region [7]. Their increased tendency to recur and less favorable prognosis have resulted in designating pilomyxoid astrocytoma as a distinct WHO grade II entity rather than simply as a rare morphologic variant of pilocytic astrocytoma [7].

Grossly, pilomyxoid astrocytomas are well-circumscribed, solid, gelatinous, or cystic lesions that are difficult to distinguish macroscopically from pilocytic astrocytoma. On microscopic examination however, unlike its close relative, pilomyxoid astrocytoma is a monophasic tumor in a predominantly myxoid background matrix (Fig. 6.2a). Embedded within the myxoid matrix are bland bipolar cells that have a tendency to form an angiocentric pattern (Fig. 6.2b). Other histological findings that may help in distinguishing this entity from pilocytic astrocytoma are its lack of protoplasmic cells, Rosenthal fibers or calcifications, and rare eosinophilic granular bodies. Neither immunohistochemistry nor molecular testing has been helpful thus far in distinguishing pilomyxoid from pilocytic astrocytoma.

Angiocentric Glioma

This entity was added to the WHO 2007 classification as a WHO grade I lesion and carries a good prognosis [2, 8]. They are cortically based, typically occurring in the frontoparietal and temporal lobes (including the hippocampal region), and present clinically with seizures. Microscopically, angiocentric gliomas are variably infiltrative and characterized by monomorphous bipolar cells with a prominent angiocentric growth pattern (Fig. 6.3a). They also frequently display subpial palisading. As for most astrocytic neoplasms, GFAP is diffusely positive. There is also an intracytoplasmic dot-like pattern of staining with epithelial membrane antigen (EMA) (Fig. 6.3b).

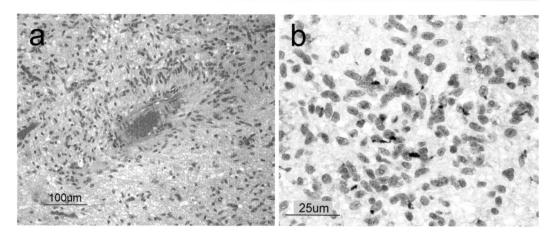

Fig. 6.3 (a) Angiocentric glioma showing elongated astrocytic tumor cells organizing around a blood vessel (angiocentric pattern). H&E, original magnification ×100.

(b), A dot-like staining pattern with epithelial membrane antigen (EMA) immunohistochemistry is a characteristic feature of angiocentric glioma. Original magnification ×400

Diffuse Astrocytoma

Diffuse astrocytomas (WHO grade II) are infiltrating glial tumors that occur throughout the pediatric CNS. Unlike in adults, diffuse astrocytomas in children rarely progress to higher grade lesions. Grossly, this tumor forms an ill-defined and occasionally cystic mass that causes enlargement and distortion of the involved anatomical structures.

Microscopically, diffuse astrocytomas are composed of hypercellular sheets of cells with oval to elongate nuclei within a fibrillar background (Fig. 6.4a). The entrapment of nonneoplastic neurons (Fig. 6.4b) and features such as perineuronal, perivascular, subpial, and subependymal aggregates of neoplastic cells (the so-called secondary structures) are evidence of their infiltrative growth. The presence of atypical nuclei that are angular, hyperchromatic, and mildly pleomorphic can help differentiate these neoplasms from reactive astrocytes. Mitoses, however, are rare or absent. GFAP is the main immunohistochemical stain that highlights the neoplastic astrocytic cells. Neurofilament is helpful for highlighting the infiltrative nature of the tumor cells (Fig. 6.4c).

Morphological variants of diffuse astrocytomas include protoplasmic and gemistocytic variants. The former is a rare hypocellular, mucoid, and microcystic lesion that is predominantly composed of cells with small nuclei, low content of glial filaments, and scant GFAP expression. The gemistocytic variant shows a predominant population of cells with abundant eosinophilic cytoplasm, nuclei that are displaced to the periphery and strong, consistent GFAP expression.

Recently, a study applying whole-genome sequencing to low-grade gliomas found a high rate (53 %) of either intragenic duplication of the tyrosine kinase domain of the FGFR1 or rearrangements of MYB in WHO grade II diffuse gliomas [9]. In a similar analysis of grade II gliomas, 28 % were shown to have partial duplication of the transcription factor MYBL1 [10]. Given the availability of specific therapeutic inhibitors of such pathways, histopathological diagnosis with supplemental molecular analysis of tumors may one day offer more patient-specific treatments and prognostication for these tumors.

Anaplastic Astrocytoma

Anaplastic astrocytomas (WHO grade III) show increased cellularity, nuclear pleomorphism, and hyperchromasia when compared to WHO grade II diffuse astrocytomas. Grossly, it is difficult to differentiate between diffuse astrocytoma WHO grade II and anaplastic astrocytoma.

The presence of mitoses is a key distinguishing feature that favors a diagnosis of anaplastic

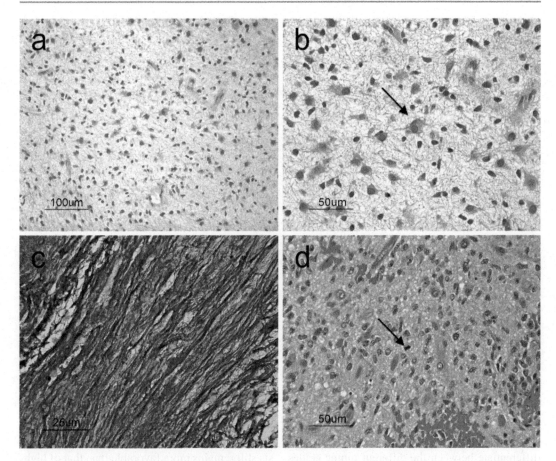

Fig. 6.4 (a) At low power, diffuse astrocytoma can be recognized as areas of hypercellularity within the brain. H&E, original magnification ×100. (b), On higher power, entrapped neurons (*arrows*) can be seen demonstrating the infiltrative nature of the tumor. H&E, original magni-fication ×200. (c), Neurofilament immunostain highlighting the infiltrative nature of the tumor. H&E, original magnification ×400. (d), Anaplastic astrocytoma showing markedly increased cellularity, nuclear pleomorphism, and mitosis (*arrow*). H&E, original magnification ×200

astrocytoma over the lower grade astrocytic neoplasms already discussed (Fig. 6.4d). Though the finding of pyknotic nuclei is still consistent with this category, geographic areas of necrosis or microvascular proliferation are usually indicative of glioblastoma.

Glioblastoma

Glioblastoma (GBM) is a malignant astrocytic tumor (WHO grade IV) that can occur throughout the CNS. It is less common in the pediatric population than in adults. As its former name "glioblastoma multiforme" suggests, the tumor exhibits tremendous phenotypic heterogeneity from one region of the tumor to another. Grossly, it usually shows areas of necrosis, hemorrhage,

peritumoral edema as well as occasional pseudo-capsule formation, in addition to a yellowish discoloration from myelin breakdown. GBMs also exhibit variable architectural patterns and cellular morphologies at the microscopic level that include multinucleated giant cells, small cells, granular cells, and lipidized cells. In addition to sharing features such as hypercellularity, diffuse infiltration, pleomorphism, and mitoses with anaplastic astrocytoma, GBMs also show either necrosis, typically with pseudopalisading of tumor cells (Fig. 6.5a) or microvascular proliferation (Fig. 6.5b).

Exome sequencing of pediatric supratentorial/hemispheric GBMs has revealed differences in the biology that governs tumorigenesis between

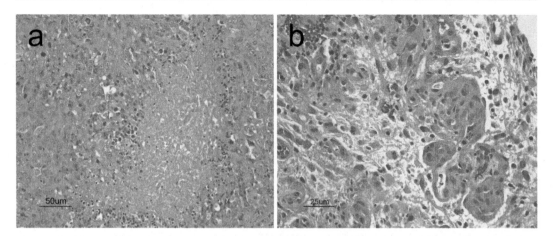

Fig. 6.5 (a), Classical palisading of the neoplastic cells around areas of necrosis. H&E, original magnification ×200. (b) vascular-endothelial proliferation. H&E, original magnification ×400

pediatric/young adult GBMs and those seen in adults. In the young age group somatic mutations in the H3.3-ATRX-DAXX chromatin remodeling pathway can be found. Mutations in the tumor suppressor *TP53* are found in approximately half of GBMs and 86 % of GBMs with H3.3 or ATRX mutations. Mutations in H3.3 were also highly specific for GBMs when compared to low-grade lesions and thus provide additional tools to help differentiate between the different tumor grades in small biopsies [11]. Although extremely rare in the pediatric population, IDH1 mutations may be encountered in the adolescent age group [12].

Pleomorphic Xanthoastrocytoma

Pleomorphic Xanthoastrocytoma (PXA) is a relatively rare astrocytic, low-grade tumor (WHO grade II) with distinctive morphologic features. It is a supratentorial lesion that classically involves the superficial cortex and leptomeninges of the temporal lobe of children and young adults with medically refractory epilepsy. Grossly, PXAs are discrete lesions with leptomeningeal involvement and may be cystic lesions. Microscopically, as its name suggests, PXAs are composed of highly pleomorphic, fibrillary astrocytes, some of which may show lipidization (Fig. 6.6a). Large, bizarre, multinucleated cells are an additional feature. Reticulin positivity is a characteristic feature (Fig. 6.6b). Eosinophilic granular bodies, perivascular infil-

tration by lymphocytes, and a solid component within the subarachnoid space are key features that can help with diagnosis. Due to its significant pleomorphism, differentiation of PXA from more malignant astrocytic tumors such as anaplastic astrocytoma or GBM is critical given the difference in prognosis. In fact, even when PXAs show "anaplastic features" (5 or more mitoses per 10 high power fields) or necrosis, the prognosis still remains more favorable than that of high-grade gliomas [13]. The neoplastic cells in PXA are positive for S100 and variably positive for GFAP and CD34 [14]. There may also be focal areas with a neuronal phenotype suggesting a multipotential precursor cell as its cell of origin [15]. Approximately two-thirds of PXAs harbor the V600E BRAF mutation [16].

Embryonal Tumors

Medulloblastoma

Medulloblastoma (WHO grade IV) is the most common malignant pediatric brain tumor. It characteristically occurs in the cerebellum and in the roof of the 4th ventricle, where it forms a well-circumscribed, soft, gray mass presenting as cerebellar dysfunction and obstructive hydrocephalus with cranial nerve findings. It has a tendency to infiltrate the leptomeninges and form spinal "drop metastases" via the CSF.

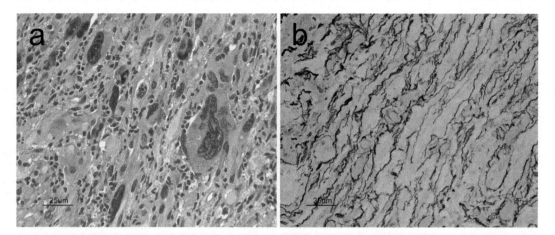

Fig. 6.6 (a) PXA showing pleomorphic fibrillary astrocytes, including large bizarre cells. H&E, original magnification ×400. (b), PXA typically exhibits an extensive reticulin network. Reticulin, original magnification ×400

Histologically, it is divided into classic medulloblastoma (majority of cases) and less common variants that include desmoplastic/nodular medulloblastoma, medulloblastoma with extensive nodularity, anaplastic medulloblastoma, and large cell medulloblastoma.

As discussed in Chap. 12, medulloblastomas can also be divided into four distinct molecular subgroups with some enrichment for the histological types. Here we will discuss the histologic variants.

The classic medulloblastoma subtype makes up approximately 70 % of all medulloblastomas and forms sheets of small round blue cells (high nucleus-to-cytoplasmic ratio) containing variable numbers of Homer-Wright (neuroblastic) rosettes characterized by a fibrillary core (Fig. 6.7a,b) and rarely differentiating ganglioneuronal elements. Medulloblastomas usually exhibit a high mitotic rate, numerous apoptotic bodies, and small areas of necrosis. The tumor cells show positivity for neuronal immunohistochemical markers such as synaptophysin, NeuN, anti-Hu, and neuron-specific enolase in addition to focal positivity with glial markers like GFAP [17].

Nodular/desmoplastic medulloblastoma is the second most common histopathological variant of medulloblastomas. Grossly, it has a firm consistency and unlike the classic form that tends to occur in the vermis, it arises in the cerebellar hemispheres. Microscopically, pale zones showing neurocytic differentiation and apoptosis are surrounded by more cellular zones that are reticulin-rich and highly proliferative (Fig. 6.7c,d). The differentiated nodules may be highlighted using neuronal markers such as synaptophysin. Nodular/desmoplastic medulloblastomas are associated with Gorlin syndrome and activation of the sonic hedgehog pathway [17].

Medulloblastoma with extensive nodularity is a rare variant, usually seen in infants, with a favorable prognosis. It is qualitatively differentiated from the nodular/desmoplastic type variant by having a predominant lobular architecture with large elongated reticulin-free zones that contain small round neurocytic cells in a fibrillary background. The internodular component of reticulin-rich areas that is commonly seen in desmoplastic medulloblastoma is largely reduced [18].

Anaplastic/large cell medulloblastomas are thought to be more aggressive variants. Anaplastic medulloblastomas show marked nuclear enlargement, nuclear pleomorphism, nuclear molding, high mitotic count, prominent necrosis, and apoptosis (Fig. 6.7e). Large cell medulloblastoma has discohesive, monomorphic large cells with round nuclei, open chromatin, and prominent nucleoli (Fig. 6.7f). The features of "anaplastic" and "large cell" may coexist in the same tumor [2].

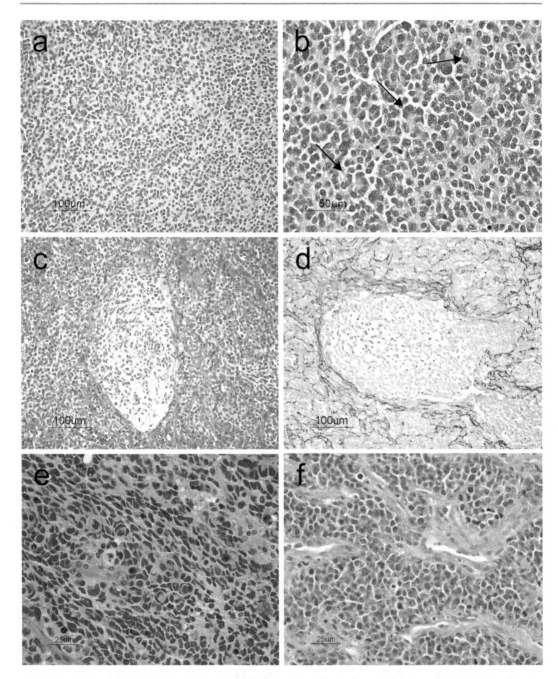

Fig. 6.7 (a) Small round blue cells characteristic of medulloblastoma. H&E, original magnification ×100. (b) Tumor cells arranged in Homer-Wright rosettes (*arrows*). H&E, original magnification ×200. (c), Desmoplastic medulloblastoma showing pale nodular areas in between more cellular internodular regions. H&E, original magnification ×100. (d) Reticulin-rich internodular regions in desmoplastic medulloblastoma. Reticulin, original magnification ×100. (e) Anaplastic medulloblastoma showing markedly pleomorphic cells, cell molding, and prominent apoptosis. H&E, original magnification ×400. (f) Large cell medulloblastoma showing large anaplastic cells with prominent nucleoli and vesicular chromatin. Note the prominent apoptosis. H&E, original magnification ×400

Other variants include medulloblastomas with melanotic or myogenic differentiation that can be highlighted by melanocytic and myogenic markers, respectively. Although histologically distinctive, these variants do not have any known prognostic significance at this time [2].

Even among histologically similar medulloblastomas, genomic approaches have helped further subclassify these tumors into clinical and biologically distinct groups. Four subgroups are currently recognized: WNT, SHH, Group 3, and Group 4. Not only will these groups provide better prognostic information for patients, but these also help stratify tumors into classes driven by distinct molecular pathways, which have the potential to be translated clinically into more patient-specific therapies [19]. These classes are discussed in more detail in Chap. 12.

Supratentorial Primitive Neuroectodermal Tumor

Supratentorial Primitive Neuroectodermal Tumor (sPNETs) (WHO grade IV) are tumors morphologically similar to medulloblastomas but that reside in the cerebral hemispheres rather than the cerebellum of children and adolescents. Compared to medulloblastomas, sPNETs are less frequently encountered and carry a worse prognosis. This tumor is mostly situated deep within the hemisphere. Usually, they are soft and pink-red to purple in color with or without cystic changes or hemorrhages. Microscopically, they resemble medulloblastomas exhibiting sheets of poorly differentiated small round blue cells with hyperchromatic nuclei and a high nucleus-to-cytoplasmic ratio (Fig. 6.8a). Homer-Wright rosettes are found with variable frequency. Areas of necrosis, abundant mitoses, and apoptosis can be seen [2]. Immunohistochemistry may demonstrate areas of divergent differentiation including neuronal, glial or, more rarely, mesenchymal. When large ganglion cells are seen disbursed throughout neuroblastic differentiation, the term ganglioneuroblastoma may be used [2].

Similar and very rare primitive embryonal tumors include those with predominant neural

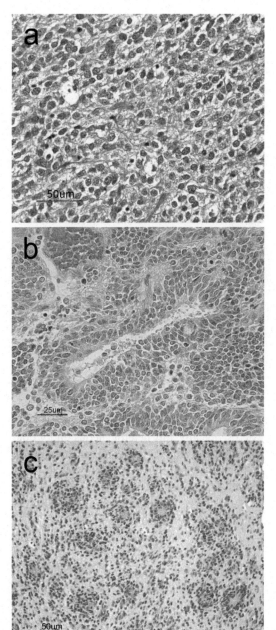

Fig. 6.8 (**a**) sPNET showing a cellular neoplasm with hyperchromatic, anaplastic nuclei, and numerous apoptotic bodies. H&E, original magnification ×200. (**b**) Medulloepithelioma showing the characteristic tubular structures mimicking the primitive neural tube. H&E, original magnification ×400. (**c**) Embryonal tumor with abundant neuropil and true rosettes demonstrating the biphasic architecture with hypercellular regions abutting hypocellular fibrillary regions. H&E, original magnification ×200

tube formation termed medulloepithelioma (Fig. 6.8b). A newly described variant is the so-called "embryonal tumor with abundant neuropil and true rosettes" (Fig. 6.8c) that shows focal areas of hypercellularity, broad bands of neuropil and rosettes with slit-like lumens and has an extremely poor outcome [20]. This tumor is characterized by frequent amplifications at chromosome 19q13 [21].

Genetic analysis of childhood PNET tumors has also been able to further subclassify these tumors into three distinct molecular subgroups with significantly different clinical outcomes based on their expression of LIN28 and OLIG2 [22]. These subgroups are discussed in more detail in Chap. 12.

Atypical Teratoid/Rhabdoid Tumor

Atypical Teratoid/Rhabdoid Tumor (ATRT) is a high-grade (WHO grade IV) tumor that can occur both supra- and infratentorially [2]. It commonly affects children below the age of 3 years and like other embryonal tumors, ATRT creates a soft pink mass with foci of necrosis. Microscopically, this heterogeneous tumor consists of large pale cells, areas of undifferentiated PNET-like small round blue cells, and areas with classic rhabdoid cells with pleomorphic eccentrically placed nuclei with vesicular chromatin and prominent nucleoli that are displaced from the center of the cell by an eosinophilic filamentous inclusion in the cytoplasm (Fig. 6.9a). Mitoses are usually abundant and the MIB-1 proliferative index is typically very high (up to 80 %). Necrotic areas are common, as are apoptotic bodies. Immunohistochemical studies may show tumor cell positivity for vimentin, EMA, smooth muscle actin as well as focally for GFAP, cytokeratin, neurofilament, and synaptophysin. They are typically negative for desmin. Typically, the tumor cells are immuno-negative for INI-1 (Fig. 6.9b) and show 22q11.2 deletions involving the hSNF5/IN1 gene [23]. This feature is diagnostically very useful in distinguishing ATRT from sPNET, choroid plexus carcinoma, and medulloblastoma which it may mimic [2].

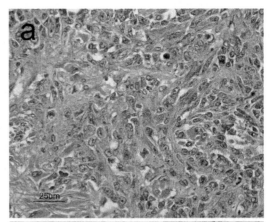

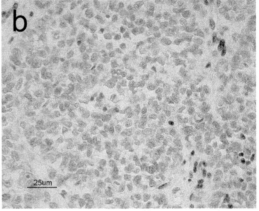

Fig. 6.9 (**a**) ATRT showing sheets of large pleomorphic cells, some of which exhibits globular cytoplasmic eosinophilic material that push the nucleus to the cell edges. Note the prominent nucleoli within vesicular nuclei. H&E, original magnification ×400. (**b**) In ATRT, the tumor cells are negative for INI-1. Original magnification ×400

Ependymomas

Ependymal tumors comprise a group of tumors with variable biological and morphological patterns and include ependymoma, anaplastic ependymoma, myxopapillary ependymoma, and subependymoma. The two most common entities in the pediatric population are ependymoma (WHO grade II) and its anaplastic variant (WHO grade III).

Ependymoma

Ependymoma (WHO grade II) most commonly occurs in the fourth ventricle in children but can be seen throughout the neuraxis. Grossly, ependymomas are usually well-circumscribed, soft masses with or without cystic changes. They commonly show a solid, fibrillary pattern with the formation of perivascular pseudorosettes (Fig. 6.10a). The latter structures are zones of fibrillary eosinophilic process, free of nuclei, abutting blood vessels. Less commonly, this tumor shows true ependymal rosettes. The cells usually have bland uniform nuclei with granular chromatin and show immunoreactivity with GFAP, vimentin, and S100. Dot-like immunopositivity for EMA is a helpful diagnostic feature but is not always present. Ultrastructural examination is often important in distinguishing the ependymal from astrocytic lineage of the neoplastic cells.

The finding of abnormal cilia, intracytoplasmic lumens with microvilli, and long junctional complexes points to an ependymal lineage (Fig. 6.10b). Morphological variants of ependymoma include cellular, clear cell, papillary, and tanycytic types.

Anaplastic Ependymomas

Anaplastic ependymomas (WHO grade III) are more aggressive appearing tumors that, although grossly well demarcated, tend to have invasive foci and high-grade cytology. Grading however remains controversial. While some authors report prognostic significance of some histological features [24, 25], others have not found a correlation [26, 27]. A more recent study reported that the current histological grading scheme may predict event-free survival, but does not correlate with overall survival [28]. This study emphasized the importance of vascular-endothelial proliferation with endothelial layering (Fig. 6.11a), high mitotic rate, palisading necrosis, and marked hypercellularity with nuclear pleomorphism and/or hyperchromasia as high-grade features. Continued refinement of these criteria for grading ependymal tumors will hopefully allow better prognostication of this group of tumors in the future.

Similar to the molecular subclassification of medulloblastomas, molecular analysis of ependymomas has led to the discovery of subgroups with different clinical outcomes [29]. Gains in chromosome 1q are common in pediatric and

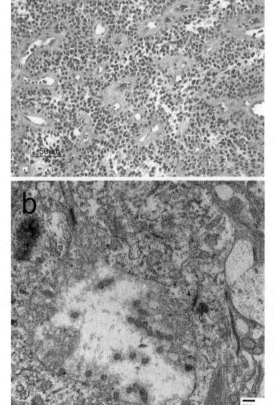

Fig. 6.10 (a) Ependymoma showing small bland cells within a fibrillary background. Note the perivascular nuclear-free zones which are characteristic low-power appearance of ependymoma. H&E, original magnification ×200. (b) Ultrastructural features of an ependymoma showing microvilli in lumina and long intracellular junctions

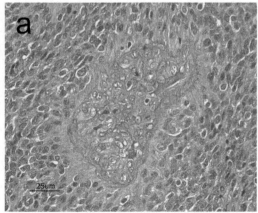

Fig. 6.11 (a) Anaplastic ependymoma showing vascular-endothelial proliferation. H&E, original magnification ×400

high-grade (WHO grade III) cases. More specifically, gains of 1q21.1–32.1 are associated with
tumor recurrence. Gains of 1q25 represent
another independent poor prognostic marker for
recurrence-free and overall survival [30].

Choroid Plexus Tumors

Choroid plexus papillomas (CPP, WHO grade I)
constitute 2–4 % of pediatric CNS tumors.
Choroid plexus carcinomas (CPC, WHO grade
III) are five times less common. Both occur in
areas where choroid plexus is normally found
[31], mainly in the lateral and third ventricles
[32] and to a lesser degree in the fourth ventricle
(the commonest location in adults).

Choroid Plexus Papilloma

Grossly, CPP forms an enlarged cauliflower-like
mass well delineated from the native choroid
plexus. Microscopically, it exhibits a normal choroid plexus-like histology with true fibrovascular
cores (Fig. 6.12a). The tumor cells typically reside
on a basement membrane (Fig. 6.12b), a feature
that is helpful in distinguishing it from papillary
ependymoma. In contrast to normal choroid plexus
papillae, however, the lining epithelial cells show
mild nuclear atypia, crowding, pseudostratifica-
tion, and more complex papillary architecture
(Fig. 6.12c). CPP tumor cells can exhibit a wide
variety of cellular changes including oncocytic
change, mucinous degeneration, and melanization.
Immunohistochemical studies show that the lining
epithelium is positive for cytokeratin, transthyretin,
vimentin, and CK7 and focally for GFAP and
EMA. They are usually negative for CK20 [33].

Atypical Choroid Plexus Papilloma

In between choroid plexus papillomas and carcinomas is a relatively new entity termed "atypical
CPP." It is essentially similar to CPP but with
increased mitotic activity. Two or more mitoses
per ten random high-power fields are required for
the diagnosis of this entity. In addition, atypical
features including increased cellularity, nuclear
pleomorphism, blurring of the papillary pattern,
and necrosis are commonly seen [34].

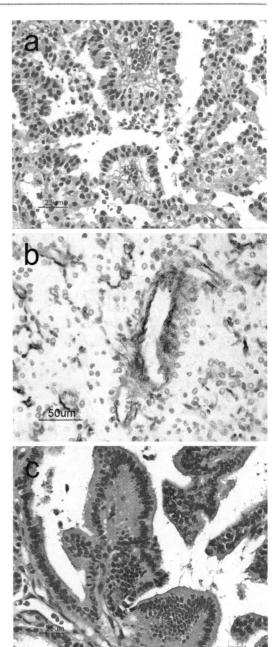

Fig. 6.12 (a) Choroid plexus papilloma showing the
papillary architecture where the papillae are formed by
fibrovascular stroma with overlying columnar epithelium.
H&E, original magnification ×400. (b) Immunohistochemical staining for laminin highlighting the basement membrane in CPP. Original magnification ×200. (c)
The epithelial cells lining the papillae are slightly crowded
and exhibit minor atypical changes such as mild nuclear
pleomorphism, hyperchromasia, and occasional mitoses.
H&E, original magnification ×400

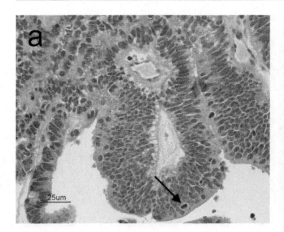

Fig. 6.13 (a) Higher-power view of a choroid plexus carcinoma showing nuclear atypia, increased cell density compared with CPP, and frequent mitoses (*arrow*). H&E, original magnification ×400

Choroid Plexus Carcinoma

CPCs usually occur in children under 3 years of age and demonstrate more hemorrhage, necrosis, and invasiveness than CPP. Microscopically, sheets of frankly anaplastic, highly cellular tumor cells with areas of necrosis and frequent mitoses (Fig. 6.13a) are commonly associated with foci that are still reminiscent of a papilloma. Typically, 5–10 mitoses per ten high-power fields are seen. Otherwise, the papillary structures are usually blurred by more solid patterns. The neoplastic cells are usually immunopositive for EMA, cytokeratin, and S100. CPCs can create poorly differentiated patterns that may be confused with embryonal tumors like ATRT, but they retain their immunoreactivity to INI1. Patients with CPC who have absence of TP53 dysfunction have a favorable prognosis and can be successfully treated without radiation therapy [35].

Neuronal and Mixed Neuroglial Tumors

Ganglioglioma

Grossly, gangliogliomas are well-demarcated solid or cystic masses that are often associated with calcifications. This tumor typically exhibits variable degrees of two distinct neoplastic cell populations: glial and neuronal/gangliocytic

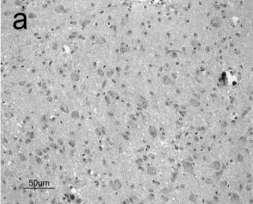

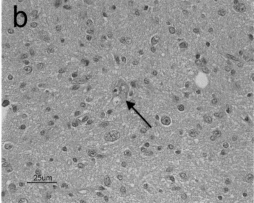

Fig. 6.14 (a) Ganglioglioma showing scattered ganglion cells within a rich fibrillary background. H&E, original magnification ×200. (b) Ganglion cells are large cells with prominent nucleoli and abundant eosinophilic cytoplasm, some contain basophilic Nissl substance in the periphery of the cytoplasm. Note the binucleation, a feature very rare in normal, non-neoplastic neurons (*arrow*). H&E, original magnification ×400

(Fig. 6.14a). When the tumor is composed solely of neuronal/gangliocytic components, it is referred to as "gangliocytoma, WHO grade I." When a neoplastic glial component is also present, the term ganglioglioma is used and the tumor is graded based upon the glial component; a pilocytic-like glial component is given a WHO grade of I while an anaplastic glial component leads to a WHO grade III designation. Criteria for grade II ganglioglioma have been suggested, but this is not currently an official WHO category [36].

Microscopically, there are ganglion cells with large vesicular nuclei, prominent nucleoli, and abundant cytoplasm where Nissl basophilic mate-

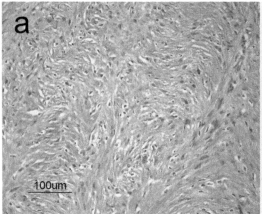 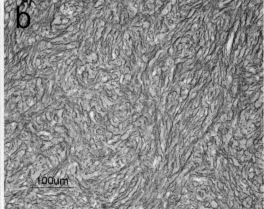

Fig. 6.15 (**a**) Desmoplastic infantile ganglioglioma/ astrocytoma showing fascicles of spindled astrocytes within a desmoplastic stroma. H&E, original magnifica- tion ×100. (**b**) Reticulin staining highlighting desmopla- sia. All pictures, original magnification ×100

rial is present. These neoplastic or atypical ganglion cells show abnormal clustering, pleomorphism, and bi- or multi-nucleation or exhibit large bizarre nuclei (Fig. 6.14b). Eosinophilic granular bodies are typically present and Rosenthal fibers can be seen. Calcifications and perivascular inflammation within a prominent capillary net- work are common features. Mitotic figures are rare in low-grade gangliogliomas (MIB-1 < 3 %), but are present in the anaplastic variant.

The neuronal/gangliocytic cells are high- lighted by immunohistochemistry for NeuN, syn- aptophysin, or chromogranin. The glial component is highlighted by GFAP. Ultrastructural examina- tion may be used to confirm the presence of both glial and neuronal/gangliocytic components. The former shows glial processes with intracytoplas- mic dense fascicles of intermediate filaments, while the latter shows microtubules, electron dense neurosecretory vesicles, and neuritic-type processes.

Anaplastic ganglioglioma can be mistaken for anaplastic astrocytomas that have infiltrated sur- rounded brain tissue and entrapped nonneoplastic neurons. Recent studies suggest that the BRAFV600E mutation is found more commonly in ganglioglioma than anaplastic astrocytoma (18 % vs 3 %) and thus may be used to differentiate between these two entities in difficult cases [16].

Desmoplastic Infantile Astrocytoma/ Ganglioglioma

This is a unique and rare pediatric low-grade glioneuronal tumor (WHO grade I) [37]. It usu- ally affects the supratentorial compartment of children less than 18 months of age. Grossly, it is large, well demarcated, superficial, and typically cystic with involvement of multiple lobes and an attachment to the overlying dura. Desmoplastic infantile astrocytomas are characterized as lesions of low cellularity within a remarkably reticulin-rich desmoplastic stroma containing fascicles, storiform, or whorled patterns of spin- dled strongly GFAP immunopositive astrocytes (Figs. 6.15a,b). A cortical component without desmoplasia may be observed. This component is usually nodular and often formed by small astro- cytes with oval nuclei and eosinophilic cyto- plasm. If a population of abnormal binucleated ganglion cells is present, then the tumor is labeled desmoplastic infantile ganglioglioma. The gan- glion cells can be difficult to detect without the use of immunohistochemical markers such as synaptophysin and chromogranin. Desmoplastic Infantile Astrocytoma/Ganglioglioma (DIA/G) usually has only rare mitoses and low (<5 %) MIB-1 proliferative index. Although the vast majority of these tumors are benign, some reports suggest that a more aggressive and malignant behavior is possible when the small cell component shows features of a poorly differentiated embryonal tumor including a high mitotic rate, microvascular proliferation, and necrosis [38].

Dysembryoplastic Neuroepithelial Tumor

Dysembryoplastic Neuroepithelial Tumor (DNETs) are low-grade cortically based tumors (WHO grade I) that have a predilection for the temporal and frontal lobes and often present with a clinical history of chronic seizures. It should not demonstrate mass effect on the surrounding brain tissue. Grossly, it is a well-defined cortical neoplasm that exhibits multinodular, cystic, and/ or gelatinous features. Different patterns have been described whose prognostic significance is unclear. These are "typical," "complex," and "nonspecific" [39]. In the simple form, the main constituent is the classic glioneuronal element. This is made up of bland monotonous oligodendroglial-like cells that flank axons, which run perpendicular to the cortical surface. Interspersed are mucinous spaces containing characteristic "floating neurons" with large bland nuclei and prominent nucleoli (Fig. 6.16a). These axons can be highlighted with synaptophysin or neurofilament staining. The oligodendroglial-like cells show positive immunohistochemical reactivity with S100, MAP2, and Olig2. In addition, a subpopulation of cells may be positive for neuronal markers such as NeuN or synaptophysin. GFAP stains the glial components.

Complex is a term that is used when the tumor has adjacent glial nodules in addition to the specific glioneuronal element. More diffuse glial components can also be seen. These often mimic a low-grade glioma but may also show some atypical features like nuclear atypia, occasional mitoses, microvascular-like proliferation, or ischemic necrosis [2]. Lastly, a controversial "nonspecific" variant has been proposed that lacks the classic histological features. It comprises mainly glial elements and would otherwise be characterized as a "low-grade glioma." Diagnosis as a nonspecific DNET is thus made based on clinicopathological correlation of a child with a radiological stable, well-circumscribed lesion with an associated history of chronic seizures.

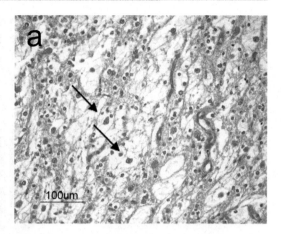

Fig. 6.16 (**a**) DNET showing bundles of axons lined with oligodendroglial cells and microcystic changes in a myxoid background with floating neurons (*arrows*). H&E, original magnification ×100

Non-neuroepithelial Tumors

Craniopharyngioma

Craniopharyngiomas (WHO grade I) usually affect the suprasellar region where they are thought to arise from Rathke's pouch remnants. It has two variants, adamantinomatous and papillary. The former is most common in the pediatric population where it accounts for 5–10 % of intracranial tumors making it the most common form of non-neuroepithelial neoplasm [40]. It usually has solid, firm, and cystic components with contents that resemble motor oil due to the nature of the mixture of blood, proteins, and cholesterol crystals. The tumor exhibits poor circumscription and has sheets, nests, and trabeculae of epithelial cell sheets in a fibrous stroma. The epithelium demonstrates a characteristic morphology where the peripheral cells show nuclear palisading while the central cells form a loose "stellate reticulum" (Fig. 6.17a). Also present are characteristic areas of "wet keratin" that frequently calcify (Fig. 6.17b). The presence of one of the latter two features (the stellate reticulum or the wet keratin) is diagnostic of craniopharyngioma [1]. In addition, cystic changes, xanthogranulomatous reaction, and cholesterol clefts are frequent findings in a craniopharyngioma. Variable degrees of necrosis can be seen and do not indicate a malig-

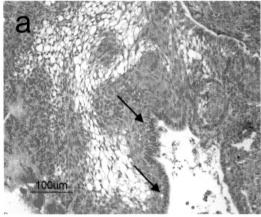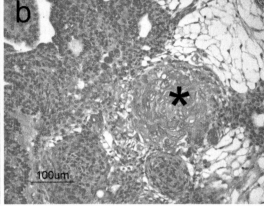

Fig. 6.17 (**a**) Craniopharyngioma showing palisaded epithelial cells, the loose stellate reticulum (*arrows*). H&E, original magnification ×100. (**b**) Characteristic wet keratin (*asterisk*) of craniopharyngioma. H&E, original magnification ×100

nant nature. Craniopharyngioma can be associated with piloid gliosis in the surrounding brain tissue where Rosenthal fibers are prominent. The latter can be confused with low-grade astrocytic neoplasms, particularly on frozen section.

References

1. Burger P, Scheithauer BW. Diagnostic pathology: neuropathology. 1st ed. Salt Lake City: Lippincott Williams & Wilkins and Amirsys; 2011.
2. Louis D, Ohgaki H, Wiestler OD, Cavenee WK. WHO classification of tumours of the central nervous system. 4th ed. Lyon: International Agency for Research on Cancer; 2007.
3. Hayostek CJ, Shaw EG, Scheithauer B, O'Fallon JR, Weiland TL, Schomberg PJ, et al. Astrocytomas of the cerebellum. A comparative clinicopathologic study of pilocytic and diffuse astrocytomas. Cancer. 1993;72(3):856–69.
4. Pollack IF, Claassen D, al-Shboul Q, Janosky JE, Deutsch M. Low-grade gliomas of the cerebral hemispheres in children: an analysis of 71 cases. J Neurosurg. 1995;82(4):536–47.
5. Tomlinson FH, Scheithauer BW, Hayostek CJ, Parisi JE, Meyer FB, Shaw EG, et al. The significance of atypia and histologic malignancy in pilocytic astrocytoma of the cerebellum: a clinicopathologic and flow cytometric study. J Child Neurol. 1994;9(3):301–10.
6. Korshunov A, Meyer J, Capper D, Christians A, Remke M, Witt H, et al. Combined molecular analysis of BRAF and IDH1 distinguishes pilocytic astrocytoma from diffuse astrocytoma. Acta Neuropathol. 2009;118(3):401–5.
7. Tihan T, Fisher PG, Kepner JL, Godfraind C, McComb RD, Goldthwaite PT, et al. Pediatric astrocytomas with monomorphous pilomyxoid features and a less favorable outcome. J Neuropathol Exp Neurol. 1999;58(10):1061–8.
8. Wang M, Tihan T, Rojiani AM, Bodhireddy SR, Prayson RA, Iacuone JJ, et al. Monomorphous angiocentric glioma: a distinctive epileptogenic neoplasm with features of infiltrating astrocytoma and ependymoma. J Neuropathol Exp Neurol. 2005;64(10):875–81.
9. Zhang J, Wu G, Miller CP, Tatevossian RG, Dalton JD, Tang B, et al. Whole-genome sequencing identifies genetic alterations in pediatric low-grade gliomas. Nat Genet. 2013;45:602–12.
10. Ramkissoon LA, Horowitz PM, Craig JM, Ramkissoon SH, Rich BE, Schumacher SE, et al. Genomic analysis of diffuse pediatric low-grade gliomas identifies recurrent oncogenic truncating rearrangements in the transcription factor MYBL1. Proc Natl Acad Sci U S A. 2013;30.
11. Schwartzentruber J, Korshunov A, Liu XY, Jones DT, Pfaff E, Jacob K, et al. Driver mutations in histone H3.3 and chromatin remodelling genes in paediatric glioblastoma. Nature. 2012;482(7384):226–31.
12. Jha P, Suri V, Singh G, Purkait S, Pathak P, Sharma V, et al. Characterization of molecular genetic alterations in GBMs highlights a distinctive molecular profile in young adults. Diagn Mol Pathol. 2011;20(4):225–32.
13. Giannini C, Scheithauer BW, Burger PC, Brat DJ, Wollan PC, Lach B, et al. Pleomorphic xanthoastrocytoma: what do we really know about it? Cancer. 1999;85(9):2033–45.
14. Reifenberger G, Kaulich K, Wiestler OD, Blumcke I. Expression of the CD34 antigen in pleomorphic xanthoastrocytomas. Acta Neuropathol. 2003;105(4):358–64.
15. Giannini C, Scheithauer BW, Lopes MB, Hirose T, Kros JM, VandenBerg SR. Immunophenotype of

pleomorphic xanthoastrocytoma. Am J Surg Pathol. 2002;26(4):479–85.

16. Schindler G, Capper D, Meyer J, Janzarik W, Omran H, Herold-Mende C, et al. Analysis of BRAF V600E mutation in 1,320 nervous system tumors reveals high mutation frequencies in pleomorphic xanthoastrocytoma, ganglioglioma and extra-cerebellar pilocytic astrocytoma. Acta Neuropathol. 2011;121(3): 397–405.

17. Ellison DW, Dalton J, Kocak M, Nicholson SL, Fraga C, Neale G, et al. Medulloblastoma: clinicopathological correlates of SHH, WNT, and non-SHH/WNT molecular subgroups. Acta Neuropathol. 2011;121(3): 381–96.

18. Giangaspero F, Perilongo G, Fondelli MP, Brisigotti M, Carollo C, Burnelli R, et al. Medulloblastoma with extensive nodularity: a variant with favorable prognosis. J Neurosurg. 1999;91(6):971–7.

19. Northcott PA, Shih DJ, Peacock J, Garzia L, Sorana Morrissy A, Zichner T, et al. Subgroup-specific structural variation across 1,000 medulloblastoma genomes. Nature. 2012;25.

20. Eberhart CG, Brat DJ, Cohen KJ, Burger PC. Pediatric neuroblastic brain tumors containing abundant neuropil and true rosettes. Pediatr Dev Pathol. 2000;3(4):346–52.

21. Pfister S, Remke M, Castoldi M, Bai AH, Muckenthaler MU, Kulozik A, et al. Novel genomic amplification targeting the microRNA cluster at 19q13.42 in a pediatric embryonal tumor with abundant neuropil and true rosettes. Acta Neuropathol. 2009;117(4):457–64.

22. Picard D, Miller S, Hawkins CE, Bouffet E, Rogers HA, Chan TS, et al. Markers of survival and metastatic potential in childhood CNS primitive neuroectodermal brain tumours: an integrative genomic analysis. Lancet Oncol. 2012;13(8):838–48.

23. Judkins AR, Mauger J, Ht A, Rorke LB, Biegel JA. Immunohistochemical analysis of hSNF5/INI1 in pediatric CNS neoplasms. Am J Surg Pathol. 2004;28(5):644–50.

24. Merchant TE, Jenkins JJ, Burger PC, Sanford RA, Sherwood SH, Jones-Wallace D, et al. Influence of tumor grade on time to progression after irradiation for localized ependymoma in children. Int J Radiat Oncol Biol Phys. 2002;53(1):52–7.

25. Figarella-Branger D, Civatte M, Bouvier-Labit C, Gouvernet J, Gambarelli D, Gentet JC, et al. Prognostic factors in intracranial ependymomas in children. J Neurosurg. 2000;93(4):605–13.

26. Agaoglu FY, Ayan I, Dizdar Y, Kebudi R, Gorgun O, Darendeliler E. Ependymal tumors in childhood. Pediatr Blood Cancer. 2005;45(3):298–303.

27. Robertson PL, Zeltzer PM, Boyett JM, Rorke LB, Allen JC, Geyer JR, et al. Survival and prognostic factors following radiation therapy and chemotherapy for ependymomas in children: a report of the Children's Cancer Group. J Neurosurg. 1998;88(4):695–703.

28. Tihan T, Zhou T, Holmes E, Burger PC, Ozuysal S, Rushing EJ. The prognostic value of histological

grading of posterior fossa ependymomas in children: a Children's Oncology Group study and a review of prognostic factors. Mod Pathol. 2008;21(2):165–77.

29. Witt H, Mack SC, Ryzhova M, Bender S, Sill M, Isserlin R, et al. Delineation of two clinically and molecularly distinct subgroups of posterior fossa ependymoma. Cancer Cell. 2011;20(2):143–57.

30. Kilday JP, Mitra B, Domerg C, Ward J, Andreiuolo F, Osteso-Ibanez T, et al. Copy number gain of 1q25 predicts poor progression-free survival for pediatric intracranial ependymomas and enables patient risk stratification: a prospective European clinical trial cohort analysis on behalf of the Children's Cancer Leukaemia Group (CCLG), Societe Francaise d'Oncologie Pediatrique (SFOP), and International Society for Pediatric Oncology (SIOP). Clin Cancer Res. 2012;18(7):2001–11.

31. Rickert CH, Paulus W. Epidemiology of central nervous system tumors in childhood and adolescence based on the new WHO classification. Childs Nerv Syst. 2001;17(9):503–11.

32. Wolff JE, Sajedi M, Brant R, Coppes MJ, Egeler RM. Choroid plexus tumours. Br J Cancer. 2002;87(10):1086–91.

33. Gyure KA, Morrison AL. Cytokeratin 7 and 20 expression in choroid plexus tumors: utility in differentiating these neoplasms from metastatic carcinomas. Mod Pathol. 2000;13(6):638–43.

34. Jeibmann A, Hasselblatt M, Gerss J, Wrede B, Egensperger R, Beschorner R, et al. Prognostic implications of atypical histologic features in choroid plexus papilloma. J Neuropathol Exp Neurol. 2006;65(11):1069–73.

35. Tabori U, Shlien A, Baskin B, Levitt S, Ray P, Alon N, et al. TP53 alterations determine clinical subgroups and survival of patients with choroid plexus tumors. J Clin Oncol. 2010;28(12):1995–2001.

36. Luyken C, Blumcke I, Fimmers R, Urbach H, Wiestler OD, Schramm J. Supratentorial gangliogliomas: histopathologic grading and tumor recurrence in 184 patients with a median follow-up of 8 years. Cancer. 2004;101(1):146–55.

37. Pommepuy I, Delage-Corre M, Moreau JJ, Labrousse F. A report of a desmoplastic ganglioglioma in a 12-year-old girl with review of the literature. J Neurooncol. 2006;76(3):271–5.

38. De Munnynck K, Van Gool S, Van Calenbergh F, Demaerel P, Uyttebroeck A, Buyse G, et al. Desmoplastic infantile ganglioglioma: a potentially malignant tumor? Am J Surg Pathol. 2002;26(11):1515–22.

39. Daumas-Duport C, Varlet P, Bacha S, Beuvon F, Cervera-Pierot P, Chodkiewicz JP. Dysembryoplastic neuroepithelial tumors: nonspecific histological forms—a study of 40 cases. J Neurooncol. 1999;41(3):267–80.

40. Adamson TE, Wiestler OD, Kleihues P, Yasargil MG. Correlation of clinical and pathological features in surgically treated craniopharyngiomas. J Neurosurg. 1990;73(1):12–7.

Basic Science of Pediatric Brain Tumors

7

Stephen C. Mack, Vijay Ramaswamy, Xin Wang,
Marc Remke, Patrick Sin-Chan, Tiffany Sin Yu Chan,
Kelsey C. Bertrand, Diana Merino, Kory Zayne,
Annie Huang, and Michael D. Taylor

Medulloblastoma

A small fraction of medulloblastomas (MBs) have inherited disorders with germline mutations, which have revealed the first pathways that underlie MB tumorigenesis. It is known that prominent tumor suppressor genes such as *TP53*

S.C. Mack, B.Sc. (✉) • X. Wang, B.H.Sc. (Hon).
K.C. Bertrand, M.D. • K. Zayne, B.Sc.
M.D. Taylor, M.D.
Department of Developmental and Stem Cell Biology,
The Hospital for Sick Children, Toronto, ON, Canada
e-mail: stephen.mack@mail.utoronto.ca

V. Ramaswamy, M.D., F.R.C.P.C.
Division of Neurosurgery, Hospital for Sick Children,
Toronto, ON, Canada

M. Remke, M.D.
Department of Laboratory Medicine and Pathobiology,
The Hospital for Sick Children, Toronto, ON, Canada

P. Sin-Chan, M.Sc.
Arthur and Sonia Labatt Brain Tumour Research Centre,
The Hospital for Sick Children, Toronto, ON, Canada

T.S.Y. Chan, B.Sc.
Department of Cell Biology/Arthur and Sonia Labatt
Brain Tumour Research Centre, The Hospital for Sick
Children, Toronto, ON, Canada

D. Merino, B.Sc.
Department of Genetics and Genome Biology,
The Hospital for Sick Children, Toronto, ON, Canada

A. Huang, M.D., Ph.D.
Department of Cell Biology, The Hospital for Sick
Children, Toronto, ON, Canada

and *APC*, when germline mutated in patients with Li-Fraumeni syndrome and Turcot syndrome, respectively, predispose to MB. Furthermore, the identification of Gorlin's syndrome, in patients harboring mutations in the patched-1 (*PTCH1*) gene, has led to the identification of aberrant sonic hedgehog signaling (SHH) in a subset of MBs (Fig. 7.1).

Integrated genomic studies have revealed that MB comprises at least four molecular variants, which are genetically and clinically distinct. These four subgroups are termed WNT, Sonic Hedgehog (SHH), Group 3, and Group 4 [1] have significant prognostic value, and can be further subdivided into additional relevant molecular subtypes. The delineation of these four core subgroups underscores the heterogeneity that exists between MB patients. The WNT subgroup is characterized by activation of the WNT pathway, which commonly harbors mutations in β-catenin (*CTNNB1*). Patients with WNT activated tumors tend to have a favorable prognosis and occur primarily outside the infant age group. The SHH subgroup is characterized by activation of the Sonic Hedgehog (SHH) pathway and is more common in infants with desmoplastic tumors and in adults. Group 3 MBs have a poor prognosis and are commonly associated with metastatic disease. *MYC* amplification is common in Group 3 MBs, and survival in these patients is poor. Group 4 MBs have an intermediate prognosis and are commonly associated with isochromosome 17q and *MYCN* amplification.

K. Scheinemann and E. Bouffet (eds.), *Pediatric Neuro-oncology*,
DOI 10.1007/978-1-4939-1541-5_7, © Springer Science+Business Media New York 2015

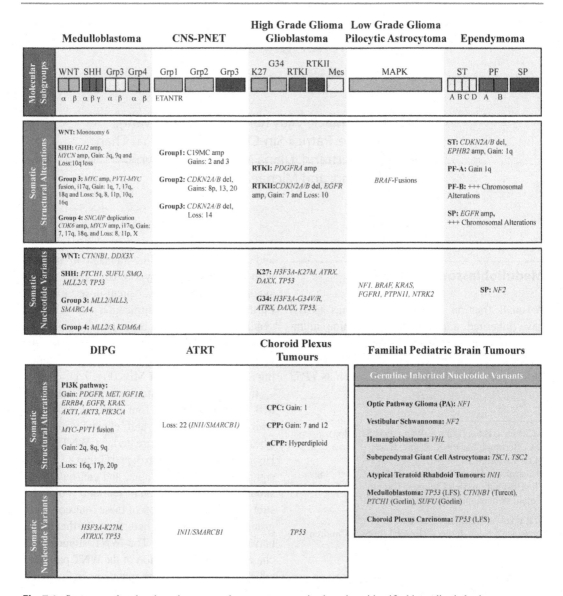

Fig. 7.1 Summary of molecular subgroups and recurrent genomic alterations identified in pediatric brain tumors

There have been a number of chromosomal alterations reported in MB. The most commonly reported cytogenetic abnormality is isochromosome 17q (i17q), involving the loss of chromosome 17p and gain of 17q, which is found in 30–40 % of all primary MB tumors. This is also a genomic feature of the Group 4 subgroup, which is observed in more than 80 % of cases. Other less common aberrations include gains on chromosomes 1q, 3q, 7, and 17q, as well as loss on chromosome 5q, 9q, 10q, 11, 17p, and 22 [2].

Recent publications highlight the importance of examining the mutational landscape of MB according to subgroup affiliation [3, 4]. WNT subgroup MBs remain the most genomically balanced of the four subgroups without any focal recurrent somatic copy number alterations (SCNAs). The most common mutation observed in this subset is in *CTNNB1*, which highlights the important role of WNT signaling in this subgroup, and less frequently in *DDX3X*. Many groups have sought to identify the cell of origin for this subgroup. It has been suggested to be the progenitor cells of the lower rhombic lip. Further, a mouse model harboring activated Ctnnb1 in the Blbp expressing radial glial cells has been shown to generate MBs that are characteristic of WNT tumors [5].

SHH subgroup is the best characterized of the four subgroups, with the distinctive feature of activated SHH signaling. Somatic mutations targeting the SHH receptor *PTCH1* and downstream genes, such as *SUFU*, are found exclusively in this subgroup. SCNAs targeting the PI3K signaling cascade have also been known to be aberrant in this subgroup. Most animal models of SHH MBs involve the inactivation of patched1 in either the cerebellar granule neuron precursors (CGNP; marked by Atoh1) or neural stem cells (NSC; marked by GFAP) [6].

Group 3 and 4 MBs are currently the least understood. Group 3 MB is associated with the worst prognosis and characterized by high-level amplification of the proto-oncogene *MYC*. Research examining somatic mutations have identified dysregulation of the epigenome in both Group 3 and 4 MBs. These events, although occurring across all MBs, are enriched in chromatin-associated genes such as *MLL2*, *MLL3*, *SMARCA4*, *and KDM6A*. These newly identified mutations point to the importance of the chromatin structure in MB pathogenesis. Efforts have also identified novel fusion proteins such as *PVT1-MYC* and novel mechanisms such as the tandem duplication of *SNCAIP* in Group 3 and 4 MBs, respectively. The biological and clinical relevance of these novel pathogenic mechanisms will need to be further studied. Although no transgenic models of Group 3 and 4 diseases exist, several orthotopic

transplantation models are currently being studied. The activation of Myc with p53 inactivation generates medulloblastomas with characteristic Group 3 features [7].

Pediatric High-Grade Glioma

Pediatric Glioblastoma

Whole-exome sequencing of pediatric glioblastoma (GBM) cases has revealed somatic recurrent mutations in a gene called *H3F3A*, which encodes a replication-independent histone variant H3.3 [2] (Fig. 7.1). Heterozygous mutations in *H3F3A* are present in 31 % of pediatric GBMs and result in amino acid substitutions within the N-terminal histone tail, specifically a lysine to methionine (K27M), a glycine to arginine (G34R), or a glycine to valine (G34V) substitution [2]. These mutations, which occur specifically in pediatric GBMs, and often with *TP53* mutations (54 % of cases), are situated at sites which are important for post-translational modification of histone 3 (H3) and regulation of global chromatin structure. Recurrent mutations in *ATRX* and *DAXX* have also been reported in 31 % of pediatric GBMs and present always in tumors harboring a G34R/V mutation [2]. The ATRX and DAXX proteins are important for H3.3 incorporation at peri-centrometic heterochromatin and telomeres [2]. Together somatic mutations in the H3.3-ATRX-DAXX chromatin remodeling pathway have been identified in 44 % of pediatric GBMs [2]. Epigenomic differences between subsets of pediatric GBM patients were demonstrated in a study examining DNA methylation signatures in a series of 59 childhood and 77 adult GBM patients [8]. Here they identified robust, epigenetically distinct subgroups defined by GBM mutations and gene expression-defined classes. The subgroups were classified as: (1) *IDH1* mutated (adults), (2) H3.3-K27 mutated, (3) H3.3-G34 mutated, (4) RTKI (*PDGFRα* amplified, proneural), (5) mesenchymal, and (6)

RTKII (classic). Copy number events also defined subgroups of pediatric GBM, specifically *PDGFRα* amplifications in the RTKI subgroup, whole chromosome 7 gains, chromosome 10 loss, *CDKN2A* homozygous deletions, and *EGFR* amplifications in RTKII pediatric GBMs [8]. Additional copy number events have been observed in comprehensive copy number studies of high-grade gliomas, including chromosome 8p12 loss in ~16 % of cases, encompassing a potential tumor suppressor gene, *ADAM3A*, *MYCN* amplifications (5 %), and chromosome 1q gain [9].

Diffuse Intrinsic Pontine Glioma

The vast majority (up to 78 %) of diffuse intrinsic pontine gliomas (DIPGs) harbors heterozygous H3.3-K27M mutations [10] (Fig. 7.1). *TP53* mutations have also been observed in up to 77 % of patients and are often concurrent with *H3F3A* mutations, *PDGFRA* gene amplifications, and *MYC-PVT1* gene fusions. *ATRX* mutations have also been reported in older DIPG patients, albeit at lower frequency (9 %), further highlighting aberrant chromatin structure in DIPG patients. The copy number landscape of DIPGs pinpoints other pathways relevant to disease formation, namely the PI3K pathway which is affected in ~47 % of DIPGs, involving *PDGFRa, MET, IGF1R, ERRB4, EGFR, KRAS, AKT1, AKT3, and PIK3CA* focal gains [11]. Gross copy number events have also reported to be enriched in DIPGs, specifically gains of chromosomes 2q, 8q, and 9q and losses of 16q, 17p, and 20p [11].

Pediatric Low-Grade Glioma

Non-diffuse Low-Grade Glioma: Pilocytic Astrocytomas

Spontaneous pilocytic astrocytomas (PAs) occur typically in the cerebellum, and in the absence of *NF1* mutations. The most common genetic alteration in spontaneous PAs results in increased activity of the MAPK pathway, through a tandem

duplication event on chromosome 7q34, which forms an in-frame fusion of *KIAA1549* with *BRAF* [12] (Fig. 7.1). Adding to this, genome sequencing studies of low-grade gliomas have shown that the MAPK pathway is affected in nearly all tumors and that PAs may represent a single pathway-driven disease [13]. Several other, albeit less frequent, genetic alterations convergent upon BRAF activation have been reported including *FAM131B-BRAF, RNF130-BRAF, CLCN6-BRAF, MKRN1-BRAF, and GNAI1-BRAF* fusions, all of which result in N-terminal loss of the *BRAF* regulatory region [13]. The significance of *BRAF* alterations is further highlighted by the presence of somatic mutations. These findings are supported functionally, in which PAs are generated by ectopic activation of BRAF in murine neural progenitor cells [14]. Recurrent, somatic, and activating mutations in PAs have also been identified at lower frequencies in other genes such as *KRAS, FGFR1, PTPN11, and NTRK2* fusions, however all of which lead to downstream MAPK activation [13].

Diffuse Low-Grade Glioma: Diffuse Grade II Astrocytomas, Ganglioglioma, Angiocentric Glioma, and Pleomorphic Xanthoastrocytoma

Diffuse low-grade gliomas are also affected by BRAF alterations; however, these occur mostly in the setting of *BRAF-V600E* mutations [15]. In the case of diffuse Grade II gliomas, recurrent amplifications of *MYC* and intragenic duplications of *FGFR1* have been reported, and shown to be largely mutually exclusive [16]. Copy number profiling in diffuse Grade II gliomas has identified other candidates, such as a partial duplication of the *MYBL1* transcription factor in 28 % of cases, which results in loss of its C-terminus negative regulatory domain [17]. In the same pathway, *MYB* amplifications have also been observed at lower frequency, in addition to deletion-truncation breakpoints in the regulatory terminus of *MYB*, seen preferentially in angiocentric gliomas [17]. Loss of chromosome 9, encompassing the *CDKN2A/p14ARF/CDKN2B* locus, has been reported in ~50 % of pleomorphic xanthoastrocytomas, along with less frequent loss of chromosome 17 [18].

Desmoplastic Infantile Astrocytomas/ Ganglioglioma

Desmoplastic infantile astrocytomas (DIA)/gan-gliogliomas (DIG) displayed only a few nonre-current genomic imbalances or normal karyotypes. Only loss of chromosome 9p and 22q was recurrently observed in a limited number of studies to date [19]. Characteristic genomic imbalances were not observed when DIA were compared with DIG [19]. *BRAF V600E* mutation, *EGFR* and *MYCN* amplification have been described in single cases.

Central Nervous System Germ Cell Tumors

Several studies have investigated cytogenetic alterations in central nervous system germ cell tumors (CNS-GCTs). A study of 15 malignant CNS-GCTs revealed recurrent gains of 12p12 which is also commonly amplified in adult tes-ticular germ cell tumors [20]. Recurrent gains of 1q and 8q and recurrent losses on chromosome 11, 18, and 13 were also detected. The genomic alterations identified in this series were almost identical to those found in gonadal and extrago-nadal germ cell tumors. Moreover, there were no differences in the cytogenetic profiles of germi-nomas compared to non-germinomatous CNS-GCT. This suggests strongly that the pathogenesis of CNS-GCTs is similar to systemic GCTs. At a transcriptional level, there are several differences between germinomas and non-germinomatous germ cell tumors. Genes responsible for self-renewal (*OCT4, NANOG,* and *KLF4*) and immune response are more highly expressed in germinomas whereas genes involved in neuronal differentiation, Wnt/β-catenin pathway, invasive-ness, and epithelial-mesenchymal transition are more commonly observed in malignant non-germinomatous germ cell tumors. The transcrip-tional profiles of non-germinomatous germ cell tumors closely resemble the profiles observed in embryonic stem cells consistent with their more undifferentiated nature.

Craniopharyngioma

Craniopharyngiomas are thought to arise from squamous-cell rests along the path of the primitive craniopharyngeal duct and adenohypophysis. The adenohypophysis arises from Rathke's pouch. As such it is believed that these squamous-cell rests represent the cell of origin for craniopharyngioma, and it is generally felt that adamantinomatous cra-niopharyngioma represents a developmental anomaly. The rare papillary histological variant more common in adults appears to arise from the adenohypophysis; however, this remains to be con-firmed. Recent studies have shown activating muta-tions in exon 3 of the β-catenin gene (*CTNNB1*) to be common in adamantinomatous craniopharyngi-oma suggesting a likely role for Wnt signaling in the pathogenesis of craniopharyngioma [21].

Central Nervous System Primitive Neuroectodermal Tumors

Primitive neuroectodermal tumors of the central nervous system (CNS-PNET) are a heteroge-neous group of pediatric neoplasms composed of poorly differentiated neuroepithelial cells with varying degrees of divergent neural, astrocytic, and ependymal differentiation. Using global profiling, Picard et al. (2012) identified that CNS-PNETs comprise three distinct molecular groups: primitive-neural (Group 1), oligoneural (Group 2), and mesenchymal (Group 3) [22] (Fig. 7.1). Group 1 tumors are enriched in primitive-neural genes (*CD133, CRABP1, LIN28,* and *ASCL1*) and display activation of SHH and WNT signal-ing. Group 2 tumors are composed of genes with roles in oligoneural differentiation (*OLIG1/2, SOX8/10,* and *BCAN*) and exhibit down-regulation of SHH components. Lastly, Group 3 tumors comprise genes involved in epithelial and mesenchymal differentiation (*COL1A2, COL5A, FOXJ1,* and *MSX1*) and display up-regulation of genes involved in TGF-β and PTEN signaling. Copy number analyses reveal that Group 2 tumors have frequent gains of chromosome 8p,

13, and 20, whereas Group 3 have frequent loss of chromosome 14. Also Group 2 and 3 tumors have frequent chromosome 9p loss centered on the *CDKN2A/2B* locus. In 2000, Eberhart et al. [23] described a new CNS-PNET variant (termed "embryonal tumor with abundant neuropil and true rosettes" or ETANTR), which, based on gene expression profiling, are subgroups with Group 1 CNS-PNETs [22, 24]. Hallmark cytogenetic features of ETANTRs include frequent gains of chromosome 2 and 3, and focal amplification of an miRNA amplicon on chr19q13.41, which encompasses the oncogenic C19MC miRNA cluster [24]. Li et al. (2009) identified that chr19q13.41 amplification characterizes CNS-PNET variants labeled as ETANTRs, medulloepithelioma, supratentorial PNET with ependymal differentiation, and ependymoblastoma, suggesting that these tumors represent closely related molecular entities [24]. Although the mechanisms by which C19MC miRNAs mediate oncogenesis remain unclear, these miRNAs are implicated in cell survival, transformation, activation of noncanonical WNT-JNK2 signaling, and inhibition of differentiation of human neural stem cells [25]. Furthermore, ETANTRs are also distinguished by the presence of distinct primitive markers, including the RNA binding protein, Lin28 [22].

Ependymoma

Using gene expression profiling, ependymomas have been divided into three principal molecular subgroups, which are separated largely according to anatomical location: (1) supratentorial (ST), (2) posterior fossa (PF), and (3) spinal cord [26]. These three subgroups have been further divided into molecularly and biologically distinct subtypes of ST and PF ependymoma as defined by diverse clinical and genomic features [27–29] (Fig. 7.1). In the case of PF ependymoma, three studies have independently reported the existence of two principle subgroups of disease [27–29]. These PF subgroups termed Group A and B are transcriptionally, clinically, and biologically distinct entities. Group A PF ependymomas occur in

young patients, invade laterally along the cerebellar-pontine angle, and are associated with increased tumor recurrence and decreased survival. Conversely, Group B PF ependymomas occur in older patients, grow along the midline, and are associated with a favorable prognosis. In addition, to the clinical differences, Group A and B are delineated by distinct genomic alterations. Group A PF ependymomas harbor chromosome 1q gain, which has been reported as a poor prognosis marker of ependymoma, but are largely characterized by balanced genomes [29]. In contrast, Group B ependymomas are defined by increased genomic instability as evidenced by increased numerical chromosome gains and losses. Group A ependymomas are characterized largely by pathways involved in angiogenesis (HIF-1α signaling, VEGF pathway), PDGF signaling, MAPK signaling, EGFR signaling, TGF-β signaling, tyrosine-receptor kinase signaling, RAS signaling, and integrin/ECM signaling, while Group B ependymomas are overrepresented by pathways involving ciliogenesis and microtubule assembly.

While these subgroup gene signatures may represent unique tumorigenic pathways, *Taylor* et al. (2005) proposed that these were potential marks of anatomically distinct cells of origin giving rise to different subgroups of ependymoma [26]. They suggested that ependymoma might originate from radial glia, a primitive neural and multipotent precursor important for neurogenesis and neuronal migration. Further evidence implicating radial glia as cells of origin of ependymoma was demonstrated by *Johnson* et al. (2010), in which over-expression of *EPHB2* in *p16/INK4A*-deficient RGCs led to the formation of the first mouse model of supratentorial ependymoma [27].

Chromosome 22 loss has been shown to be the most frequent genomic alteration in ependymoma with a frequency ranging from 26 to 71 % [30]. Further, chromosome 22q loss has been observed preferentially in spinal versus intracranial ependymoma, and in adult versus pediatric cases [30]. *NF2* is thought to be the candidate tumor suppressor gene of this region, as patients with neurofibromatosis type II develop a variety of central nervous system tumors including ependymoma, schwannoma, and meningioma [30]. However, *NF2* has been shown to be mutated exclusively in spinal ependymomas, thus suggesting alternate mechanisms of down-regulation, or another putative 22q tumor suppressor gene in the case of intracranial ependymoma. Other recurrent gross chromosomal abnormalities in ependymoma involve losses of chromosome 1p, 3, 6q, 9p, 10q, 13q, 16p, 17, 21, and 22q and gains of 1q, 4q, 5, 7, 8, 9, 12q, and 20 [30].

The telomerase pathway and its role in ependymoma pathogenesis have also been studied by several groups. Specifically, the expression of hTERT, the enzyme responsible for telomere extension, and its cofactor nucleolin have both been shown to be independent predictors of ependymoma patient survival [31]. *Castelo-Branco* et al. (2013) suggest that a possible mechanism leading to hTERT over-expression could be due to epigenetic silencing of repressor regions in the promoter of *hTERT* by DNA hypermethylation [32].

As novel ependymoma targets are discovered, evaluation, validation, and prioritization of candidates will require accurate preclinical models of ependymoma. Atkinson et al. (2011) demonstrate the utility and promise of this approach in ST-Group D ependymomas, generated by *EPHB2* over-expression and *CDKN2A/Ink4a* deletion in forebrain radial glia [33]. They performed a compound library screen of 7890 compounds, in both tumor and matched normal neural stem cells, and identified inhibitors of thymidylate synthase (TYMS) and dihydrogolate reductase, namely 5-FU as highly and specifically active in ST ependymoma cells.

Choroid Plexus Tumors

Choroid plexus tumors (CPTs) are classified as three distinct entities according to pathological examination: choroid plexus papillomas (CPPs, Grade I), atypical choroid plexus papillomas (aCPPs, Grade II), and choroid plexus carcinomas (CPCs, Grade III). CPCs are considered a hallmark tumor of the Li-Fraumeni syndrome

(LFS). Germline and somatic mutations in *TP53*, a classical tumor suppressor gene involved in DNA repair, cellular differentiation, and apoptosis, are commonly found in CPCs [34]. The frequency of *TP53* mutations is much higher in the carcinomas (~50 %) than papillomas (~5 %), which may contribute to the aggressiveness and poor outcome of these malignant tumors [35] (Fig. 7.1). No CPPs, or aCPPs, harbored germline mutations in *TP53*, while at least 36 % of CPCs harbored a germline TP53 mutation [35].

CPTs are characterized by a high degree of chromosomal imbalances. Generally, CPPs are characterized by extensive chromosomal gains, and CPCs by both gains and losses, yet CPCs demonstrate greater imbalances per tumor than CPPs [36]. CPPs exhibit recurrent gains in chromosomes 7 and 12, while CPCs exhibit gains and losses throughout the genome with a higher frequency of chromosome 1 gains. Association of chromosomal aberrations with survival revealed a significant association between gain of 9p and loss of 10q with improved survival [36]. Cytogenetics studies in aCPPs, although limited, have revealed variable aneuploidy phenotypes characterized by polyploidy.

Atypical Teratoid Rhabdoid Tumors

Atypical teratoid rhabdoid tumors (ATRT) are of mesenchymal origin and are characterized by biallelic loss of *SMARCB1/INI1*, which encodes the SNF5 protein, a core subunit of the SWI/SNF chromatin remodeling complex [37] (Fig. 7.1). *SNF5* is a tumor suppressor gene located on chromosome 22q11.23 and is inactivated by a variety of genetic lesions including homozygous deletions and nonsense, missense, and frameshift mutations. The SWI/SNF complex is an ATP-dependent regulator of gene expression which acts by remodeling chromatin and repositioning nucleosomes through catalyzing the insertion and removal of histone proteins. Despite being extremely aggressive, SNF5-deficient cancers are diploid and genomically stable, highlighting the importance of this gene as a central driver of ATRT tumorigenesis [38]. Mechanistically, inactivation of SNF5 has been linked to broad repression of polycomb repressor complex 2 (PRC2) regulated genes [39]. Specifically loss of SNF5 leads to up-regulation of EZH2, the core enzymatic component of the PRC2 complex, and subsequent loss of the tumor suppressors such as p16^{INK4a}. ATRT development is also affected by the Sonic Hedgehog (SHH) signaling pathway. SNF5 localizes to Gli1-regulated promoters of the SHH pathway, thus repressing Gli1targets [40]. Hence, loss of Snf5 leads to up-regulation of Gli1 targets and activation of the Hh-Gli pathway driving oncogenesis [40].

References

1. Taylor MD, Northcott PA, Korshunov A, Remke M, Cho YJ, Clifford SC, et al. Molecular subgroups of medulloblastoma: the current consensus. Acta Neuropathol. 2012;123(4):465–72.
2. Schwartzentruber J, Korshunov A, Liu XY, Jones DT, Pfaff E, Jacob K, et al. Driver mutations in histone H3.3 and chromatin remodelling genes in paediatric glioblastoma. Nature. 2012;482(7384):226–31.
3. Northcott PA, Shih DJ, Peacock J, Garzia L, Morrissy AS, Zichner T, et al. Subgroup-specific structural variation across 1,000 medulloblastoma genomes. Nature. 2012;488(7409):49–56.
4. Jones DT, Jager N, Kool M, Zichner T, Hutter B, Sultan M, et al. Dissecting the genomic complexity underlying medulloblastoma. Nature. 2012;488(7409): 100–5.
5. Gibson P, Tong Y, Robinson G, Thompson MC, Currle DS, Eden C, et al. Subtypes of medulloblastoma have distinct developmental origins. Nature. 2010;468(7327):1095–9.
6. Yang ZJ, Ellis T, Markant SL, Read TA, Kessler JD, Bourboulas M, et al. Medulloblastoma can be initiated by deletion of Patched in lineage-restricted progenitors or stem cells. Cancer Cell. 2008;14(2): 135–45.
7. Pei Y, Moore CE, Wang J, Tewari AK, Eroshkin A, Cho YJ, et al. An animal model of MYC-driven medulloblastoma. Cancer Cell. 2012;21(2):155–67.
8. Sturm D, Witt H, Hovestadt V, Khuong-Quang DA, Jones DT, Konermann C, et al. Hotspot mutations in H3F3A and IDH1 define distinct epigenetic and biological subgroups of glioblastoma. Cancer Cell. 2012;22(4):425–37.
9. Paugh BS, Qu C, Jones C, Liu Z, Adamowicz-Brice M, Zhang J, et al. Integrated molecular genetic profiling of pediatric high-grade gliomas reveals key differences with the adult disease. J Clin Oncol. 2010;28(18):3061–8.
10. Wu G, Broniscer A, McEachron TA, Lu C, Paugh BS, Becksfort J, et al. Somatic histone H3 alterations in pediatric diffuse intrinsic pontine gliomas and nonbrainstem glioblastomas. Nat Genet. 2012;44(3): 251–3.
11. Paugh BS, Broniscer A, Qu C, Miller CP, Zhang J, Tatevossian RG, et al. Genome-wide analyses identify recurrent amplifications of receptor tyrosine kinases and cell-cycle regulatory genes in diffuse intrinsic pontine glioma. J Clin Oncol. 2011;29(30): 3999–4006.
12. Jones DT, Kocialkowski S, Liu L, Pearson DM, Backlund LM, Ichimura K, et al. Tandem duplication producing a novel oncogenic BRAF fusion gene defines the majority of pilocytic astrocytomas. Cancer Res. 2008;68(21):8673–7.
13. Jones DT, Hutter B, Jager N, Korshunov A, Kool M, Warnatz HJ, et al. Recurrent somatic alterations of FGFR1 and NTRK2 in pilocytic astrocytoma. Nat Genet. 2013;45(8):927–32.
14. Gronych J, Korshunov A, Bageritz J, Milde T, Jugold M, Hambardzumyan D, et al. An activated mutant BRAF kinase domain is sufficient to induce pilocytic astrocytoma in mice. J Clin Invest. 2011;121(4): 1344–8.
15. Schindler G, Capper D, Meyer J, Janzarik W, Omran H, Herold-Mende C, et al. Analysis of BRAF V600E mutation in 1,320 nervous system tumors reveals high mutation frequencies in pleomorphic xanthoastrocytoma, ganglioglioma and extra-cerebellar pilocytic astrocytoma. Acta Neuropathol. 2011;121(3): 397–405.
16. Zhang J, Wu G, Miller CP, Tatevossian RG, Dalton JD, Tang B, et al. Whole-genome sequencing identifies genetic alterations in pediatric low-grade gliomas. Nat Genet. 2013;45(6):602–12.
17. Ramkissoon LA, Horowitz PM, Craig JM, Ramkissoon SH, Rich BE, Schumacher SE, et al. Genomic analysis of diffuse pediatric low-grade gliomas identifies recurrent oncogenic truncating rearrangements in the transcription factor MYBL1. Proc Natl Acad Sci USA. 2013;110(20):8188–93.
18. Weber RG, Hoischen A, Ehrler M, Zipper P, Kaulich K, Blaschke B, et al. Frequent loss of chromosome 9, homozygous CDKN2A/p14(ARF)/CDKN2B deletion and low TSC1 mRNA expression in pleomorphic xanthoastrocytomas. Oncogene. 2007;26(7):1088–97.
19. Kros JM, Delwel EJ, de Jong TH, Tanghe HL, van Run PR, Vissers K, et al. Desmoplastic infantile astrocytoma and ganglioglioma: a search for genomic characteristics. Acta Neuropathol. 2002;104(2): 144–8.
20. Schneider DT, Zahn S, Sievers S, Alemazkour K, Reifenberger G, Wiestler OD, et al. Molecular genetic analysis of central nervous system germ cell tumors with comparative genomic hybridization. Mod Pathol. 2006;19(6):864–73.
21. Sekine S, Shibata T, Kokubu A, Morishita Y, Noguchi M, Nakanishi Y, et al. Craniopharyngiomas of ada-

mantinomatous type harbor beta-catenin gene mutations. Am J Pathol. 2002;161(6):1997–2001.

22. Picard D, Miller S, Hawkins CE, Bouffet E, Rogers HA, Chan TS, et al. Markers of survival and metastatic potential in childhood CNS primitive neuroectodermal brain tumours: an integrative genomic analysis. Lancet Oncol. 2012;13(8):838–48.

23. Eberhart CG, Brat DJ, Cohen KJ, Burger PC. Pediatric neuroblastic brain tumors containing abundant neuropil and true rosettes. Pediatr Dev Pathol. 2000;3(4): 346–52.

24. Li M, Lee KF, Lu Y, Clarke I, Shih D, Eberhart C, et al. Frequent amplification of a chr19q13.41 microRNA polycistron in aggressive primitive neuroectodermal brain tumors. Cancer Cell. 2009;16(6): 533–46.

25. Viswanathan SR, Powers JT, Einhorn W, Hoshida Y, Ng TL, Toffanin S, et al. Lin28 promotes transformation and is associated with advanced human malignancies. Nat Genet. 2009;41(7):843–8.

26. Taylor MD, Poppleton H, Fuller C, Su X, Liu Y, Jensen P, et al. Radial glia cells are candidate stem cells of ependymoma. Cancer Cell. 2005;8(4): 323–35.

27. Johnson RA, Wright KD, Poppleton H, Mohankumar KM, Finkelstein D, Pounds SB, et al. Cross-species genomics matches driver mutations and cell compartments to model ependymoma. Nature. 2010;466(7306): 632–6.

28. Wani K, Armstrong TS, Vera-Bolanos E, Raghunathan A, Ellison D, Gilbertson R, et al. A prognostic gene expression signature in infratentorial ependymoma. Acta Neuropathol. 2012;123(5):727–38.

29. Witt H, Mack SC, Ryzhova M, Bender S, Sill M, Isserlin R, et al. Delineation of two clinically and molecularly distinct subgroups of posterior fossa ependymoma. Cancer Cell. 2011;20(2):143–57.

30. Mack SC, Taylor MD. The genetic and epigenetic basis of ependymoma. Childs Nerv Syst. 2009;25(10): 1195–201.

31. Tabori U, Ma J, Carter M, Zielenska M, Rutka J, Bouffet E, et al. Human telomere reverse transcriptase expression predicts progression and survival in pediatric intracranial ependymoma. J Clin Oncol. 2006;24(10):1522–8.

32. Castelo-Branco P, Choufani S, Mack S, Gallagher D, Zhang C, Lipman T, et al. Methylation of the TERT promoter and risk stratification of childhood brain tumours: an integrative genomic and molecular study. Lancet Oncol. 2013;14(6):534–42.

33. Atkinson JM, Shelat AA, Carcaboso AM, Kranenburg TA, Arnold LA, Boulos N, et al. An integrated in vitro and in vivo high-throughput screen identifies treatment leads for ependymoma. Cancer Cell. 2011;20(3):384–99.

34. Kamaly-Asl ID, Shams N, Taylor MD. Genetics of choroid plexus tumors. Neurosurg Focus. 2006;20(1):E10.

35. Tabori U, Shlien A, Baskin B, Levitt S, Ray P, Alon N, et al. TP53 alterations determine clinical subgroups and survival of patients with choroid plexus tumors. J Clin Oncol. 2010;28(12):1995–2001.

36. Rickert CH, Wiestler OD, Paulus W. Chromosomal imbalances in choroid plexus tumors. Am J Pathol. 2002;160(3):1105–13.

37. Wilson BG, Roberts CW. SWI/SNF nucleosome remodellers and cancer. Nat Rev Cancer. 2011;11(7): 481–92.

38. Lee RS, Stewart C, Carter SL, Ambrogio L, Cibulskis K, Sougnez C, et al. A remarkably simple genome underlies highly malignant pediatric rhabdoid cancers. J Clin Invest. 2012;122(8):2983–8.

39. Wilson BG, Wang X, Shen X, McKenna ES, Lemieux ME, Cho YJ, et al. Epigenetic antagonism between polycomb and SWI/SNF complexes during oncogenic transformation. Cancer Cell. 2010;18(4):316–28.

40. Jagani Z, Mora-Blanco EL, Sansam CG, McKenna ES, Wilson B, Chen D, et al. Loss of the tumor suppressor Snf5 leads to aberrant activation of the Hedgehog-Gli pathway. Nat Med. 2010;16(12): 1429–33.

Cancer Predisposition in Children with Brain Tumors

8

Uri Tabori, Anne-Marie Laberge, Benjamin Ellezam, and Anne-Sophie Carret

Introduction

Cancer in children is a rare event. It is much less prevalent than adults for whom cancer is one of the most common chronic diseases in older age. In contrast to adults where genetic predisposition accounts to a minority of cancers and environmental and infectious as well as other chronic disease contribute to carcinogenesis, in children, germline mutations are thought to be responsible for a significant proportion of cancers. The general concept is that cancer predisposition accounts for up to 15 % of childhood cancers [1] but can approach 50–100 % in specific cancers [2]. Lymphoblastic leukemias are the most common childhood cancer, but genetic predisposition is rare in this tumor type. Brain tumors constitute the second largest group of tumors and by far the largest group of tumors associated with cancer predisposition. Germline mutations occur most commonly in tumor suppressors. These mutations are usually heterozygous and inherited in an autosomal dominant fashion. They comply with the "two-hit" concept in which in order to disrupt gene function the two copies of the gene need to be lost. This event rarely occurs in sporadic fashion. However, if one allele is already mutated in the germline, the chances of the other one are lost and by that cause cancer is exponentially high. The two-hit model was first applied to the retinoblastoma gene and is similarly important to *TP53*. Alterations in these two cardinal genes often termed "gatekeepers of our genome" are responsible to the prototype of cancer predisposition syndromes. They predispose the carrier child to a large variety of tumors with high penetrance (chances of having cancer if one is carrying the mutation) and have 50 % chance of inheriting this disorder to the offspring. Nevertheless other syndromes are inherited differently and exhibit different phenotype. For us as clinicians, it is important to recognize how to suspect and diagnose each cancer predisposition syndrome and how to address specific issues which relate the child's treatment, management of other cancer risks, and other family members. This complex approach requires a multidisciplinary team which includes geneticists, physicians with

U. Tabori, M.D. (✉)
Department of Hematology/Oncology, The Hospital for Sick Children/Institute of Medical Sciences, University of Toronto/The Arthur and Sonia Labatt Brain Tumour Research Centre, Toronto, ON, Canada
e-mail: uri.tabori@sickkids.ca

A.-M. Laberge, M.D., Ph.D.
Medical Genetics Division, Department of Pediatrics, Université de Montréal, Montréal, QC, Canada

B. Ellezam, M.D., Ph.D.
Department of Pathology, CHU Sainte-Justine, Université de Montréal, Montréal, QC, Canada

A.-S. Carret, M.D.
Department of Pediatrics, Division of Hematology/Oncology, CHU Sainte-Justine/Université de Montréal, Montréal, QC, Canada

K. Scheinemann and E. Bouffet (eds.), *Pediatric Neuro-oncology*,
DOI 10.1007/978-1-4939-1541-5_8, © Springer Science+Business Media New York 2015

expertise in the specific syndrome and its complications, genetic counselors, and social workers to name a few. Indeed, the emotional, social, and financial implications of these devastating syndromes cannot be overemphasized.

In this chapter, we will focus on the relevant clinical presentation, the genetics, specific tumor types, and the management of each of the major syndromes predisposing for brain tumors in children. We will also suggest an approach to these syndromes in the perspective of the pediatric oncologist. We do not aim to cover all syndromes and focus our efforts on the most relevant and common syndromes. In order to simplify the clinical approach, we divided the syndromes into ones in which tumors are just a part of the phenotype and ones in which cancer is the only manifestation of the condition.

Systemic Syndromes Associated with Brain Tumors: Neurofibromatosis Type 1

Neurofibromatosis 1 (NF1) is an autosomal dominant multisystemic disorder. Diagnostic criteria include the presence of at least two of the following: multiple café au lait spots (>6 measuring >5 mm in prepubertal individuals and >15 mm in postpubertal individuals), axillary freckling, Lisch nodules, optic gliomas, neurofibromas of any type, distinctive osseous lesions (sphenoid dysplasia or tibial pseudarthrosis), or a first-degree relative with NF1 [3]. Other manifestations of NF1 include macrocephaly, learning disabilities, vasculopathies that can lead to hypertension, renal artery stenosis, cerebral aneurysms, and scoliosis. Individuals with NF1 are at higher risk of developing a variety of cancers including malignant nerve sheath tumors (which can arise from neurofibromas) and leukemias, especially chronic myelomonocytic leukemia and other solid tumors.

The clinical presentation of NF1 is extremely variable, even within the same family. Some have only pigmentary lesions, while others may develop learning disabilities, renal complications, or central or peripheral nervous system tumors. Tumors and vasculopathies account for a reduction in average life expectancy of about 15 years.

Clinical Genetics

NF1 is caused by mutations in the *NF1* gene. The gene encodes the protein neurofibromin which is a major inhibitor of the major oncogene *RAS*. Neurofibromin is a GTPase which catalyzes the hydrolysis of active GTP-RAS to inactive GDP-RAS [4]. Dysfunctional neurofibromin results in constitutive activation of downstream oncogenic pathways including MAPK and mammalian target of rapamycin (mTOR).

Most mutations lead to loss of function of the gene product. In about 5 % of cases, NF1 is due to deletion of the entire gene. Over 500 mutations have been identified in *NF1*, but are usually unique to a family. Mutations are inherited from an affected parent only in half of the cases. When the mutation appears to be de novo, siblings of the proband have a low risk of having inherited the disease because of the possibility of germline mosaicism in one of the unaffected parents.

Penetrance is complete, which means that a child who inherits a mutation in *NF1* will inevitably develop features of NF1, but it is impossible to predict which features will develop, even within the same family.

Genetic testing is not necessary to establish a diagnosis of NF1. It is necessary to be able to offer prenatal diagnosis. In some cases with atypical features or younger patients with some diagnostic features but not enough to establish a diagnosis, genetic testing can help clarify the situation. When indicated, genetic testing should be done by testing both mRNA and genomic DNA to detect not only mutations in the coding region but also whole gene deletions and splice site mutations. Current strategies reach a mutation detection rate of about 95 %.

Tumor Spectrum

NF1-associated tumors of the CNS include optic pathway gliomas (OPGs), brainstem gliomas, and gliomas elsewhere along the neuraxis.

Optic Pathway Gliomas
OPGs are the most prevalent CNS tumors in patients with NF1. An association between NF1

and optic pathway tumors was first described in 1968. They are almost invariant of astrocytic nature and low-grade spectrum. Although OPGs are WHO grade I tumors, morbidity can be significant and includes decreased vision, precocious puberty, and other hypothalamic-pituitary-adrenal axis disorders.

OPGs tend to arise in infancy and rarely develop after childhood years. They can be found in approximately 15 % of individuals with NF1, with around half being symptomatic [5]. It is probably largely underestimated since routine screening with brain MRI is very controversial and not evenly prescribed. A retrospective study from the Montreal Children's Hospital reported an incidence of 13 % ($n=44$) of OPGs among 331 NF1 patients. Only 8 patients of 44 with OPGs were reported symptomatic (with either deceased vision or precocious puberty), and of those, only 5 required treatment for their symptoms [6].

NF1-related OPGs have similar neuroradiologic findings as non-NF1-associated OPGs, including solid and cystic appearance and variable degree of enhancement. The coappearance of foci of abnormal signal intensity (FASI) and bilateral optic nerve involvement is highly suggestive of NF1 (see Fig. 9.4 now).

Neuropathologic studies of OPGs are limited by lack of surgical resection and biopsy material. However, NF1 OPGs are almost invariantly pilocytic or pilomyxoid lesions which are different from gliomas in other locations. Gliomas occurring in NF1 are not distinguishable from those occurring sporadically based on tissue examination alone.

Since only a minority of children with NF1 and OPG will require treatment, a conservative approach is the standard of care. Watchful observation with repeated ophthalmologic examinations (including visual fields), imaging and endocrine evaluations is recommended. Treatment should be initiated only when a combination of tumor progression by MRI and symptoms such as visual loss is observed. As in sporadic OPG, complete surgical resection is unfeasible in most cases and chemotherapy is the initial mode of treatment.

NF1-related OPGs have a superior natural history and response to therapy with longer periods of growth stability compared to sporadic OPGs. Patients with NF1 are particularly sensitive to damaging effects of ionizing radiation and are at increased risk of radiation-induced cancers [7] as well as cerebrovascular damage such as moyamoya syndrome.

Brainstem and White Matter Lesions

Use of MRI has led to more frequent identification and better delineation of signal abnormalities in asymptomatic NF1 patients. The presence of multiple, nonenhancing areas of high signal intensity, typically smaller than 5 mm without mass effect or edema, is well recognized on T2-weighted MRIs in children with NF1. These lesions are often considered to be pathognomonic of NF1 in children, although they are not currently considered to be one of the diagnostic criteria. These are not thought to have potential for malignant transformation and do not require treatment. These brainstem hyperintensities are frequent and may be difficult to distinguish from low-grade neoplasms. Focal brainstem enlargements with or without abnormal signal change or mass effect are considerably less frequent [8]. In one study 23 such brainstem lesions (~20 %) were described among 125 NF1 patients and only 6 of these patients required treatment (surgery, irradiation, or chemotherapy) [8]. Only one of the 17 untreated patients experienced radiographic and clinical deterioration.

In the brainstem, pathology data is also limited by the small number of biopsied cases, but in one recent retrospective series pilocytic and diffuse astrocytomas contributed in roughly equal proportions.

As with OPG, conservative management should be favored for brainstem lesions. Treatment may ultimately be required in those patients with documented rapid progression on serial MRIs accompanied by neurological deterioration. A biopsy may be required prior to treatment initiation since these lesions may range from low-grade to high-grade ones.

Malignant Gliomas

Astrocytomas with diffuse growth patterns are known to be more aggressive than those with pilocytic morphology, and this seems to hold true in NF1 patients as well, regardless of location. Moreover, both tumor types do not occur only in optic pathways and brainstem as NF1 patients may also have astrocytomas in the hemispheres, thalamus, cerebellum, and spinal cord.

Malignant transformation of NF1-associated gliomas is rare but well recognized. Grade III and IV diffuse astrocytomas can occur throughout the CNS, especially in adults, and share the same molecular abnormalities and poor prognosis as non-syndromic patients. Interestingly, whole genome studies have now included NF1 as one of the most frequently mutated genes in sporadic glioblastoma. Recent data suggest that NF1-associated glioblastomas appear to have better outcome than their sporadic counterparts, particularly in children. Anaplastic transformation and aggressive behavior of occasional pilocytic astrocytomas are now being recognized and this phenomenon may be more common in NF1 than in non-syndromic patients. Indeed, in a recent series of 25 such tumors, 28 % were in NF1 patients [9]. Location was supratentorial or infratentorial and did not involve optic pathways. Molecular data in this series and others suggest that anaplastic transformation of pilocytic astrocytoma involves activation of the PI3K/AKT pathway and is not related to radiation therapy in NF1 patients.

Clinical Applications

Routine screening with brain MRI is still controversial for detection of clinically relevant OPG, but ophthalmological surveillance including visual fields is recommended throughout childhood. NF1 children with OPGs, in particular, and brain tumors, in general, should avoid cranial irradiation. For the same reason, physicians should favor MRIs rather than CT scans in order to decrease exposure to radiation. Additional molecular studies are needed to better understand the malignant transformation of NF1-related high-grade gliomas. These findings will ultimately lead to the development of more targeted therapeutic agents with less morbidity and mortality for children with NF1.

Since NF1 is a systemic condition, surveillance by a dedicated NF1 team is recommended for other aspects of the syndrome in parallel to neurooncological surveillance/therapy.

Tuberous Sclerosis Complex

Tuberous sclerosis complex (TSC) is an autosomal dominant disorder seen in about 1/6,000 individuals worldwide. As with NF1, it is a multisystem disorder. Diagnosis of TSC relies on diagnostic criteria which include major and minor features. Major features include cutaneous features (facial angiofibromas, periungual fibromas, hypomelanotic macules, shagreen patch, etc.), neurologic features (cortical tuber, subependymal nodule, subependymal giant cell astrocytoma (SEGA)), as well as features affecting other organ systems (multiple retinal nodular hamartomas, cardiac rhabdomyoma(s), lymphangiomyomatosis, and renal angiomyolipoma). The diagnosis of TSC is definite in the presence of either two major features or one major and two minor features. Diagnosis is probable in the presence of one major and one minor feature and suspect in the presence of either one major or two or more minor features.

The cutaneous features occur in over 90 % of affected individuals, especially hypomelanotic macules (ash leaf spots), often present from birth but difficult to see without an ultraviolet light. Angiofibromas, ungula fibromas, and shagreen patches appear with age. Retinal lesions are also found in the majority of cases, but can be difficult to see without dilating the pupils. They only rarely affect vision. About two thirds of newborns with TSC have at least one cardiac rhabdomyoma, which would be very likely diagnostic of TSC in a child at 50 % risk of inheriting TSC from an affected parent. On the other hand, cardiac rhabdomyomas shrink over time and can be asymptomatic. Renal angiomyolipomas occur in about 75–80 % of cases over the age of 10 years and the prevalence increases with age.

Clinical Genetics

TSC can be caused by mutations in either of two different genes, *TSC1* and *TSC2*. These tumor suppressor genes are inhibitors of mTOR, which is a key component of a major pro-proliferative and metabolic pathway and is involved in many cancers. More cases have mutations in *TSC2* than in *TSC1*, with a ratio of about 3.4:1. Mutations involving large gene rearrangements are also mostly found in *TSC2*. The phenotype cannot be predicted based on the gene involved in a given patient, but those with mutations in *TSC2* seem to have more severe neurologic features and familial cases tend to have mutations in *TSC1*. Penetrance is incomplete, which means that some individuals inherit a *TSC1* or *TSC2* mutation but never develop any feature of TSC. In the majority of cases (66–75 %), TSC is due to a new mutation. Even when the mutation is not found in parents, there is a residual risk for siblings of a proband because of the risk of germline mosaicism (estimated to be about 2 %).

Testing for *TSC1* and *TSC2* is available by sequence analysis and deletion/duplication analysis, but it is not required to establishing the diagnosis. Genetic testing is helpful in atypical cases or to assess whether a seemingly unaffected first-degree relative is at risk of transmitting the disease to its offspring, since the mutation may be non-penetrant in some individuals. Even in individuals with a clear clinical diagnosis of TSC, the mutation detection rate when testing *TSC1* and *TSC2* is 85 %.

Tumor Spectrum

The main CNS neoplasm in tuberous sclerosis is SEGA, a WHO grade I tumor which affects 5–15 % of TSC patients. SEGAs usually present in the first two decades of life and are considered pathognomonic of TSC. SEGAs can be identified radiologically before they become symptomatic; they are well-circumscribed, frequently calcified, contrast-enhancing lesions. Histologically, SEGAs are composed of fascicles and nests of epithelioid, gemistocyte-like cells with cytologic and immunophenotypic features intermediate between astrocytes and neurons. They are thought to arise from subependymal hamartomatous nodules ("candle gutterings") which are disorganized collections of dysmorphic neurons and balloon cells with glioneuronal immunophenotype similar to cortical tubers. Because of their characteristic location near the foramen of Monro, SEGAs often cause increased intracranial pressure due to obstruction of CSF pathways. Early diagnosis can potentially improve chances of curative surgery. Such lesions can grow rapidly, especially in childhood, justifying serial follow-up MRIs during childhood and adolescence when the risk of SEGA is highest. Surgical resection has been the standard treatment until recent reports demonstrated that mTOR inhibitors are able to reduce tumor size in almost all patients [10]. Stopping therapy, however, results in regrowth of SEGAs in most cases. Currently, oral therapy with everolimus or sirolimus is used as initial therapy in many centers for growing SEGAs.

Clinical Applications

As with NF1, TSC is a systemic condition requiring a multimodality approach. Surveilance protocols for all clinical aspects of TSC including tumors are available. Periodic neuroimaging with improved modalities facilitates early tumor diagnosis. The initial treatment of SEGAs and length of treatment are still controversial. Nevertheless, growing evidence of improvement in neuropsychiatric, seizure control and other manifestations of TSC upon treatment with mTOR inhibitors suggest that long-term treatment with these agents may become standard of care in the near future.

Gorlin or Nevoid Basal Cell Carcinoma Syndrome

Nevoid basal cell carcinoma syndrome (NBCCS), also known as nevoid basal cell carcinoma syndrome or Gorlin syndrome, is an autosomal dominant disorder. It predisposes to skeletal overgrowth and tumor formation [11].

Diagnosis of NBCCS is made in the presence of two major criteria or one major and one minor criterion. Major criteria include the following: at least two basal cell carcinomas; odontogenic keratocysts of the jaws proven by histopathology; palmar or plantar pits; bilamellar calcification of the falx cerebri; bifid, fused, or markedly splayed ribs; or first-degree relative with NBCCS. Minor criteria include macrocephaly, facial features (cleft lip or palate, frontal bossing, coarse face, hypertelorism), other skeletal abnormalities (Sprengel deformity, pectus deformity, syndactyly) or radiological abnormalities (hemivertebrae, fusion or elongation of vertebral bodies, etc.), ovarian fibroma, or medulloblastoma.

Clinical Genetics

BCNS is an autosomal dominant condition caused by mutations in the *PTCH1* gene. *PTCH1* is a tumor suppressor in the SHH pathway which is cardinal to human development.

Large gene rearrangements may occur, so testing should include both sequencing and deletion/duplication analysis. Mutation detection rate in individuals with a clinical diagnosis of BCNS is not precisely established, but is estimated to be as high as 87 %. Genetic testing is not required to establish a diagnosis, but may impact diagnosis and management in atypical cases or in at-risk family members who want predictive testing: if a mutation is identified, surveillance would be indicated [12]. About 20–30 % of probands have a de novo mutation. Penetrance of the condition is variable, even within the same family, with some individuals having only the rib anomalies or the facial features. Assessment of the parents is recommended to determine if the condition may have been inherited. Although mutations in PTCH1 are the most common as causing the syndrome, germline mutations in SUFU, another tumor suppressor in the pathway has been reported in familial medulloblastoma [13].

Tumor Spectrum

The hallmark of NBCCS is the development of basal cell carcinomas and medulloblastomas. Additional ovarian fibromas and postradiation meningiomas have been reported.

Medulloblastoma

Since the first report of medulloblastoma in association with this heritable syndrome in 1963, several distinct characteristics have been well established. First, almost 5 % of patients with NBCCS develop medulloblastoma and, conversely, approximately 1–4 % of all medulloblastomas develop in the setting of Gorlin syndrome. Second, the age of onset of medulloblastoma in the setting of Gorlin syndrome is younger than in non-Gorlin patients, with up to 97 % presenting prior to age 5 and up to 66 % prior to age 2. Third, medulloblastoma is almost always the first tumor manifestation of Gorlin syndrome.

NBCCS medulloblastomas are mostly of desmoplastic/nodular subtype and have a better outcome than sporadic medulloblastomas. Less frequently, histology reveals medulloblastomas with extensive nodularity (MBEN), a more recently described subtype initially reported as "cerebellar neuroblastoma" which is associated with excellent outcome. Although craniospinal irradiation and chemotherapy are standards in the postoperative care of medulloblastoma, several patients with Gorlin syndrome and MBEN have been treated and cured without radiation therapy. Interestingly, a few treated MBENs may undergo maturation and show a ganglion cell-rich histology.

Although all medulloblastomas of Gorlin syndrome are PTCH1 mutants and therefore fall into molecular group 2 (SHH), not all desmoplastic medulloblastomas fall within that group as some fall into groups 3 and 4 [14]. Little published data exists on the molecular work-up of MBENs, but at least one case studied showed monosomy 9q, where PTCH1 is located.

In patients NBCCS with medulloblastoma treated with craniospinal irradiation, basal cell carcinomas usually develop in the radiation fields within a period of 9 years posttreatment. This latency period is considered much shorter than for classic radiation-induced neoplasms.

Meningioma

At least 15 cases of meningioma have been reported so far in patients with Gorlin syndrome. Although this number is small, epidemiological data suggests increased incidence of meningiomas in patients with NBCCS. Interestingly, 6 of these 15 reported cases occurred in patients who had undergone radiation therapy for medulloblastoma 15–34 years earlier. Some of these reported meningiomas were multifocal and caused increased intracranial pressure by mass effect or blockage of CSF. Molecular data is limited but at least one Gorlin-associated meningioma showed compound heterozygous mutations in PTCH1, supporting a classic two-hit event.

Clinical Applications

Because medulloblastoma is usually the first manifestation of Gorlin syndrome, it has been strongly recommended that all children with MBEN, especially those who are younger than 3 years of age, undergo formal genetic, dermatologic, and appropriate imaging to document a possible association with Gorlin syndrome. The documentation of medulloblastoma in the setting of Gorlin syndrome represents a strong argument against the use of radiation therapy, because of both the high cure rate with chemotherapy alone and well-documented high rate of radiation-induced multiple basal cell carcinoma and other types of radiation-induced second malignancies. The recent exciting novel *SHH* inhibitors currently developed for medulloblastoma [15] may offer targeted therapies for individuals with germline *PTCH1* and *SUFU* mutations and possible primary prevention of tumors.

PTEN Hamartoma Tumor Syndrome

PTEN hamartoma tumor syndrome (PHTS) is an entity that includes four distinct syndromes all associated with germline mutations in *PTEN*:

Cowden syndrome, Bannayan-Riley-Ruvalcaba syndrome, Proteus syndrome, and Proteus-like syndrome. All are associated with unregulated cell proliferation leading to the development of hamartomas. Cowden syndrome is the only entity that is known to be associated with a risk of malignancy, but it is now thought that all individuals with mutations in *PTEN* should undergo surveillance.

Cowden syndrome is an autosomal dominant disorder characterized by the presence of hamartomas, mucocutaneous features, megencephaly/macrocephaly, gastrointestinal polyps, and glycogenic acanthosis. Individuals with Cowden syndrome are at increased risk of both benign and malignant tumors of breast, thyroid, and endometrium, skin cancer, renal cell cancer, and brain tumors. Clinical diagnostic criteria have been developed but are most useful in adults when mucocutaneous lesions are present.

Clinical Genetics

Mutations in the *PTEN* gene are found in 85 % of individuals who meet diagnostic criteria for Cowden syndrome, 65 % of those with a clinical diagnosis of Bannayan-Riley-Ruvalcaba syndrome, 20 % of those with Proteus syndrome, and 50 % of those with Proteus-like syndrome. PTEN is a major tumor suppressor of the PI3K-AKT pathway. This pathway is activated in most cancers including brain tumors. Testing should include both sequencing (including promoter region if possible) and deletion/duplication analysis. Only 10–50 % of individuals with a diagnosis of Cowden syndrome and a mutation in *PTEN* have an affected parent.

Mutations in *PTEN* have also been found in 10–20 % of individuals with autism/pervasive developmental disorder and macrocephaly.

Tumor Spectrum

As mentioned above, increased risk of malignancy has only been described in Cowden syndrome with particular predisposition to cancer of breast (lifetime risk 25–50 %), thyroid (lifetime risk 10 %), and endometrium (lifetime risk unknown). Approximately 90 % of patients with CS manifest its clinical symptoms before 20 years of age. The main CNS tumor of this syndrome is Lhermitte-Duclos disease (LDD).

Cerebellar Dysplastic Gangliocytoma (Lhermitte-Duclos Disease)

This brain tumor was first described in 1991 and has features of both neoplasm and hamartoma. LDD is a rare cerebellar tumor (cerebellar dysplastic gangliocytoma) associated with Cowden syndrome, both conditions known to be associated with germline mutations in the PTEN gene. The overall incidence of LDD is about 15 % among patients with CS undergoing MRI surveillance screening, with additional patients having meningiomas (5 %) or other vascular malformations (30 %). The precise relationship between LDD, CS, and germline PTEN mutations is less clear as not all patients with LDD develop clinical manifestations of CS and many patients with LDD lack germline mutations in PTEN, especially children. In a recent series of 18 unselected LDD surgical resections, PTEN mutations were found in 15 samples, all with adult onset. The three remaining PTEN wild-type samples were from patients with childhood onset. Furthermore, not all patients with germline PTEN mutations manifest CS as described by Robinson and Cohen's review of children with LDD [16]. Although this lesion is histopathologically benign, recurrences following surgical resection are not uncommon. It can cause signs of mass effect in the posterior fossa and lead to hydrocephalus, brain herniation, and death if not treated. The prognosis has markedly improved with advances in neuroimaging and neurosurgical techniques. LDD will typically present in nonenhancing gyriform patterns of enlargement of cerebellar folia. This unique MR imaging pattern can obviate the need for a diagnostic biopsy procedure in asymptomatic patients [16]. The histogenesis of this lesion is unclear but has been ascribed to aberrant migration and hypertrophy of cerebellar granule neurons.

Clinical Applications

All individuals with PHTS, including LDD, should follow the cancer screening strategy recommended for Cowden syndrome (www.NCCN.org) [17]. With better understanding of the PTEN signaling cascade, patients will benefit from more precise diagnosis and targeted pharmacotherapies in the near future.

Fanconi Anemia

Fanconi anemia (FA) is an autosomal recessive disorder (except FANCB, which is X-linked). Fanconi anemia is characterized by the combination of multiple congenital anomalies, bone marrow failure, and predisposition to malignancies. Congenital anomalies include radial aplasia, hyperpigmentation of the skin, growth retardation, microphthalmia, and renal anomalies. Bone marrow failure usually presents as aplastic anemia in late childhood. Malignancies may be related to bone marrow failure (e.g., acute myelogenous leukemia) or may be solid tumors. FA is associated with increased risks of squamous cell carcinomas of the head and neck, esophagus, and vulva, cervical cancer, breast cancer, and brain tumors.

The diagnosis of FA rests on cytogenetic testing for increased chromosomal breakage or rearrangement in the presence of diepoxybutane (DEB) or radial figures with mitomycin C (MMC). If the result is normal in blood and clinical suspicion is high, consider testing a different tissue (e.g., fibroblasts) to ensure that lymphocyte mosaicism didn't lead to a false-negative result.

Clinical Genetics

Fanconi anemia is a genetically heterogeneous disorder: multiple genes can cause FA. Fifteen genes are known to cause Fanconi anemia. This pathway is responsible for specific DNA damage repair which involved homologous recombination. One gene is X-linked (FANCB), but in all

other cases FA is inherited in an autosomal recessive pattern. *FANCA* is the gene most often
involved, in 60–70 % of cases, followed by
FANCC (14 %) and *FANCG* (10 %). All other
genes explain ≤3 % of cases.

Current practice is to perform complementa-
tion analysis to identify the gene involved and
then proceed to sequencing analysis of that gene.
The implementation of next-generation sequencing in clinical laboratories is likely to change that
practice through the development of multi-gene
panels at a reasonable price.

Tumor Spectrum

Tumors of the CNS are uncommon in Fanconi
anemia. The rare individuals who develop
medulloblastoma in the setting of FA are usually
in the context of BRCA2 or PALB2 mutations
[18, 19]. These patients do so at a very early age,
often before the formal diagnosis of FA. In 27
patients with BRCA2 mutations, the authors
report a cumulative probability of brain tumor of
85 % by age 9 years (predominantly medulloblastomas) and any malignancy of 97 % by age
5.2 years. In this subgroup of FA, these probabil-
ities are much higher than that observed in
genetically   unclassified   patients   with
FA. Recently, germline mutations in PALB2,
another gene in FA pathway, were reported to be
associated with medulloblastomas and other
types of cancers. The possibility of specific associations between specific genotypes/mutations
and brain tumors is reported in a limited number
of patients and must be confirmed on larger
series of patients.

Clinical Applications

Patients with FA are well recognized to be highly
sensitive to both irradiation and chemotherapy
(especially alkylating agents) with increase risk
of severe toxicities. For all children diagnosed at
young age with medulloblastoma, a meticulous
clinical exam must be performed, with prompt
genetic testing especially in the presence of

cutaneous, skeletal, or neurological abnormalities consistent with FA.

Constitutional Mismatch Repair Deficiency Syndrome (Turcot Syndrome 1)

Turcot syndrome classically referred to the combination of colorectal polyposis and primary
tumors of the central nervous system. Identifying
the genetic basis for Turcot resulted in two very
distinct   cancer   predisposition   syndromes.
Mutations in the *APC* gene (see "Familial
Adenomatous Polyposis") have no other systemic manifestations while heterozygous germline mutations in any of the four mismatch repair
genes predispose to Lynch syndrome [20]. Lynch
syndrome is an autosomal dominant condition
characterized by an increased risk of colon cancer, as well as cancers of the endometrium, ovary,
stomach, small intestine, hepatobiliary tract, and
urinary tract. In individuals with Lynch syndrome, the lifetime risks for cancer are for
colorectal cancer (52–82 %), with a mean age at
diagnosis 48–62 years while the risk of brain
tumors is extremely low.

Diagnosis of Lynch syndrome is made based
on family history, using the Amsterdam Criteria:
at least three family members (one of whom is a
first-degree relative of the other two) with Lynch
syndrome-related   cancers,   two   successive
affected generations, and at least one of the cancers diagnosed before age 50 years. Importantly,
biallelic mutations in any of these genes result in
a very different and aggressive cancer predisposition syndrome named constitutional mismatch
repair deficiency syndrome (CMMR-D). These
children present with café au lait spots and frequent history of consanguinity. These families
lack the impressive family history of GI malignancies and therefore do not meet the Amsterdam
criteria.

CMMR-D results in an extremely high rate of
malignant cancers before age 18. The most frequent are brain tumors followed by hematopoietic malignancies (usually T-cell lymphomas)

and GI cancers. Survival above the second decade is uncommon among these individuals.

Clinical Genetics

The mutations described in CMMR-D involve MSH2, MSH6, PMS2, and MLH1. The mismatch repair system is one of the major DNA repair pathways in humans. Its primary function is to repair specific types of DNA errors such as single base pair mismatches and misalignments usually occurring during DNA replication. As opposed to Lynch syndrome where mutations in MLH1 and MSH2 are the most common, in CMMR-D biallelic PMS2 mutations are most frequent followed by MSH6. Penetrance of CMMR-D is extremely high reaching more than 90 % at age 20.

Tumor Spectrum

Although individuals with CMMR-D can present with leukemias and lymphomas (usually T-cell origin, but not necessarily) and premalignant and malignant GI lesions, the most common malignancy and the cause of death in these children are malignant brain tumors.

Brain tumors associated with CMMR-D are gliomas, usually malignant, and medulloblastoma/PNET. The distinction between malignant gliomas and PNET may be difficult in the setting of CMMR-D since they exhibit both neural and glial markers and immaturity. Some of the tumors have atypical morphology compatible with pleomorphic xanthroastrocytoma.

With early detection of tumors, some low-grade gliomas were identified suggesting a role for surveillance. Diagnosis of MMR deficiency can be made by immunohistochemistry for the four MMR genes. These usually demonstrate lack of stain of the mutated gene and can be used for targeted sequencing. Importantly, microsatellite instability, which is a feature of Lynch-related GI cancers, is not observed in most CMMR-D malignant brain tumors.

Although the data is anecdotal, several reports suggest that malignant gliomas in the context of CMMR-D may have favorable outcome, especially when early detection leads to complete resection. The toxicity and risk of secondary malignancies of radiation therapy or chemotherapy has not been assessed in patients with CMMR-D and brain tumors. However, treatment with temozolomide can cause an aggressive hypermutated phenotype when MMR deficiency of the tumor is observed.

Clinical Applications

The clinician should be attentive to any patient with high-grade glioma or PNET with café au lait spots since these cancers are uncommon in individuals with NF1. Family history of consanguinity or Lynch-related tumors and personal history of hematologic and GI malignancy strongly suggest CMMR-D. A surveillance protocol is available and had shown to increase survival especially when early detection of brain tumors is achieved.

Nonsyndromic Cancer Predisposition

This group of syndromes lacks other manifestations except for cancer predisposition. Therefore, phenotypic clues will not exist except for family history of specific types of cancer.

Familial Adenomatous Polyposis (Turcot Syndrome 2)

As outlined above, familial adenomatous polyposis (FAP) is a variant of Turcot syndrome which is classically described as the association of colonic adenomatous polyposis and tumors of the central nervous system. Some cases of Turcot syndrome are actually part of the FAP spectrum. In those cases, the brain tumor is most often medulloblastoma. Other cases of Turcot syndrome are actually variants of CMMR-D.

FAP is an autosomal dominant condition characterized by the development of hundreds to thousands of adenomas in the rectum and colon during childhood and adolescence. It has a prevalence of 2–3/100,000 individuals. Although FAP accounts for less than 1 % of all colorectal cancers, 95 % of individuals with FAP will have polyps by age 35 and will almost inevitably develop colorectal cancer if untreated. Extracolonic manifestations include polyps in the upper gastrointestinal tract, osteomas, dental anomalies, congenital hypertrophy of the retinal pigment epithelium (CHRPE), desmoid tumors, and other cancers.

The diagnosis of FAP is considered clinically in an individual with either more than 100 colorectal adenomatous polyps or fewer than 100 adenomatous polyps and a relative with similar type of tumors. Attenuated FAP is considered if the individual has between 10 and 100 adenomatous polyps or if he has a personal history of colorectal cancer with a family history of multiple adenomatous polyps.

Clinical Genetics

FAP is caused by germline mutations in the *APC* gene. *APC* is a tumor suppressor in the WNT pathway. Activation of this pathway has been found in many cancers including colorectal cancers and medulloblastomas [21]. In individuals with a classic phenotype, the mutation detection rate is at least 90 %. About 8–12 % of these individuals have a partial or whole deletion of the *APC* gene. In individuals with an attenuated phenotype, less than 30 % will have an identifiable mutation in *APC*. About 25 % of identified mutations are de novo.

The penetrance of adenomatous polyps is complete, but the occurrence of associated cancers including medulloblastoma is variable. No specific genotype-phenotype correlations have been established in relation to brain tumors.

Tumor Spectrum

Children with FAP are at risk of developing not only multiple gastrointestinal tract polyps (>100) with high risk of cancer transformation but also medulloblastoma, hepatoblastoma, and aggressive fibromatosis. Epidemiologic data from several FAP pedigrees suggested an increased risk of 92 times for the development of medulloblastoma in carriers. As opposed to patients with Gorlin syndrome, patients with FAP have later-onset medulloblastomas, with a median age of occurrence of 15 years as compared to 7 years for sporadic medulloblastoma. While FAP syndrome cases are characterized by APC mutations, a minority (<5 %) of sporadic medulloblastomas also harbor mutations in that gene. Interestingly, syndromic cases show truncating nonsense mutations while sporadic cases show missense mutations, but the significance of this difference is unclear. *APC* mutations in sporadic tumors cluster in the beta-catenin binding site region which suggests pathogenicity through impaired APC binding to beta-catenin. By virtue of their presumably impaired APC-beta-catenin interaction, these tumors should belong to the WNT group which has favorable outcome; however, data are lacking for this association.

Clinical Applications

Although any patient with medulloblastoma and FAP should benefit from gastrointestinal cancer surveillance, the penetrance of medulloblastoma in FAP is relatively low, so primary neuroimaging for these patients is not currently recommended. Treatment strategies follow the same rules than for sporadic medulloblastoma, despite specific molecular genetic markers.

Neurofibromatosis Type 2

Although the names are similar, neurofibromatosis type 1 and 2 are very different conditions in terms of clinical phenotypes, tumor spectrum, and at the genetic level. It is important not to confuse and associate the syndromes together.

Neurofibromatosis 2 (NF2) is an autosomal dominant disorder characterized by bilateral vestibular schwannomas. Affected individuals may also develop other CNS tumors. Diagnostic criteria for NF2 are based on a combination of unilateral vestibular schwannoma, presence of other related tumors (meningioma, schwannoma, glioma, neurofibroma, posterior subcapsular lenticular opacities), and/or a first-degree relative with NF2 [22].

Average age of onset is young adulthood (18–24 years), but age of onset can range from birth to 70 years of age. Its prevalence is estimated at 1/80,000 worldwide. Average age of death is reported to be 36 years.

Clinical Genetics

NF2 is due to mutations in the *NF2* or *MERLIN* gene. The exact function of the gene is still not completely understood. It is involved in both cytoskeletal and cell signaling pathways. At least 10–15 % of mutations are deletions. About 50 % are inherited and the other half is de novo. The mutation detection rate is over 90 % in familial cases, but only 60–70 % in simplex cases. In 25–33 % of cases, the absence of detectable mutation is explained by the presence of somatic mosaicism. When a mutation in NF2 is inherited, penetrance is 100 %.

Tumor Spectrum

Intracranial Tumors

NF2 is characterized by the development of bilateral vestibular schwannomas (Fig. 8.1) and other cranial, spinal, and peripheral schwannomas. Bilateral vestibular schwannomas are the hallmark of NF2 and are usually pathognomonic. Vestibular schwannomas affect both the seventh and the eighth cranial nerves causing hearing loss, tinnitus, and facial paresis. Management of these tumors is difficult and requires a multidisciplinary team. As opposed to sporadic unilateral acoustic tumors, both surgery and radiation therapies failed to prevent hearing loss in these individuals. Long-term follow-up is needed to address concerns about radiation-induced malignant transformation or adjacent tumor development [2]. Surgery is usually reserved to time of hearing loss to prevent facial palsy at the corre-

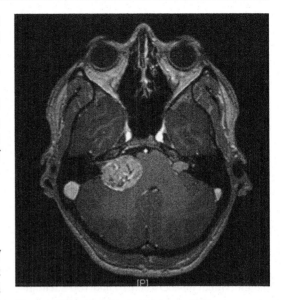

Fig. 8.1 Bilateral acoustic neuroma in NF2

sponding side. In recent years, several studies have shown encouraging tumor control using medical therapies. Specifically, bevacizumab [23] and lapatinib [24] have shown improvement in hearing and tumor control. These therapies are currently reserved for symptomatic acoustic neuromas. Novel medical therapies offer hope for these individuals in delaying/preventing these devastating long-term disabilities.

Patients with NF2 can also develop intracranial, spinal, and optic nerve sheath meningiomas, ependymomas, and gliomas of the CNS. Most meningiomas of the cerebral hemispheres and spinal canal can be safely resected while those originating from optic nerve sheath and skull base might be associated with significant surgical morbidity. Medical therapies have not shown sufficient tumor control in nonacoustic tumors. Up to 18 % of NF2 patients presented before age 15 years and with an isolated feature of the disease and no suggestive family history. NF2 patients who present in childhood tend to have a more aggressive clinical course with a variety of tumors requiring multiple interventions.

Spinal Tumors

Since the advent of MRI, spinal tumors are detected in up to 90 % of patients. However, only 25–30 % of these are symptomatic. Ependymomas are the most common tumor type. When multiple, they can appear like a string of pearls on contrast-enhanced MRI. Early onset of symptoms such as back pain, weakness, or sensory disturbances best determines the timing for spinal intervention [2].

Clinical Applications

Children presenting with bilateral acoustic neuroma or multiple meningiomas or schwannomas should be suspected of having NF2, and genetic testing is recommended. There are established screening programs for children of affected parents and of individuals with an NF2-related tumor in childhood (family history, full craniospinal MRI, extensive dermatologic and ophthalmologic examination) [22]. It will permit early diagnosis, close surveillance, and development of treatment frameworks based on molecular pathogenesis and natural history of lesions. Presymptomatic genetic testing for children at risk of NF2 is now possible in most families.

Schwannomatosis

Schwannomatosis is an autosomal dominant disorder characterized by the predisposition to develop multiple schwannomas. Suggested clinical diagnostic criteria include the presence of at least two non-intradermal schwannomas with one pathologically confirmed schwannoma or intracranial meningioma and an affected first-degree relative. These criteria exclude patients with bilateral vestibular schwannoma or having a germline mutation in NF2 which fulfill diagnostic criteria for NF2.

Clinical Genetics

Recently, schwannomatosis was found to be associated with germline mutations in *SMARCB1*. Most cases are sporadic; only 15–25 % of cases have inherited the condition

from an affected parent. Mutations in SMARCB1 are found in 40–60 % of familial cases of schwannomatosis and less than 10 % of simplex cases [25].

Tumor Spectrum

Schwannomas arising in the setting of schwannomatosis usually present in the second and third decades and are characteristically painful. Histologic examination reveals that a high proportion of tumors are hybrid neurofibroma/schwannoma. This hybrid histology is also frequently encountered in NF1 and NF2. Immunostaining for SAMRCB1 can be of diagnostic significance for these patients. A mosaic-type pattern of immunohistochemical positivity for SMARB1/INI-1 is specific for non-solitary schwannomas. Conversely, the absence of the mosaic-type pattern is a good indicator of nonfamilial tumors, which could be clinically helpful as part of genetic counseling.

Because two patients harbored a combination of *SMARCB1* and *NF2* mutations with LOH at both alleles, a four-hit mechanism involving the two tumor suppressor genes has been proposed [26]. Importantly, since the majority of schwannomatosis patients do not have a germline mutation in SMARCB1, other constitutional mutations are likely implicated in schwannomatosis tumorigenesis.

Rhabdoid Tumor Predisposition Syndrome

The rhabdoid tumor predisposition syndrome (RTPS) is an autosomal dominant disorder characterized by a predisposition to rhabdoid tumors in the kidney, other extrarenal locations, and the central nervous system [27]. There are no established criteria to diagnose RTPS. Rather, the presence of rhabdoid tumors could be enough to justify investigating further from a genetics standpoint.

Clinical Genetics

Mutations in *INII/SMARCB1* are the initiating event for the development of rhabdoid tumors. *SMARCB1* is a tumor suppressor gene located on the long arm of chromosome 22. The exact function of *SMARCB1* is unknown, but the SMARC genes are important in chromatin modification. A germline mutation can be identified in about 35 % of patients with rhabdoid tumors. The majority of these tumors seem to be de novo, but families in which multiple siblings are affected have been reported. *SMARCB1* is also implicated in schwannomatosis and families with both phenotypes have been reported. The penetrance of SMARCB1 is still unknown, but it is incomplete since asymptomatic carrier parents have been reported.

Tumor Spectrum

Rhabdoid tumors in all sites tend to present at an early age and have an extremely aggressive course. The most common location for extrarenal rhabdoid tumor is the CNS, where it is referred to as atypical teratoid/rhabdoid tumor (AT/RT). AT/RT and rhabdoid tumors of the kidney may present synchronously or at months of interval.

Atypical Teratoid/Rhabdoid Tumor of CNS

Since the first well-documented case of malignant rhabdoid tumor of the CNS published in 1986, atypical teratoid/rhabdoid tumor (AT/RT) has been recognized as a distinct pathological entity. AT/RT commonly affects very young children under 2 years of age at diagnosis. They are most commonly located in the posterior fossa (60 %), but also present supratentorially and often metastasize throughout the CNS at presentation (27 %). In the past AT/RT was often misdiagnosed as medulloblastoma or PNET. The first diagnostic clue came from the identification of deletion of chromosome 22q in these tumors. In 1999, Biegel et al. have reported germline and somatic mutations of *SMARCB1* gene, a tumor suppressor gene, which maps to 22q11.2 in

children with CNS AT/RT [28]. Most mutations result in loss of function of the gene and therefore lack of immunostaining of the corresponding antibody BAF47 is diagnostic for AT/RT. In 2008, the fourth edition of WHO classification of tumors of CNS included the newly described entity of AT/RT. AT/RT still confers poor outcome. However, the use of aggressive multimodality treatment combining extensive surgical excision with intensive systemic chemotherapy using myeloablative chemotherapy with autologous stem cell rescue, with or without brain irradiation has recently improved the prognosis [29–31]. Whether intrathecal chemotherapy can replace irradiation for young children is still unclear. The outcome of CNS AT/RT in the setting of rhabdoid predisposition syndrome has not yet been reported.

Clinical Applications

Children diagnosed with rhabdoid tumor of the kidney or with CNS AT/RT should have imaging of both the abdomen and the brain as a part of their initial work-up. Testing for germline mutations in SMARCB1 is highly recommended. A surveillance protocol has been developed for carriers [32]; however, since until recently most patients did not survive, the exact tumor spectrum and the significance of this approach in RTPS are still unknown.

Li-Fraumeni Syndrome

Li-Fraumeni syndrome (LFS) is considered the prototype of cancer predisposition syndromes. Although initially characterized by a predisposition to soft tissue sarcoma, premenopausal breast cancer, and brain tumors, individuals with LFS are at risk of developing cancer at any age and in almost any tissue.

Clinical diagnosis of classic LFS is defined by the following criteria: a proband with sarcoma diagnosed before age 45 years, and a first-degree relative with any cancer before age 45 years and a first- or second-degree relative with any cancer before age 45 years or a sarcoma at any age. In 2009, more detailed criteria were proposed to guide testing for TP53 (2009 Chompret criteria) [33]: a proband who has a tumor belonging to the LFS spectrum before age 46 and at least one first- or second-degree relative with an LFS tumor, or a proband with multiple tumors, two of which belong to the LFS spectrum and the first of which occurred before age 46 or a proband with adreno-cortical carcinoma or choroid plexus tumor, irre-spective of family history.

Clinical Genetics

LFS is inherited in an autosomal dominant fash-ion and is caused by germline mutations in the *TP53* gene. Sequencing of TP53 detects about 95 % of all mutations in TP53. Deletion analysis can identify an additional 1 % of mutations in TP53. Most mutations are inherited and the exact frequency of de novo mutations in TP53 is not established. Penetrance is high but not complete. The risk of cancer in LFS is estimated to be 50 % by age 30 years and 90 % by age 60 years, with higher risks in women than men. Mutations in CHEK2 have been reported in a few families, but it is not thought to be a major underlying cause of LFS.

Tumor Spectrum

During childhood, LFS individuals are at high risk of developing adrenocortical carcinoma, soft sarcomas including rhabdomyosarcoma, osteo-sarcoma, and leukemia. Brain tumors associated with LFS are high-grade gliomas, choroid plexus carcinoma (CPC), and medulloblastoma.

Diffuse Astrocytoma (Grade II–IV)
Malignant gliomas are the most frequent brain tumors affecting individuals with LFS. However, they tend to occur during late childhood and adult life. In the setting of LFS, both de novo glioblastoma and diffuse astrocytomas with secondary transforma-tion are reported. The prognosis for LFS-associated gliomas is just as poor as in sporadic cases.

The fact that brain tumors seem to cluster in certain families with LFS suggests that mutations in specific regions of TP53, such as those binding the minor groove of DNA, may exert some degree of organ-specific carcinogenesis. Mutations in IDH1, ubiquitous in secondary sporadic GBM, are also present in astrocytomas from LFS patients [34]. However, in all reported cases the acquired mutation was R132C, a rare occurrence in the setting of sporadic tumors (<5 %).

Choroid Plexus Carcinoma
TP53 alterations play a significant role in CPC tumorigenesis. Somatic *TP53* mutations were observed in 50 % of CPC and germline mutations in 16–36 % of patients. Therefore, the new LFS guidelines include CPC as a part of the diagnostic criteria for LFS. P53 dysfunction is associated with poor outcome in CPC; however, the signifi-cance of germline TP53 mutations on survival is still unknown.

Medulloblastoma
Medulloblastomas account for 11 % of reported LFS-associated brain tumors. *TP53* mutations are found in 5–10 % of medulloblastomas. Most LFS-associated medulloblastomas belong to the SHH group and are associated with the large cell type, anaplastic type, high degree of genomic instability, and poor outcome [35]. In contrast to CPC which occur at young age, most LFS-associated medulloblastomas occur in the second decade at older age than sporadic medulloblastomas.

Clinical Applications

Current recommendations are to screen every patient with CPC for tumor and germline *TP53* mutations. Medulloblastomas which stain posi-tive for P53 or belong to the SHH subgroup should be screened for TP53 mutations and if positive proceed to genetic counseling and germ-line testing. Since most childhood gliomas are not associated with LFS, testing should rely on family and patient history. Since surveillance protocol has been shown to improve survival for individuals with LFS [36], this protocol should be offered to all patients and family members (see Fig. 17.1 now).

Von Hippel-Lindau Disease

Von Hippel-Lindau (VHL) is an autosomal dominant disorder, and is suspected in the presence of characteristic lesions such as hemangioblastomas, multiple renal cysts and renal cell carcinoma, pheochromocytoma, and endolymphatic sac tumors.

Diagnosis of VHL is established clinically, using the following diagnostic criteria: in an individual with no family history of VHL, the presence of at least two characteristic lesions and in an individual with a positive family history of VHL, the presence of retinal angioma, spinal or cerebellar hemangioblastoma, pheochromocytoma, renal cell carcinoma, or multiple renal or pancreatic cysts.

VHL type 1 is the combination of retinal angioma, CNS hemangioblastoma, renal cell carcinoma, pancreatic cysts, and neuroendocrine tumors. It is characterized by a low risk of pheochromocytoma. VHL type 2 is associated with pheochromocytoma. VHL type 2A is the combination of pheochromocytoma, retinal angiomas, and CNS hemangioblastoma, with a low risk for renal cell carcinoma. VHL type 2B combines the characteristics of type 2A with pancreatic cysts, neuroendocrine tumors, and a high risk for renal cell carcinoma. VHL type 2C is associated with pheochromocytoma only.

Clinical Genetics

VHL is a major tumor suppressor in the hypoxia-induced factor (HIF) pathway. This oncogenic pathway is activated in many cancers and is responsible for angiogenesis in these tumors. VHL recruits ubiquitin ligase that targets HIF for degradation. In recent years, other tumor suppressive functions of VHL have been recognized, linking it to other cancer predisposition

syndromes [37]. Molecular analysis identifies mutations in 95 % of classical VHL, partial or whole gene deletions accounting for 30–40 % of cases. Mutations are inherited in about 80 % of cases and de novo in 20 %. Truncating mutations or missense mutations that are predicted to grossly disrupt protein structure are associated with VHL type 1. Other missense mutations are typically associated with VHL type 2. Penetrance is high: almost all individuals with a mutation in VHL develop symptoms by age 65.

Tumor Spectrum

Central Nervous System Hemangioblastomas

Hemangioblastomas of the CNS are the most common tumor in VHL disease, affecting 60–80 % of all patients at an average age of 33 years. The earliest case reported was at 11 years of age. In a recent series of 6 children with solitary cerebellar hemangioblastoma, only those with other suggestive features of VHL had a germline mutation [38]. Although of benign nature, these tumors are a major cause of morbidity. Symptoms related to hemangioblastomas depend on tumor location and size, the presence of associated cysts (30–80 %), and/or edema. They arise anywhere along the craniospinal: spinal cord (13–50 %), the cerebellum (44–72 %), the brainstem (10–25 %), the lumbosacral nerve roots (<1 %), and the supratentorial region (<1 %). Hemangioblastomas of the CNS often grow at several sites simultaneously with an irregular and unpredictable growth pattern. They are best assessed by gadolinium-enhanced MRI. Preoperative embolization is done at some centers to reduce tumor vascularity before resection. Most of them can be safely and completely resected by surgery. Stereotactic radiation therapy is used in case of multiple craniospinal hemangioblastomas, especially those not associated with cysts. Erythrocytosis occurs in 5–20 % of cerebral hemangioblastomas and can necessitate periodic phlebotomies, but it responds to surgical resection [39].

Retinal Hemangioblastomas

The mean age at diagnosis of retinal hemangioblastomas ("retinal angiomas") is 25 years. Only 5 % are discovered before 10 years of age. They are seen in as many as 60 % of patients. They arise in the periphery, on or near the optic disc, or both. In about 50 % of cases, they are multifocal and bilateral. At initial stages, they are detectable only by examination of dilated eyes. Despite being asymptomatic initially, they can lead to part or total loss of vision. Both peripheral and central retinal hemangioblastomas can cause exudative and tractional retinal detachment as they enlarge. Most peripheral tumors respond to laser photocoagulation or cryotherapy. Vitrectomy and enucleation might be necessary in complicated and/or advanced cases (glaucoma or severe pain). The role of radiation therapy in severely affected patients needs to be defined. Anti-VEGF therapy is still experimental.

Clinical Applications

CNS and retinal hemangioblastomas are extremely uncommon during childhood. Therefore all patients with hemangioblastomas should be considered potentially affected by VHL disease and benefit from an intensive family history and screening studies. Surveillance guidelines for VHL carriers exist and may allow for early diagnosis and treatment to prevent visual loss and other sequelae.

A Clinical Approach to Cancer Predisposition in Childhood Brain Tumors

A clinician treating children with brain tumors needs to be aware of the relatively high rate of germline mutations in this patient population. Therefore, high index of suspicion should be employed. Detailed family history of cancer is helpful in syndromes such as Li-Fraumeni; however, this should not rule out a patient since the rate of de novo mutations is high and some autosomal recessive syndromes may have uninformative family history. A child with a brain tumor and consanguineous parents should be a red flag.

Clinical examination at initial visit should focus on signs such as skin lesions and dysmorphism which can suggest a specific syndrome. In any case of suspicion, a referral to genetic counseling and testing is highly recommended, preferably before treatment initiation as this may affect the results of some functional and genetic tests. For each specific tumor, a different group of syndromes may be applied. This may guide the clinician on specific questions and clues upon physical examination (Table 8.1). Finally, some tumors are specifically associated with specific syndromes. In these cases, since the rate of germline mutations is extremely high, referral to genetic counseling is recommended even without the classical history and signs on physical examination.

Finally, the new molecular and genetic tests which are added to the pathological work may suggest somatic tumor mutations which should be traced to the germline. Examples include a young infant with desmoplastic medulloblastoma with SHH gene signature which is highly suggestive of Gorlin syndrome and a very young child with AT/RT and negative stain for BAF47 which is associated with germline mutations in *SMARCB1*.

Summary

The aim of this chapter was to give an outline and a clinical approach to the major cancer predisposition syndromes associated with pediatric brain tumors. As discussed in the introduction, we did not aim at covering all syndromes where childhood brain tumors were reported. Furthermore, next-generation sequencing reveals that the mutation spectrum uncovered by clinical associations is only the tip of the iceberg and novel genetic syndromes may be a part of our landscape and require specific individualized approach in the near future. However, the role of the clinician in suspecting, pursuing the diagnosis,

Table 8.1 Clinicians' approach to genetic predisposition syndromes in pediatric neurooncology

Tumor	Family history and other tumors	Physical findings	Genes screened	Surveillance/targeted therapies
Glioma	Consanguinity, Mideastern origin. Colon cancer, lymphoma/leukemia	Café au lait spots	MMR	Surveillance protocol available
	Multiple tumors in family members: breast cancer, brain tumors, sarcomas, ADCC, others	None	TP53	Surveillance protocol available
	First-degree members with NF1 Plexiform and other neurofibromas	Café au lait spots, short stature, developmental delay, cardiovascular and bony abnormalities	Neurofibromin	Surveillance protocol available
Medulloblastoma	Other family members with similar clinical manifestations. Basal cell carcinoma of skin	Jaw cysts, palmar/plantar pits, *spine abnormalities*, rib abnormalities, metacarpal/phalangeal abnormalities	PTCH1 PTCH2, Sufu	Surveillance protocol available
	Multiple tumors in family members: breast cancer, brain tumors, sarcomas, ADCC, others	None	TP53	Surveillance protocol available
	Aplastic anemia, multiple carcinomas in family members. Wilms, breast cancer, pancreatic cancer	Café au lait, short stature, limb abnormalities	BRCA2, PALB2	
	Family members with GI polyps and cancers, hepatoblastoma, GI polyps, desmoid tumors	Dental anomalies, hypertrophy of the retinal pigment	APC	
Choroid plexus carcinoma	Multiple tumors in family members: breast cancer, brain tumors, sarcomas, ADCC, others	None	TP53	Surveillance protocol available
Ependymoma (usually spinal)	Schwannomas, meningiomas, vestibular schwannoma		Merlin	Surveillance protocol available
Tumor-specific syndromes				
Atypical teratoid/rhabdoid tumor	Family history of schwannomas, renal and extrarenal rhabdoid tumors	None	INI1	
Hemangioblastoma	Hemangioblastomas in other CNS locations, retinal hemangioblastomas, renal cell carcinomas and cysts. Pheochromocytoma, pancreatic tumors and cysts, epididymal and broad ligament cystadenomas, endolymphatic sac tumors	None	VHL	Surveillance protocol available

Tumor	Family history and other tumors	Physical findings	Genes screened	Surveillance/targeted therapies
Dysplastic gangliocytoma of the cerebellum	Family members with breast carcinoma, thyroid follicular carcinoma, endometrial carcinoma, renal cell carcinoma	Trichilemmomas, acral keratoses, oral mucosal papillomatosis, palmoplantar keratoses	PTEN	
		Hamartomas of gastrointestinal tract, bones, brain, eyes, and genitourinary tract		
Subependymal giant cell astrocytoma (SEGA)	Renal angiomyolipoma, cardiac rhabdomyoma, pulmonary lymphangiomyomatosis, renal cell carcinoma	*Epilepsy, developmental delay, and autism spectrum.* Hypomelanotic macules, facial angiofibromas ungual fibromas, truncal connective tissue nevus ("shagreen patch"), dental enamel pits, multiple retinal nodular hamartomas (phakomas), hypopigmented iris spots	TSC1, TSC2	Targeted therapy with mTOR inhibitors available
Bilateral acoustic schwannomas	Family members with the same tumor or multiple CNS schwannomas and meningiomas. Low-grade spinal ependymomas	Posterior subcapsular "juvenile" cataracts, retinal hamartomas, epiretinal membranes	NF2, Merlin	Surveillance protocol available, targeted therapies with antiangiogenic agents

and building a patient-oriented treatment and surveillance protocols cannot be overemphasized. These qualities can improve survival of both the child and family members [36] in the world of precision medicine.

References

1. Strahm B, Malkin D. Hereditary cancer predisposition in children: genetic basis and clinical implications. Int J Cancer. 2006;119:2001–6.
2. Asthagiri AR, Parry DM, Butman JA, et al. Neurofibromatosis type 2. Lancet. 2009;373:1974–86.
3. Jett K, Friedman JM. Clinical and genetic aspects of neurofibromatosis 1. Genet Med. 2010;12:1–11.
4. Rubin JB, Gutmann DH. Neurofibromatosis type 1—a model for nervous system tumour formation? Nat Rev Cancer. 2005;5:557–64.
5. Tischkowitz M, Rosser E. Inherited cancer in children: practical/ethical problems and challenges. Eur J Cancer. 2004;40:2459–70.
6. Segal L, Darvish-Zargar M, Dilenge ME, et al. Optic pathway gliomas in patients with neurofibromatosis type 1: follow-up of 44 patients. J AAPOS. 2010;14:155–8.
7. Sharif S, Ferner R, Birch JM, et al. Second primary tumors in neurofibromatosis 1 patients treated for optic glioma: substantial risks after radiotherapy. J Clin Oncol. 2006;24:2570–5.
8. Ullrich NJ, Raja AI, Irons MB, et al. Brainstem lesions in neurofibromatosis type 1. Neurosurgery. 2007;61:762–6; discussion 766–7.
9. Rodriguez EF, Scheithauer BW, Giannini C, et al. PI3K/AKT pathway alterations are associated with clinically aggressive and histologically anaplastic subsets of pilocytic astrocytoma. Acta Neuropathol. 2011;121:407–20.
10. Krueger DA, Care MM, Holland K, et al. Everolimus for subependymal giant-cell astrocytomas in tuberous sclerosis. N Engl J Med. 2010;363:1801–11.
11. Bree AF, Shah MR. Consensus statement from the first international colloquium on basal cell nevus syndrome (BCNS). Am J Med Genet A. 2011;155A:2091–7.
12. Lo Muzio L. Nevoid basal cell carcinoma syndrome (Gorlin syndrome). Orphanet J Rare Dis. 2008;3:32.
13. Brugieres L, Remenieras A, Pierron G, et al. High frequency of germline SUFU mutations in children with desmoplastic/nodular medulloblastoma younger than 3 years of age. J Clin Oncol. 2012;30:2087–93.
14. Taylor MD, Northcott PA, Korshunov A, et al. Molecular subgroups of medulloblastoma: the current consensus. Acta Neuropathol. 2012;123:465–72.
15. Rudin CM, Hann CL, Laterra J, et al. Treatment of medulloblastoma with hedgehog pathway inhibitor GDC-0449. N Engl J Med. 2009;361:1173–8.
16. Robinson S, Cohen AR. Cowden disease and Lhermitte-Duclos disease: an update. Case report and review of the literature. Neurosurg Focus. 2006;20:E6.
17. Blumenthal GM, Dennis PA. PTEN hamartoma tumor syndromes. Eur J Hum Genet. 2008;16:1289–300.
18. Alter BP, Rosenberg PS, Brody LC. Clinical and molecular features associated with biallelic mutations in FANCD1/BRCA2. J Med Genet. 2007;44:1–9.
19. Reid S, Schindler D, Hanenberg H, et al. Biallelic mutations in PALB2 cause Fanconi anemia subtype FA-N and predispose to childhood cancer. Nat Genet. 2007;39:162–4.
20. Kohlmann W, Gruber SB. Lynch syndrome. In: Pagon RA, Bird TD, Dolan CR, et al., editors. GeneReviews. Seattle: University of Washington; 2004.
21. Jasperson KW, Burt RW. APC-associated polyposis conditions. In: Pagon RA, Bird TD, Dolan CR, et al., editors. GeneReviews. Seattle: University of Washington, Seattle; 1998.
22. Evans DG, Baser ME, O'Reilly B, et al. Management of the patient and family with neurofibromatosis 2: a consensus conference statement. Br J Neurosurg. 2005;19:5–12.
23. Plotkin SR, Stemmer-Rachamimov AO, Barker II FG, et al. Hearing improvement after bevacizumab in patients with neurofibromatosis type 2. N Engl J Med. 2009;361:358–67.
24. Karajannis MA, Legault G, Hagiwara M, et al. Phase II trial of lapatinib in adult and pediatric patients with neurofibromatosis type 2 and progressive vestibular schwannomas. Neuro Oncol. 2012;14:1163–70.
25. Plotkin SR, Blakeley JO, Evans DG, et al. Update from the 2011 International Schwannomatosis Workshop: from genetics to diagnostic criteria. Am J Med Genet A. 2013;161:405–16.
26. Sestini R, Bacci C, Provenzano A, et al. Evidence of a four-hit mechanism involving SMARCB1 and NF2 in schwannomatosis-associated schwannomas. Hum Mutat. 2008;29:227–31.
27. Anderson J. Malignant rhabdoid tumors: a familial condition? Pediatr Blood Cancer. 2011;56:1–2.
28. Versteege I, Sevenet N, Lange J, et al. Truncating mutations of hSNF5/INI1 in aggressive paediatric cancer. Nature. 1998;394:203–6.
29. Chi SN, Zimmerman MA, Yao X, et al. Intensive multimodality treatment for children with newly diagnosed CNS atypical teratoid rhabdoid tumor. J Clin Oncol. 2009;27:385–9.
30. Hilden JM, Meerbaum S, Burger P, et al. Central nervous system atypical teratoid/rhabdoid tumor: results of therapy in children enrolled in a registry. J Clin Oncol. 2004;22:2877–84.
31. Tekautz TM, Fuller CE, Blaney S, et al. Atypical teratoid/rhabdoid tumors (ATRT): improved survival in children 3 years of age and older with radiation therapy and high-dose alkylator-based chemotherapy. J Clin Oncol. 2005;23:1491–9.
32. Teplick A, Kowalski M, Biegel JA, et al. Educational paper: screening in cancer predisposition syndromes:

guidelines for the general pediatrician. Eur J Pediatr. 2011;170:285–94.

33. Tinat J, Bougeard G, Baert-Desurmont S, et al. 2009 version of the Chompret criteria for Li Fraumeni syndrome. J Clin Oncol. 2009; 27:e108–9; author reply e110.

34. Watanabe T, Vital A, Nobusawa S, et al. Selective acquisition of IDH1 R132C mutations in astrocytomas associated with Li-Fraumeni syndrome. Acta Neuropathol. 2009;117:653–6.

35. Zhukova N, Ramaswamy V, Remke M, et al. Subgroup-specific prognostic implications of TP53 mutation in medulloblastoma. J Clin Oncol. 2013;31:2927–35.

36. Villani A, Tabori U, Schiffman J, et al. Biochemical and imaging surveillance in germline TP53 mutation carriers with Li-Fraumeni syndrome: a prospective observational study. Lancet Oncol. 2011;12:559–67.

37. Kaelin Jr WG. The von Hippel-Lindau tumour suppressor protein: O2 sensing and cancer. Nat Rev Cancer. 2008;8:865–73.

38. Fisher PG, Tontiplaphol A, Pearlman EM, et al. Childhood cerebellar hemangioblastoma does not predict germline or somatic mutations in the von Hippel-Lindau tumor suppressor gene. Ann Neurol. 2002;51:257–60.

39. Lonser RR, Glenn GM, Walther M, et al. von Hippel-Lindau disease. Lancet. 2003;361:2059–67.

Low Grade Glioma

Katrin Scheinemann and Juliette Hukin

Epidemiology

Low grade gliomas are the most common brain tumors in the pediatric population comprising around 30–50 % of all newly diagnosed brain tumors [1].

Predisposing factors are hereditary phakomatosis like neurofibromatosis (NF) 1 and 2 as well as tuberous sclerosis (TS). Around 15–20 % of all patients with NF 1 will develop an optic pathway glioma, accounting for around 80 % of all tumors in this location. Another 4 % of patients with underlying NF 1 will develop a low grade glioma outside the optic pathway. Between 6 and 14 % of all TS patient will develop a subependymal giant cell astrocytoma (SEGA).

Most children have a few months to year's history of subtle symptoms mainly related to chronic hydrocephalus (posterior fossa or tectal location or SEGA). Visual symptoms are very common for the optic pathway glioma (OPG) group including nystagmus, esotropia, scotoma, visual field defect, or decreased visual acuity. Within the suprasellar location patients often present with endocrinopathies including growth hormone deficiency and diencephalic syndrome. Brainstem lesions may present with Parinaud syndrome (near light dissociation, retraction nystagmus, and limited up gaze), unexplained vomiting without headache, postural hypotension, dysphagia, hoarse voice, and/or obstructive or central apnea.

Location

LGG can occur anywhere within the central nervous system (CNS), and the most common location is within the posterior fossa (around 20–25 %) [1]. Other common locations are brainstem or midline location (optic pathway, suprasellar, tectal, thalamic). Locations within the cerebral hemispheres are more commonly of neuronal origin-like dysembryoplastic neuroepithelial tumor (DNET), presenting with temporal lobe seizures. Primary spinal location is described at around 5 %.

Leptomeningeal disease is described in around 3–10 %, but could be underreported as staging (MRI spine and lumbar CSF) for nonsymptomatic patients is not standard of care. It seems to occur more often in a progressive setting.

LGG are the typical CNS tumor in patients with neurofibromatosis type I or patients with tuberous sclerosis. The classical location of a low grade glioma in patients with neurofibromatosis

K. Scheinemann, M.D. (✉)
Department of Pediatrics, Division of Hematology/
Oncology, McMaster Children's Hospital,
McMaster University, Hamilton, ON, Canada
e-mail: kschein@mcmaster.ca

J. Hukin, M.B.B.S., F.R.C.P.C.
Division of Neurology and Oncology,
British Columbia Children's Hospital, Vancouver,
BC, Canada

K. Scheinemann and E. Bouffet (eds.), *Pediatric Neuro-oncology*,
DOI 10.1007/978-1-4939-1541-5_9, © Springer Science+Business Media New York 2015

type I is within the optic pathway; pathological confirmation is not necessary in the case of classical imaging findings. Subependymal giant cell astrocytoma (SEGA), the classic tumor in tuberous sclerosis patients, is characteristically found in the lateral and third ventricles.

Imaging Findings

Standard of care for imaging these tumors is magnetic resonance imaging (MRI) plus gadolinium [2]. Classically these tumors are hypointense on T1 and hyperintense on T2 images. Contrast enhancement is quite variable and can change over time—the significance of this is still unclear.

Magnetic resonance spectroscopy has not proven to be of any major benefit as the pattern is similar to the normal brain. Functional MRI may be helpful for operative planning.

Typically posterior fossa juvenile pilocytic astrocytomas (JPA) present with a combination of a large cystic component with an enhancing mural nodule (Fig. 9.1).

Within the brainstem an exophytic tumor component is suggestive of a low grade glioma (Fig. 9.2).

For optic pathway glioma, classically the intraorbital portion of the optic nerve shows some tortuosity and thickening (Fig. 9.3).

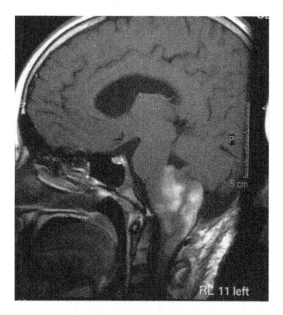

Fig. 9.2 Exophytic brainstem low grade glioma. Reprinted from Warmuth-Metz M. Neoplasms, Brain, Posterior Fossa, Pediatric. In: Baert AL (ed). Encyclopedia of Diagnostic Imaging. Berlin, Germany: Springer-Verlag; 2008:1231–1237. With permission from Springer Verlag

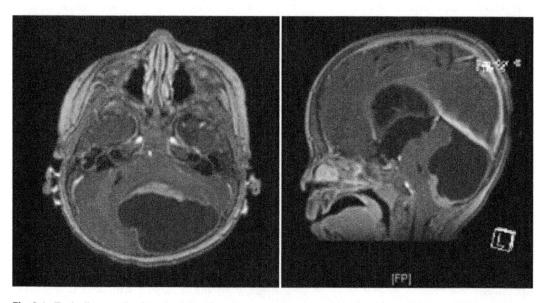

Fig. 9.1 Typically posterior fossa juvenile pilocytic astrocytomas

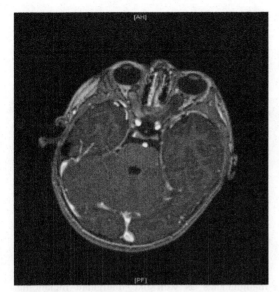

Fig. 9.3 Optic pathway glioma

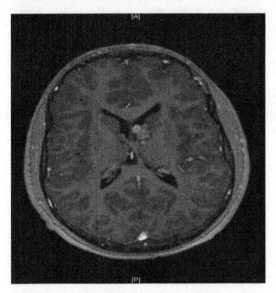

Fig. 9.4 Subependymal giant cell astrocytoma

Subependymal giant cell astrocytomas have the appearance of "snowballs" sitting in the ventricles (Fig. 9.4).

Pathology

Low grade gliomas are grade I or II tumors as per the WHO grading system of astrocytic, oligodendroglial, and mixed glial–neuronal origin. They

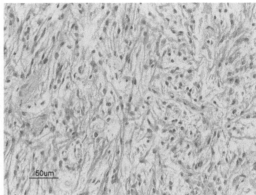

Fig. 9.5 Juvenile pilocytic astrocytoma. Courtesy of Cynthia E. Hawkins

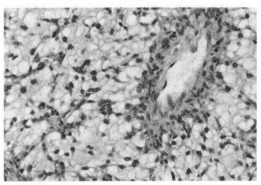

Fig. 9.6 Pilomyxoid astrocytoma (PMA). Reprinted from Louis DN, Ohgaki H, Wiestler OD, Cavenee WK, Burger PC, Jouvet A, Scheithauer BW, Kleihues P. The 2007 WHO classification of tumours of the central nervous system. Acta Neuropathologica, 2007; 114: 97–109. With permission from Springer Verlag

represent a heterogeneous group of tumors and as per the 2007 World Health Organization (WHO) classification of primary CNS tumors include the most common ones [3]:

(a) Juvenile pilocytic astrocytoma (JPA), characterized through Rosenthal fibers (Fig. 9.5)
(b) Pilomyxoid astrocytoma (PMA), first named in 1999 by Tihan et al., describing a tumor typically located in the hypothalamic/chiasmatic region, affecting predominantly infants and younger children and appears to have a less favorable prognosis [4]. They are characterized histologically by a prominent myxoid matrix and angiocentric arrangement of monomorphous, bipolar tumor cells (Fig. 9.6).

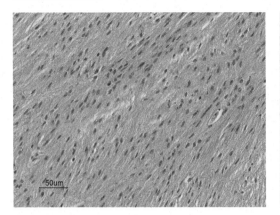

Fig. 9.7 Fibrillary astrocytomas. Courtesy of Cynthia E. Hawkins

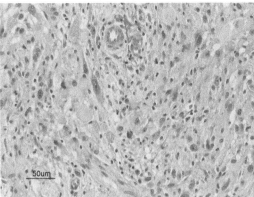

Fig. 9.8 Pleomorphic xanthoastrocytomas. Courtesy of Cynthia E. Hawkins

(c) Diffuse (fibrillary, gemistocytic, protoplasmic) astrocytoma, this subtype is the most common in the adult population. Fibrillary astrocytomas stain positively for glial fibrillary acidic protein (GFAP). Some pediatric series describe fibrillary astrocytoma as the second most common subtype [1] (Fig. 9.7).

(d) Pleomorphic xanthoastrocytomas (PXA) are typically superficial cortical tumors with a large cystic component arising from cortex. They are uncommon, but important to recognize as usually WHO grade II tumors. The neoplasm consists of sheets of large pleomorphic cells with abundant pink cytoplasm and focal perivascular collections of lymphocytes. Cytoplasmic vacuolization due to the presence of lipid accumulation is often present in the bizarre cells, although it is not a prominent feature of this case. Rosenthal fibers and eosinophilic granular bodies are sometimes found. Mitotic activity, microvascular proliferation, and necrosis are usually absent. They can often be cured with a gross total resection alone (Fig. 9.8).

The WHO grading is very important for treatment and prognosis. As WHO grade II tumors tend to have a more aggressive behavior, the role of adjuvant treatment has to be considered carefully as the risk of further progression is higher.

Despite being the most frequent brain tumor in childhood, there are hardly any data on molecular biology available. Currently the main focus is on BRAF gene mutations [5, 6], which were initially described in 2005 and have been described in other malignancies as well like malignant melanoma. BRAF is a proto-oncogene that works as a downstream target for the RAS protein. The RAS (MAPK) signaling pathway plays a significant role in cell growth, differentiation, and apoptosis. So mutations or duplications of the BRAF gene will lead to oncogenic activation (Fig. 9.9).

The majority of LGA (low grade astrocytoma) have the KIAA-1549 fusion gene as demonstrated below (Fig. 9.10).

The clinical relevance of this finding has been studied in a paper by Hawkins et al. [7]. They correlated tumor samples with BRAF alterations with clinical data retrospectively and the fusion of the BRAF-KIAA-1549 has been identified as a positive predictive marker in an incompletely resected LGA independent of their location, pathology, or age. This pathway could serve as a possible drug target for treatment.

Spontaneous growth arrest can be observed in LGA. It has been speculated that the lack of telomere maintenance is responsible for this biological behavior [7]. Telomeres are found at the terminal end of each chromosome. They are protective, but get shortened which each mitotic cycle until a growth arrest state. This study demonstrated that the telomeres of younger astrocytoma patients were significantly longer resulting in a more aggressive behavior and further recurrence. The conclusion was made that telomere maintenance could function as a biological prognostic marker.

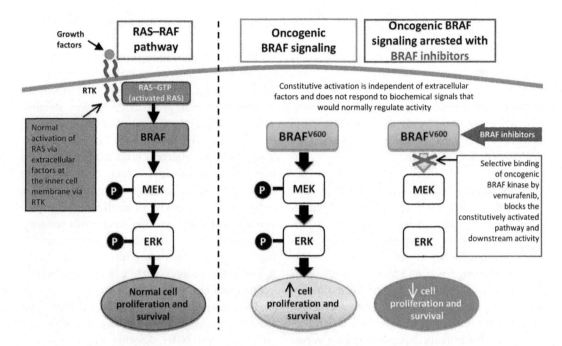

Fig. 9.9 BRAF gene. Reprinted from Ascierto PA, Kirkwood JM, Grob J-J, et al. The role of BRAF V600 mutation in melanoma. Journal of Translational Medicine 2012; 10(1):85. With permission from BioMed Central Ltd.

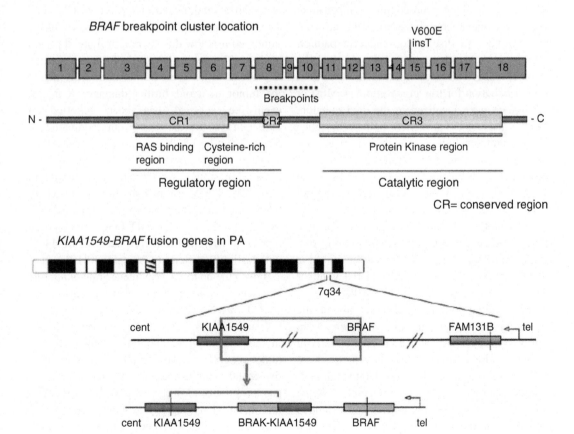

Fig. 9.10 Graphic breakpoint of the BRAF gene. Reprinted from Cin H, Meyer C, Herr R, et al. Oncogenic FAM131B–BRAF fusion resulting from 7q34 deletion comprises an alternative mechanism of MAPK pathway activation in pilocytic astrocytoma. Acta Neuropathol 2011; 121(6): 763-774. With permission from Springer Verlag

Treatment

Surgery is the main treatment modality and curative when complete removal is possible with acceptable functional outcome [8]. This mainly applies to tumors within the cerebellum or hemispheric tumors.

Since surgery for deep-seated tumors is often restricted to debulking procedures or image-guided biopsies, focal radiation therapy was traditionally applied to such tumors. Over the years the lower age limit for radiation as a first-line adjuvant therapy has been changed to older children (over 10 years of age), but between different study groups no consensus has been reached in regard to the optimal age to continue deferral of radiation. This is likely dependent at least in part to the degree of dysfunction from the tumor and the potential radiation volume. Also more knowledge not only about neurocognitive impairment but also vascular complications, e.g., cavernomas, Moyamoya disease, or endocrinopathies, has emerged. Merchant et al. [9] published the largest prospective series on late effects for conformal radiation for low grade gliomas. Most of the tumors were localized in the diencephalon. Most of these patients needed multiple hormone replacements including growth hormone, thyroid, glucocorticoid, and gonadotropin-releasing hormone replacement. IQ decline was more severe with younger age at radiation and did not plateau 5 years post radiation treatment.

Merchant et al. described in a prospective series disease control with a 5-year event-free survival at 87.4±4.4 %, but raised the concerns of higher rates of vasculopathy in the younger age group less than 5 years of age [10].

After initial anecdotal observations in the 1970s, chemotherapy has gained an important role as primary treatment of LGG, particularly in young children. Most of the early series were using a single-agent approach with either alkylating or platinum-based chemotherapies. More recently, combination therapies over extended periods were developed to potentially address the biological pattern of these slow growing tumors.

The initial indication for the use of chemotherapy was a salvage approach in the setting of a progressive tumor following radiation treatment. However, several prospective studies demonstrated safety and efficacy of chemotherapy as the first-line treatment for LGG. The primary goal with this approach is to avoid or at least postpone radiotherapy, which will then be reserved for recurrent/progressive tumors. Since radiation therapy is known to affect neurocognitive and endocrine function and growth and may trigger malignant transformation, there is increasing interest in considering repeated chemotherapy at further progression of LGG, particularly in young children.

The most commonly used combination (North America and Europe) is still carboplatin and vincristine (CV). Another well-established regimen is TPCV (thioguanine, procarbazine, lomustine, and vincristine), which has been tested in a randomized study versus CV [11]. The treatment adapts to the natural growth of the tumor, so it is low dose over a prolonged period of time (52 weeks). The goal of the treatment is to prevent further growth and stabilize the size of the tumor to avoid further damage. A 5-year event-free survival has been reported at 39 % ± 4 % for the CV group compared to 52 ± 5 % for the TPCV group in patients less than 10 years of age ($p = 0.1$). Response rate in both arms were similar with progressive disease in 32 %. The TPCV arm had slightly more toxicity when allergic reactions to carboplatin were excluded. The German HIT-LGG study group reports a 10-year event-free survival of 44 % with a slightly different CV regimen [12].

Given the up to 30 % incidence rate of allergic reaction to carboplatin, the Canadian group started a trial with monotherapy vinblastine as a CV substitute [13]. Nine children were enrolled in the original trial, and none showed further tumor progression. This resulted into a prospective weekly vinblastine phase II trial for relapsed and progressive low grade gliomas [14]. With minimal toxicity the 5-year event-free survival was 42.3 % ± 7.2 %, comparable to so far published up-front chemotherapy regimens.

In the meantime the Canadian Pediatric Brain Tumor Consortium (CPBTC) has completed a weekly vinblastine trial for chemotherapy-naïve children with progressive LGG as the frontline therapy.

The second-line chemotherapy has also been established for salvage therapy following further progression after initial chemo- or radiotherapy [15]. Thirty-eight patients received the second-line chemotherapy often within the same group (vinca-alkaloid) and the 5-year event-free survival was reported as 37.5 ± 8 % with similar toxicity compared to the first line.

With regard to the use of newer chemotherapeutic agents, bevacizumab-based therapy has been investigated in recurrent low grade gliomas [16]. The majority of patients received a combination with irinotecan with acceptable toxicities. Overall objective response was observed in 86 % of the patients with the initial treatment and no patient showed progression on treatment, only after discontinuation, but all were salvageable with bevacizumab again. These results have led to conduct a first-line chemotherapeutic trial with bevacizumab/vinblastine versus vinblastine monotherapy.

Targeted treatment is currently being studied in low grade astrocytomas within the setting of neurofibromatosis type I or tuberous sclerosis. mTor pathway inhibitors are currently being tested in phase I/II trials for the treatment of SEGA [17]. The big advantage of mTor inhibitor like sirolimus or everolimus is the oral delivery. However it has been observed that the SEGAs regrow on stopping the inhibitor, thus committing the child to long-term therapy or alternatively providing an opportunity for an easier surgical resection once the tumor has partially responded to the inhibitor.

Outcome

Over the years quite a few prognostic markers have been established. Gross total resection has been identified as a very strong positive predictive marker with an overall survival of around 100 % [8].

This is also confirmed for the group of primary spinal location with a difference of a 5-year event-free survival of 88 % ± 13 % for GTR compared to 34 % ± 11 % for less than GTR [18].

On the other hand intra- and perioperative death in infants with suprasellar tumor location has been reported most likely related to severe hypothalamic-pituitary dysfunction.

In some series underlying NF 1 has been a positive prognostic factor for treatment response. These results have been controversially discussed as many OPG in this patient population get diagnosed by surveillance MRI for their underlying NF 1 and so potentially the treatment indication could have been different. The German HIT-LGG study group did perform a separate analysis of their NF 1 patient population [19]. One hundred and nine patients were included, 76 % of them with an OPG. Within the chemotherapy group (CV regimen) a 5-year event-free survival of 73 % was reported.

As negative prognostic markers, young age (<1 year), midline location, and histology other than juvenile pilocytic subtype have been identified [12].

There is a huge difference between overall and progression-free survival in this tumor. Whereas overall survival is over 90 % at 5 years, progression-free survival is reported in different studies at around 40–50 % for nonsurgical tumors. Even in the setting of posterior fossa location with subtotal resection, the 5-year event-free survival is only around 63 % [8].

Whereas malignant transformation from low- to high grade astrocytoma is very common in the adult population, it is a rare phenomenon in the pediatric world [20]. The long-term risk is less than 10 % for patients with a WHO grade II tumor. The molecular changes observed in this transformation as similar to adult glioblastoma with TP53 overexpression and abnormalities in the retinoblastoma tumor-suppressor pathway. Radiation therapy as the primary treatment modality could not be identified as a risk factor in this study. However there are occasional case reports of malignant transformation of JPA but only following radiation.

Over the past few years long-term morbidity has become a major focus of research as the overall survival is excellent in this tumor group.

Benesch et al. [21] reviewed a group of 78 long-term survivors of pediatric low grade gliomas over a 20-year time period. Overall survival of this group has been 79 %. Chronic medical problems included neurological sequelae, neuroendocrine issues, visual deficits, hearing impairment, and others. The severity of the long-term side effects was mainly influenced by location (midline) and treatment (radiotherapy).

From a neurodevelopmental point of view this group has been understudied for a long period of time given the overall outcome and the "mild" unimodal treatment. Newer research has identified issues with lower IQ, overall adaptive behavior, internalizing symptoms, and adaptive skills independent of location even in the group of cerebellar location [22]. Hypothalamic involvement, chronic hydrocephalus, and volume of radiation are likely contributory causes.

But how do all of these results influence the quality of life from the perspective of the patient? In a German study 49 survivors of pediatric low grade glioma and their parents were assessed with a quality of life questionnaire tool [23]. The survivors rated their quality of life, physical well-being, and self-esteem higher than their healthy peers, but their parents had a different impression. This demonstrates the coping mechanism of children with a chronic disease.

Future Directions

As low grade gliomas are a very heterogeneous group of tumors, treatment has to be modified for certain risk groups.

For tumors which can be gross or near totally resected and show WHO grade I histology, a watch-and-follow approach seems to be justified.

Patients less than 1 year of age with a suprasellar lesion seem to comprise a high risk population, most likely reflecting the biological behavior of a WHO grade II tumor requiring more intense treatment. Patients with low grade medullary lesions should be considered for adjuvant therapy early following resection, in view of the critical function of this location.

Also patients with WHO grade II histology seem to fit into a higher risk group, where adjuvant treatment is more likely required.

Further targeted treatment especially in the patients with NF 1 with better understanding of the affected pathway should be implemented in pilot treatment protocols.

The role of radiotherapy in these tumors given the increasing number of long-term sequelae and no superior role in tumor growth control needs to be rediscussed and defined.

A further discussion is warranted regarding the primary endpoint of treatment: radiological response versus symptoms response as sometimes findings on MRI can be very subtle and volume calculation changes very difficult.

An interdisciplinary team approach (e.g., ophthalmology, endocrinology, and neuropsychology) as practiced at many centers should be considered the standard of care.

A further point of discussion is follow-up care in this patient population given that many of them have residual tumors. Surveillance MRI frequency has not been established yet, as the question remains as to whether these tumors will undergo malignant transformation during adulthood.

As overall pediatric low grade glioma can be considered a chronic disease, interventions and follow-ups have to be balanced with long-term morbidity.

References

1. Sievert AJ, Fisher MJ. Pediatric low-grade gliomas. J Child Neurol. 2009;24(11):1397–408.
2. Panigrahy A, Blüml S. Neuroimaging of pediatric brain tumors: from basic to advanced magnetic resonance imaging (MRI). J Child Neurol. 2009;24(11):1343–65.
3. Louis DN, Ohgaki H, Wiestler OD, Cavenee WK, Burger PC, Jouvet A, Scheithauer BW, Kleihues P. The 2007 WHO classification of tumours of the central nervous system. Acta Neuropathol. 2007;114: 97–109.
4. Tihan T, Fisher PG, Kepner JL, Godfraind C, McComb RD, Goldthwaite PT, Burger PC. Pediatric

astrocytomas with monomorphous pilomyxoid features and a less favourable outcome. J Neuropathol Exp Neurol. 1999;58:1061–8.

5. Pfister S, Janzarik WG, Remke M, Ernst A, Werft W, Becker N, Toedt G, Wittmann A, Kratz C, Olbrich H, Ahmadi R, Thieme B, Joos S, Radlwimmer B, Kulozik A, Pietsch T, Herold-Mende C, Gnekow A, Reifenberger G, Korshunov A, Scheurlen W, Omran H, Lichter P. BRAF gene duplication constitutes a mechanism of MAPK pathway activation in low-grade astrocytomas. J Clin Invest. 2008;118(5):1739–49.

6. Hawkins C, Walker E, Mohamed N, Zhang C, Jacob K, Shirinian M, Alon N, Kahn D, Fried I, Scheinemann K, Tsangaris E, Dirks P, Tressler R, Bouffet E, Jabado N, Tabori U. BRAF-KIAA1549 fusion predicts better clinical outcome in pediatric low-grade astrocytoma. Clin Cancer Res. 2011;17(14):4790–8.

7. Tabori U, Vukovic B, Zielenska M, Hawkins C, Braude I, Rutka J, Bouffet E, Shire J, Malkin D. The role of telomere maintenance in the spontaneous growth arrest of pediatric low-grade gliomas. Neoplasia. 2006;8(2):136–42.

8. Wisoff JH, Sanford RA, Heier LA, Sposto R, Burger PC, Yates AJ, Homes EJ, Kun LE. Primary neurosurgery for Pediatric low-grade gliomas: a prospective multi-institutional study from the Children's Oncology Group. Neurosurgery. 2011;68(6):1548–54.

9. Merchant TE, Conklin HM, Wu S, Lustig RH, Xiong X. Late effects of conformal radiation therapy for pediatric patients with low-grade glioma: prospective evaluation of cognitive, endocrine and hearing deficits. J Clin Oncol. 2009;27(22):3691–7.

10. Merchant TE, Kun LE, Wu S, Xiong X, Sanford RA, Boop FA. Phase II trial of conformal radiation therapy for pediatric low-grade glioma. J Clin Oncol. 2009;27(22):3598–604.

11. Ater JL, Zhou T, Holmes E, Mazewski CM, Booth TN, Freyer DR, Lazarus KH, Packer RJ, Prados M, Sposto R, Vezina G, Wisoff JH, Pollack IF. Randomized study of two chemotherapy regimens for treatment of low-grade glioma in young children: a report from the Children's Oncology Group. J Clin Oncol. 2012;30(21):2641–7.

12. Gnekow AK, Falkenstein F, von Hornstein S, Zwiener I, Berkefeld S, Bison S, Warmuth-Metz M, Hernaiz Driver P, Soerensen N, Kortmann RD, Pietsch T, Faldum A. Long-term follow up of the multicenter, multidisciplinary treatment Study HIT-LGG-1996 for low-grade glioma in children and adolescents of the German Speaking Society of Pediatric Oncology and Hematology. Neuro Oncol. 2012;14(10):1265–84.

13. Lafay-Cousin L, Holm S, Qaddoumi I, Nicolin G, Bartels U, Tabori U, Huang A, Bouffet E. Weekly vinblastine in pediatric low-grade glioma patients with carboplatin allergic reaction. Cancer. 2005;103(12):2636–42.

14. Bouffet E, Jakacki R, Goldman S, Hargrave D, Hawkins C, Shroff M, Hukin J, Bartels U, Foreman N, Kellie S, Hilden J, Etzel M, Wilson B, Stephens D, Tabori U, Baruchel S. Phase II study of weekly vinblastine in recurrent or refractory pediatric low-grade glioma. J Clin Oncol. 2012;30(12):1358–63.

15. Scheinemann K, Bartels U, Tsangaris E, Hawkins C, Huang A, Dirks P, Fried I, Bouffet E, Tabori U. Feasibility and efficacy of repeated chemotherapy for progressive pediatric low-grade gliomas. Pediatr Blood Cancer. 2011;57(1):84–8.

16. Hwang EI, Jakacki RI, Fisher MJ, Kilburn LB, Horn M, Vezina G, Rood BR, Packer RJ. Long-term efficacy and toxicity of bevacizumab-based therapy in children with recurrent low-grade gliomas. Pediatr Blood Cancer. 2013;60:776–82.

17. Lam C, Bouffet E, Tabori U, Mabbott D, Taylor M, Bartels U. Rapamycin (sirolimus) in tuberous sclerosis associated pediatric central nervous system tumors. Pediatr Blood Cancer. 2010;54(3):476–9.

18. Scheinemann K, Bartels U, Huang A, Hawkins C, Kulkarni AV, Bouffet E, Tabori U. Survival and functional outcome of childhood spinal cord low-grade gliomas. J Neurosurg Pediatr. 2009;4(3):254–61.

19. Hernaiz Driever P, von Hornstein S, Pietsch T, Kortmann R, Warmuth-Metz M, Emser A, Gnekow AK. Natural history and management of low-grade glioma in NF-1 children. J Neurooncol. 2010;100:199–207.

20. Broniscer A, Baker SJ, West AN, Fraser MM, Proko E, Kocak M, Dalton J, Zambetti GP, Ellison DW, Kun LE, Gajjar A, Gilbertson RJ, Fuller CE. Clinical and molecular characteristics of malignant transformation of low-grade glioma in children. J Clin Oncol. 2007;28(6):682–9.

21. Benesch M, Lackner H, Sovinz P, Suppan E, Schwinger W, Eder HG, Dombusch HJ, Moser A, Triebl-Roth K, Urban C. Late sequelae after treatment of childhood low-grade gliomas: a retrospective analysis of 69 long-term survivors treated between 1983 and 2003. J Neurooncol. 2006;78:199–205.

22. Ris MD, Beebe DW. Neurodevelopmental outcomes of children with low-grade gliomas. Dev Disabil Res Rev. 2008;14:196–202.

23. Musial-Bright L, Panteli L, Driver Hernaiz P. Pediatric low-grade glioma survivors experience high quality of life. Childs Nerv Syst. 2011;27:1895–902.

High-Grade Glioma

Magimairajan Issai Vanan, Vivek Mehta, and David D. Eisenstat

Introduction

Gliomas are primary brain tumors derived from the glial cell (astrocytic and/or oligodendroglial) lineage. These tumours are historically separated into low- or high-grade categories according to the World Health Organization (WHO) classification system. Low-grade astrocytomas (WHO grades I and II) constitute approximately 50 % of primary supratentorial tumors of childhood and are more common than high-grade astrocytomas (WHO grades III and IV) [1, 2]. High-grade gliomas (HGGs) are less common in the pediatric age group when compared to adults [1] constituting 3–7 % of all childhood brain tumors [2, 3], are a histologically heterogeneous group of tumors, and are classified, according to the putative cell of origin, as: astrocytic tumors (anaplastic astrocy-

toma (AA), glioblastoma (GBM), giant cell GBM, and gliosarcoma), oligodendroglial tumors (anaplastic oligodendroglioma), or oligoastrocytic (mixed) tumors (anaplastic oligoastrocytoma). Other rare HGG varieties include anaplastic ganglioglioma, which appears to have a more favorable prognosis than other HGGs and anaplastic pleiomorphic xanthoastrocytoma [1]. Special categories of HGG include diffuse intrinsic pontine gliomas [DIPG, WHO grade IV; discussed in a separate chapter] and gliomatosis cerebri (grade III). All of these HGG tumors are characterized by their highly invasive nature leading to difficulty in treatment and they are poorly responsive to even the most aggressive therapies. Surgery and Radiation therapy (RT) are the usual modes of therapy, especially for AAs and GBM and prognosis is better in children than adults [2]. The optimal use and selection of chemotherapy, given concurrently with RT and/or in the adjuvant setting, remain to be determined.

M.I. Vanan, M.D., M.P.H., F.A.A.P.
Departments of Pediatrics and Child Health, Oncology and Cell Biology, Cancer Care Manitoba, Manitoba Institute of Cell Biology, University of Manitoba, Winnipeg, MB, Canada

V. Mehta, M.D., M.Sc.
Division of Neurosurgery, Department of Surgery, Stollery Children's Hospital/University of Alberta, Edmonton, AB, Canada

D.D. Eisenstat, M.D., M.A., F.R.C.P.C. (✉)
Departments of Pediatrics, Medical Genetics and Oncology, Stollery Children's Hospital, University of Alberta, Edmonton Clinic Health Academy, Edmonton, AB, Canada
e-mail: eisensta@ualberta.ca

Epidemiology

Gliomas are the most common childhood tumors of the central nervous system (CNS), accounting for 53 % of tumors in children ages 0–14 years and 37 % in adolescents aged 15–19 years [2]. HGGs comprise ~17 % of childhood and ~8 % of adolescent brain tumors when including DIPG [2]. HGGs are at least 20 times more common in adults than in children, particularly GBM, which is the most common primary malignant brain tumor in adults. GBM comprises approximately 3 % of all brain and CNS tumors reported among 0–19 year olds [2]. In the pediatric population HGGs seem to affect boys and girls equally [2].

Etiology and Associations

The causes of gliomas remain largely unknown, although certain familial cancer predisposition syndromes are associated with an increased risk of HGG. Li–Fraumeni syndrome (LFS), a dominantly inherited syndrome involving the p53 tumor suppressor gene, is characterized by one or more cancer occurrences in children including HGGs. *p53* mutations are rare in sporadic pediatric CNS tumors lacking a typical family history. In addition to LFS, neurofibromatosis type I (NF-I, with mutations in the neurofibromin gene, which is also a tumor suppressor gene) and familial cancer syndromes involving the DNA mismatch repair (MMR) genes can predispose to HGG [4]. These disorders include: (i) Turcot syndrome, type I (HNPCC, hereditary non-polyposis colorectal cancer) with MSH6 gene mutations; (ii) Turcot syndrome, type II with APC gene mutations; and (iii) BRCA syndrome with BRCA1 or BRCA2 gene mutations. As well, patients with multiple enchondromatosis are at increased risk of HGG. However, to date, the most robust association linked to the development of malignant gliomas is prior exposure to therapeutic ionizing radiation.

Clinical Features

The presentation of HGG varies and depends largely on the age of the patient, the anatomic location of the tumor, and the associated effects on the structures surrounding the tumor. Compared with low-grade gliomas (LGG), HGGs tend to have a shorter interval of symptoms. The signs and symptoms can be broadly divided into three categories:

(a) *General and Non-localizing Features:* Constitutional symptoms such as developmental delay, failure to thrive, behavioral or mood changes, declining school performance, changes in handwriting, and loss or regression of previously attained milestones.

(b) *Increased Intracranial Pressure* (ICP): Children with HGG frequently present with symptoms related to raised ICP, including headache, nausea, and vomiting, which are all classically worse in the morning attributed to increased cerebrovenous pooling during sleep. Clinical signs include papilledema, Parinaud's syndrome ("setting sun" sign), anisocoria (pupillary size inequality), ataxia, and head tilt. In the infantile period when the sutures are still open, the signs may include delayed closure of the fontanelles, or a bulging anterior fontanelle with separation of sutures and increased head circumference usually due to concurrent hydrocephalus.

(c) *Localizing Signs*: Localizing neurological deficits depend on the site of the tumor. HGGs that originate supratentorially often present with hemiparesis or progressively worsening seizures, although seizures are a less common presenting sign in HGG than in LGG. Cortical gliomas can present with dysphasia, hemisensory loss, early handedness, or change in handedness apart from the nonspecific signs described above. Midline gliomas can present with cranial neuropathies (visual loss, diplopia, facial palsy, etc.). Dissemination of malignant gliomas into the cerebrospinal fluid is less common than for medulloblastoma and other neural tumors but is being recognized more frequently, particularly as patients survive longer. In a large German series approximately 3 % of patients with HGGs had metastatic disease at presentation [5]. Though a delay in diagnosis is a frequent occurrence, the impact on overall survival may not be significant although the quality of survival may be affected by inordinate delays [6].

Diagnostic Evaluation

Imaging Studies

Neuroimaging examinations in HGG are used to determine the size and site of origin of the lesion, establishing a primary diagnosis (DIPG), and planning treatment. Various neuroimaging modalities are being used for selecting a site for stereotactic biopsy, guiding resection, radiation therapy planning, application of experimental therapeutics (such as convection-enhanced delivery or CED), and delineation of tumor from functionally important brain parenchyma.

CT Scans

Computed tomographic (CT) scans are usually the first imaging procedure done in patients with raised ICP or seizures in the emergency room. HGG can be identified on computed tomographic (CT) scans as irregular isodense or hypodense white matter lesions. There is overlap in anatomical localization of pediatric supratentorial HGG and LGG (grade II). Both grade II and grade III lesions tend to be ill-defined, being hypodense masses on CT studies. Calcification or cystic changes may be seen. Anaplastic astrocytoma often shows enhancement, at least focally. GBM characteristically presents as a ring-enhancing lesion in post-contrast-enhanced CT images. CT scans are used rarely for routine surveillance and follow-up of pediatric patients due to poor anatomic delineation of tumor to adjacent brain and to potential radiation exposure and long-term cancer risk. However, CT scan is very helpful for rapid assessment of ventricular status and to determine whether intracranial or intra-tumoral bleeding has occurred in the inpatient or emergency room setting.

MRI

Magnetic resonance imaging (MRI) is currently the modality of choice for localization and assessment of HGG. MRI provides valuable information about secondary phenomena such as mass effect, edema (pseudoresponse vs. progression during therapy), hemorrhage, necrosis (radiologic), and signs of increased ICP. In addition, MRI provides excellent tissue contrast and high spatial resolution. Standard (conventional) MRI sequences obtained during routine imaging include T1-weighted (pre- and post-contrast images, usually with gadolinium), T2-weighted, and

fluid-attenuated inversion recovery (FLAIR) images. Examples of two patients with HGG are shown (Fig. 10.1).

Conventional MRI features of HGG are varied and can resemble LGG. These tumors are usually solitary or rarely can be multifocal. Cortical tumors usually have an irregularly enhancing rim surrounding a necrotic core or can be poorly margined with diffuse infiltration into white matter tracts such as the corpus callosum and anterior and posterior commissures. On pre-contrast T1-weighted sequences, these tumors are iso- or hypointense. Post-contrast T1-weighted sequences typically show an irregular enhancing rim surrounding a non-enhancing area of central necrosis. Intratumoral hemorrhage may be present in grade IV tumors. The enhancing rim typically represents highly proliferative, invasive, and radio-resistant tumor cells. T2-weighted and FLAIR sequences usually show a heterogeneous mass with variable signal intensity surrounded by bright areas representing a zone of vasogenic edema. It is important to note that infiltrating malignant tumor cells extend far beyond the area of enhancement. Giant cell glioblastoma and gliosarcoma tend to be more demarcated than other glioblastomas. In gliomatosis cerebri at least three cerebral lobes are typically involved, and these tumors are usually bilateral and extend into deep gray matter structures. Gliomatosis may extend to involve the posterior fossa or even the spinal cord. Lesions are characteristically hyperintense on T2 and FLAIR MR imaging. Imaging of the neuraxis is indicated when there is concern for disseminated disease throughout the brain and spinal cord.

Functional Neuroimaging

Conventional MRI which gives information based largely on tumor structure and anatomic location is increasingly being supplemented by methods commonly referred to by the collective term "functional imaging" [7]. A range of functional imaging techniques for brain tumors that provide information on cellularity, tissue ultrastructure, metabolism, and vascularity are available and best acquired as part of a multimodal protocol. There has been an increased interest in using functional

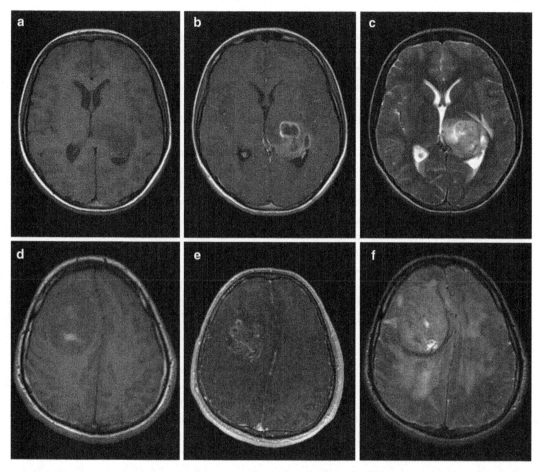

Fig. 10.1 (**a–c**) A 12-year-old female with GBM. (**a**) Axial T1, (**b**) axial T1 with gadolinium, (**c**) axial T2. (**d–f**) A 15-year-old male with malignant glioma. (**d**) Axial T1, (**e**) axial T1 with gadolinium, and (**f**) axial T2. Both tumors demonstrate minimal contrast enhancement

imaging to assist in the diagnosis, management, and determination of treatment response of HGG. Some of the commonly used functional imaging techniques and their clinical uses are:

(a) *Diffusion MRI* with two different techniques: diffusion-weighted imaging (DWI) and diffusion tensor imaging (DTI). DWI uses apparent diffusion coefficient (ADC) histograms and has been valuable in the grading of gliomas (especially LGG). Low ADC values correlate with high cellularity and proliferation, most often seen in aggressive tumors. DTI has been shown to be useful in discriminating LGG from HGG and also in presurgical evaluation and radiosurgical planning of white matter tracts surrounding the tumor

(DT tractography). Fractional anisotropy (FA) using DTI may prove helpful for the assessment of treatment-induced white matter changes in children during follow-up.

(b) *Perfusion MRI* (pMRI) provides a surrogate for neo-angiogenesis, which is a key feature of many malignant gliomas. An indirect measurement of pMRI, the relative cerebral blood volume (rCBV), has been shown to correlate with tumor vascularity and HGGs tend to have higher rCBV values than low-grade tumors.

(c) *Functional MRI* (fMRI) is a commonly used technique for identifying the eloquent gray matter in cortical HGGs prior to surgery. This approach may be limited to older children and adolescents.

(d) *Magnetic resonance spectroscopy* (MRS) measures the chemical composition of tissue and provides semiquantitative information about major cellular metabolites. A common pattern in brain tumors is a decrease in *N*-acetylaspartate (NAA), a neuron-specific marker, a decrease in creatine (Cr), and an increase in choline (Cho), lactate (Lac), and lipids (L). The concentration of Cho is a reflection of the turnover of cell membranes (due to accelerated synthesis and destruction) and is more elevated in regions with a high neoplastic activity. Lactate is the end product of nonoxidative glycolysis and a marker of hypoxia and possibly necrosis in tumor tissue. Tumor hypoxia is now recognized as a major promoter of tumor angiogenesis and invasion. MRS may be used in distinguishing tumor from non-tumor masses (abscess, infections, and metabolic disorders) or from radiation necrosis and in characterizing tumor grade (high grade vs. low grade). Multivoxel MRS imaging (MRSI) has the advantage of improved characterization of heterogeneous tumors but is technically more demanding, may be less reproducible, and is not widely available except in tertiary or quaternary treatment centers.

(e) *Positron emission tomography* using fluoro-deoxyglucose or F^{18} (FDG-PET) is another noninvasive molecular imaging modality that aids in the diagnosis of malignant tumors and may distinguish active tumor from radionecrosis. Besides F^{18}, other radioisotopes, such as C^{11}, are under the increasing use in adults and children.

Functional imaging techniques are becoming more widely available in clinical practice and have an important role in aiding the clinical management of children with HGG. They are increasingly used preoperatively to differentiate between tumor and non-tumor pathology (MRS, pMRI), high- and low-grade tumors (MRS, DWI), and primary HGG and metastatic lesions to the brain (MRS). These adjunct studies may also improve diagnostic accuracy of a biopsy by determining the most abnormal region of the tumor (MRS, DWI) and to define tumor margins for both surgi-cal resection and radiation fields (fMRI, DTI). In the intraoperative and postoperative periods, functional imaging is most commonly used to identify eloquent areas of the brain especially in cortical tumors (fMRI, DTI) and for treatment planning for surgery, stereotactic radiosurgery, and radiation therapy (DT tractography). Monitoring for therapy-induced white matter changes and related toxicities (DTI), radiation necrosis versus residual/recurrent tumor, (MRS, DWI), and especially treatment response monitoring, including pseudoresponse (PsR) and pseudoprogression (PsP), is enhanced by these MRI- or PET-related imaging modalities [7]. The Response Assessment in Neuro-Oncology (RANO) criteria uses conventional MRI to assess treatment response of patients with gliomas (Table 10.1) [8]. Pediatric RANO (RAPNO) criteria are under development [9].

Pathology

Pediatric HGGs are less common than many other brain tumors occurring in infancy, childhood, and adolescence. Based upon the CCG-945 study and others, central neuropathology review can often result in a reclassification of HGG to an LGG or other histopathological entity [10–12].

Morphology

Macroscopically HGGs, particularly GBM, tend to have a heterogeneous appearance, forming obvious masses, often containing areas of hemorrhage and/or necrosis. They typically have a mottled tan, red, and brown coloration with alternating firm and softened zones. Gliosarcomas may be quite firm in consistency, due to the presence of sarcomatous components.

Histology

Microscopically, HGGs are distinguished from LGG by the presence of four important histologic criteria: nuclear atypia, mitotic activity (WHO

Table 10.1 Response Assessment in Neuro-Oncology (RANO)

First progression	Definition
Progressive disease <12 weeks after completion of chemoRT	• Progression can only be defined using diagnostic imaging if there is new enhancement outside of the radiation field (beyond the high-dose region or 80 % isodose line) or if there is unequivocal evidence of viable tumor on histopathologic sampling (e.g., solid tumor areas [i.e., > 70 % tumor cell nuclei in areas], high or progressive increase in MIB-1 proliferation index compared with prior biopsy, or evidence for histologic progression or increased anaplasia in tumor)
	• Given the difficulty of differentiating true progression from pseudoprogression, clinical decline alone, in the absence of radiographic or histologic confirmation of progression, will not be sufficient for definition of progressive disease in the first 12 weeks after completion of concurrent chemoRT
Progressive disease >or equal to 12 weeks after completion of chemoRT	• New contrast-enhancing lesion outside of radiation field on decreasing, stable, or increasing doses of corticosteroids
	• Increase by >or equal to 25 % in the sum of the products of perpendicular diameters between the first post-radiotherapy scan, or a subsequent scan with smaller tumor size, and the scan at 12 weeks or later on stable or increasing doses of corticosteroids
	• Clinical deterioration not attributable to concurrent medication or comorbid conditions is sufficient to declare progression on current treatment but not for entry onto a clinical trial for recurrence
	• For patients receiving antiangiogenic therapy, a significant increase in T2/FLAIR non-enhancing lesion may also be considered progressive disease. The increased T2/FLAIR must have occurred with the patient on stable or increasing doses of corticosteroids compared with baseline scan or best response after initiation of therapy and not been a result of comorbid events (e.g., effects of radiation therapy, demyelination, ischemic injury, infection, seizures, postoperative changes, or other treatment effects)

Based on data from Ref. [8]

grades III and IV), necrosis (grade IV), and/or microvascular proliferation (grade IV). Tumor grade is established based on the area of the greatest anaplasia. AAs (grade III) are hypercellular astrocytomas that in addition to nuclear atypia have increased mitotic activity. Vascular proliferation and necrosis are absent. Cells with large pleiomorphic or multiple nuclei may be present. GBM (grade IV), in addition to findings listed for AA, display necrosis (typically pseudopalisading necrosis) or microvascular proliferation. Atypical mitotic figures may be present. Gliosarcoma (grade IV) is a biphasic high-grade glioma with both malignant astrocytic (GBM) and sarcomatous components. The sarcomatous portion is frequently fibrosarcoma, though it may include malignant fibrous histiocytoma, chondrosarcoma, osteosarcoma, leiomyosarcoma, rhabdomyosarcoma, or even liposarcoma. Trichrome and reticulin stains are frequently helpful. Gliomatosis cerebri (GC, grade III) is most frequently astrocytic tumors, though infrequently may contain oligodendroglial elements. Nuclei

tend to be elongated and hyperchromatic, and pleiomorphic forms are not uncommon. Secondary structures are frequently present. Mitotic activity is variable. Areas resembling GBM may be present in some cases.

Immunohistochemistry

Expression of the intermediate filament *glial fibrillary acidic protein* (GFAP) reflects the glial origin of these tumors and sometimes the extent of cytoplasmic development and is present in the intervening fibrillary matrix of these lesions. *S100* often shows diffuse nuclear and cytoplasmic positivity, and another intermediate filament *vimentin* is similarly positive. The proliferation marker *Ki-67* (or *MIB-1*) is variably positive, reflecting the low (grade II) to brisk (grades III and IV) proliferative activity of these lesions, respectively. *Neurofilament* staining of intratumoral neuritic processes provides evidence of the infiltrative pattern of these neoplasms.

Pancytokeratin is often positive at least focally in higher grade lesions, showing cross-reactivity with glial intermediate filaments. More specific cytokeratin antibodies are usually negative. Sarcomatous portions of gliosarcoma, though not positive for GFAP, are consistently vimentin positive and tend to take on the staining properties of the particular sarcoma element present (muscle, fat, cartilage, etc.). Gliomatosis is variably positive for GFAP and S100 expression [1]. It may sometimes be a challenge for the neuropathologist to distinguish pediatric HGG from supratentorial primitive neuroectodermal tumors (sPNET), mandating central review for patients entered on a clinical trial.

Molecular Biology

In adults, GBM is typically classified as either primary or secondary based on clinical and biological features. The vast majority of GBM (approximately 90 %) develop rapidly de novo in middle-aged or elderly patients, without clinical or histological evidence of a less malignant precursor lesion (primary glioblastomas). Secondary GBM progress stepwise from low-grade diffuse astrocytoma (grade II) or anaplastic astrocytoma (grade III). Histologically, primary and secondary glioblastomas may be indistinguishable, but they differ in their genetic and epigenetic profiles. Isocitrate dehydrogenase IDH1 mutations are classically seen only in secondary glioblastoma [13] and associated with a hypermethylation phenotype [14].

Based on the histological similarity and recurrent genomic aberrations, pediatric GBM (pGBM) were historically thought to more closely resemble the secondary adult GBM (aGBM). PDGFRA mutations and focal amplifications are often present. Paugh et al. discovered somatic activating mutations in 14.3 % of pediatric non-brainstem HGG [15]. In another study using FISH, PDGFRA amplification was noted in 29.3 % pediatric and 20.9 % adult HGG, but amplification was not prognostic in children [16]. EGFR amplification and EGFRvIII and PTEN mutations are less common in pGBM than aGBM

[17, 18]. MGMT methylation as assessed by MGMT overexpression [19, 20] or methylation-specific PCR assays [21] has been correlated with improved EFS but has not yet been validated as either an independent predictive or prognostic marker for pediatric HGG when compared to adult GBM [22].

Rapid advances in the field of genomics (exome and whole genome sequencing studies) and international collaborative efforts (providing access to a large number of pediatric tumors) have led to greater understanding of HGG in children and adults. It is now clear that in the majority of cases described to date, pGBM is biologically distinct from aGBM [23, 24]. The majority of pediatric GBM arise de novo and have characteristic clinical, genetic, and epigenetic features. Recurrent somatic driver mutations in the H3F3A gene, which encodes the replication-independent histone 3 variant (H3.3), lead to amino acid substitutions at key residues, namely lysine (K) 27 (K27M) and glycine 34 (G34R/V), identify distinct subgroups of pediatric GBM, and are seen in 30–45 % of cases [23–25]. H3.3 K27M mutations are more frequent in subcortical regions such as the thalamus and brainstem, whereas the H3.3 G34R/V lesions tend to be in hemispheric locations [26]. IDH1/2 mutations are very rare in childhood GBM (<10 %) [27]. Moreover mutations in H3F3A and IDH1 are mutually exclusive anatomically and across specific age groups: in children (K27M mutations), adolescents (G34R/V mutations), and young adult patients (IDH1 mutations) locations [26].

Whole exome sequencing studies of pediatric GBM identified mutations in α-thalassemia/mental retardation syndrome X-linked (ATRX) and death domain-associated protein (DAXX) genes in 45 % of cases [6]. These genes encode two subunits of a chromatin-remodeling complex required for H3.3 incorporation in pericentric heterochromatin and telomeres. ATRX and/or DAXX mutations have a strong association with TP53 mutations and alternative lengthening of telomeres (ALT) [23, 24]. IDH1/2 mutations lead to overproduction of 2-hydroxyglutarate (2-HG) which inhibits demethylases required for modification of histones and DNA and may thereby block differentiation and tumorigenesis. The H3F3A mutations (K27M leading to transcriptional derepression and G34R leading to altered gene expression, such as of MYCN; [28] are hypothesized to induce epigenetic reprogramming leading to tumorigenesis [29], although the exact mechanisms remain to be fully elucidated. Very recently, mutations were identified in SETD2, a H3K36 trimethyltransferase, in pediatric HGGs localized to the cerebral hemispheres. SETD2 mutations are specific to HGG in children (15 %) and adults (8 %). In HGG these mutations are mutually exclusive with H3F3A mutations but sometimes overlap with IDH1 mutations [30].

Of interest, activating BRAF mutations such as BRAF V600E are also present in 15–20 % of pediatric HGG (reviewed in [31]). The genetic differences of HGGs across the age spectrum are summarized in Table 10.2 [32].

Therapy

Treatment of HGGs requires a multidisciplinary approach and involves surgery, radiation therapy (RT), and chemotherapy.

Surgery

Patients presenting with signs of increased ICP may require emergent neurosurgical intervention to relieve obstructive hydrocephalus with several alternatives in addition to tumor debulking: placement of external ventricular drain (EVD) or a ventriculoperitoneal shunt (VP shunt) or by means of a third ventriculostomy, and the latter via the use of a neurosurgical endoscope. The use of preoperative corticosteroids, usually dexamethasone, can significantly decrease peritumoral edema, thus decreasing focal symptoms and often eliminating the need for emergency surgery. Tumor resection is safer when performed 1–2 days following reduction in edema and ICP by these means. Seizures are treated with anticonvulsants. Prophylactic anticonvulsants in patients who do not present with seizures are not recommended, and antiseizure medications are usually tapered and discontinued in the postoperative period.

The main goals of tumor surgery include obtaining tissue for histopathologic diagnosis and whenever possible, to achieve a gross total resection (GTR). The *extent of resection* (EOR) in HGGs has two important limitations. First, these highly infiltrative tumors invade the surrounding brain tissue, beyond the margins of the visible tumor in neuroimaging. Hence, even in the case of a GTR of all visible tumors, microscopic disease is present beyond the surgical margins, and surgery alone is not considered curative. The second limitation derives from the growth pattern and the anatomic location of the tumor. Multifocal or diffusely infiltrative tumors, deep-seated tumors, and tumors adjacent to or within eloquent areas of the brain may limit the possible extent of resection or even preclude any attempt of surgery beyond a biopsy. Preoperative functional imaging techniques (fMRI, DTI) and intraoperative MRI scans help in achieving the maximum resection possible with minimal impact on postoperative neurologic ability. The diagnostic yield of stereotactic biopsy in deep-seated lesions is greatly improved by functional imaging (MRS, DWI) to localize the tumor tissue.

The extent of resection (EOR) along with age at diagnosis and the grade of the tumor are considered to be the most important prognostic factors in pediatric HGG. If a GTR cannot be achieved, surgical debulking to achieve a maximum possible resection with preservation of neurologic function should be attempted. Aggressive cytoreduction will not only relieve the signs and symptoms due to mass effect but will also reduce the residual tumor volume to be treated by adjuvant therapies (RT, chemotherapy) and may also improve tolerance to RT. In the CCG945 study overall, children with HGGs who underwent GTRs (defined as >90 % resection) had a 5-year progression-free survival (PFS) of 35 % in comparison with 17 % in the group that underwent subtotal resection (STR) (p=0.006). Patients with GBM (grade IV) who underwent GTR had a 5-year PFS of 26 % in comparison

Table 10.2 Integrated genomic classification of GBM

Subgroup	K27	G34	RTKI	IDH	Mesenchymal	RTKII (classic)
Clinical features						
Age distribution in years (median, range)	10.5 (5–23) child/adolescent	18 (9–42) adolescent/young adult	36 (8–74) adolescent/young adult, with another peak in adult/elderly	40 (13–71) young adult/adult	47 (2–85) adult, with a smaller peak in childhood	58 (36–81) adult/elderly
Tumor location	Midline/deep - ST 70–80 % (thalamus, basal ganglia) - IT 60 % (brainstem, spinal cord)	Cortical T>P>O	Cortical F>P>T	Cortical F>>>T>P	Cortical F=P>T	Cortical F=T>P
Gender ratio (M/F)	~ 1:1	~ 1:1	~ 1:1	1:1.7	~ 1:1	1.46:1
Histology	GBM	GBM	GBM	GBM	GBM	GBM
Survival	Very poor	Poor	Poor/fair	<10 % long-term survivors	<10 % long-term survivors	<10 % long-term survivors
Genomic features						
Mutations/cytogenetics	H3F3A (K27M)	H3F3A (G34R/V)	PDGFRA (ampl/mut) CDKN2A/B (del)	IDH1(R132H)	— Copy number variations (low)	EGFR(ampl) Chr 7 (gain) Chr 10q (loss) CDKN2A(del)
TP53	+++	+++	–	+++	+	++
ATRX	++	+++	–	++	–	–
DAXX	+	+++	–	–	–	–
ALT	NR	+++	NR	NR	NR	NR
SETD2	–	–	+	+		
Gene expression signature	Proneural	Mixed	Proneural	Proneural	Mesenchymal	Classical
Immunohistochemistry (FOXG1/OLIG2)	FOXG1/OLIG2+	FOXG1+/OLIG2-	FOXG1+/OLIG2+	FOXG1+/OLIG2+	FOXG1+/OLIG2+	FOXG1+/OLIG2+
Epigenetic features						
DNA methylation	CHOP+	CHOP+		G-CIMP+		

ALT alternative lengthening of telomeres, CHOP CpG island *hypomethylator* phenotype, F frontal lobe, G-CIMP GBM CpG island methylator phenotype, IT infratentorial, O occipital lobe, P parietal lobe, ST supratentorial, T temporal lobe
Adapted from Refs. [24, 32, 57]

with 4 % in those who underwent subtotal resections (STRs) ($p=0.046$). In the same study, patients with AA (grade III) who underwent GTRs had a 5-year PFS of 44 % in comparison with 22 % in those who underwent STRs ($p=0.055$) [33].

Radiation Therapy

Most patients (especially children >3 years old) with HGG require external radiotherapy to achieve local control of microscopic or macroscopic residual disease. Adjuvant RT has been shown to be a very effective treatment modality with rapid symptomatic improvement and increased EFS and overall survival (OS) when offered at doses greater than or equal to 5,400 cGy as delivered in ~30 fractions over 6 weeks. Three-dimensional conformal treatment planning techniques including intensity-modulated radiation therapy (IMRT) are well tolerated and may have decreased side effects by decreasing the exposure of adjacent brain. Adaptation of these techniques has resulted in reduction of the margins used by radiation oncologists, including the gross target volume (GTV), the clinical target volume (CTV) to treat microscopic disease extending beyond the GTV, and the planning target volume (PTV). The CTV is anatomically confined and is usually limited to 2 cm. The PTV compensates for movement and uncertainties regarding daily positioning of the patient and setup of equipment and software; usually the PTV ranges from 0.3 to 0.5 cm. The use of palliative re-irradiation in relapsed cases can help by improving symptom control, but its impact regarding extending survival has yet to be established. Concern regarding long-term toxicities of radiation to the developing CNS (cognition, growth, endocrinopathies, and second malignancies) has led to the implementation of chemotherapeutic strategies to delay or obviate the need for RT and radiosensitization to decrease the dose of RT. *Proton beam* RT (protons) may be less effective than conventional RT (photons) due to the highly invasive nature of HGG and proton RT is currently not recommended for the adjuvant treatment of pedi-

atric HGG. Brachytherapy, stereotactic radiosurgery, and fractionated stereotactic radiosurgery as alternatives to conventional RT are presently under study and may prove useful in selected relapsed patients.

Chemotherapy

In children, multi-agent adjuvant chemotherapy added to postoperative radiation results in a significant but modest improvement in event-free survival (EFS) compared with postoperative radiation alone. Historically, HGGs in children have been treated by using traditional cytotoxic drugs either as single agents or in various combinations, schedules, and doses. However, no particular chemotherapeutic regimen has clearly demonstrated superiority, and thus, the most effective agent(s) remains to be determined. To date, the Children's Cancer Group (CCG) study CCG-943 is the only study to show a clear survival advantage associated with adjuvant chemotherapy in pediatric HGG. In this study following surgical resection patients were randomized to RT alone (standard arm) or RT plus prednisone, CCNU/lomustine, and vincristine chemotherapy. Children in the chemotherapy arm showed a significant survival advantage (33 % 5-year EFS) when compared to RT alone [34]. These results have never been improved over the subsequent two decades. The follow-up CCG study CCG-945 enrolled 172 children in a phase III RCT comparing the nitrosourea-containing chemotherapy arm of CCG-943 to a new regimen known as "8-in-1" (eight drugs in one day) given pre- and post-RT; neither arm of the study was superior [35]. Subsequent to CCG-945, commonly used adjuvant chemotherapy regimens using lomustine included PCV (procarbazine, CCNU, and vincristine) and TPCH (6-thioguanine, procarbazine, lomustine, and hydroxyurea). The Children's Oncology Group phase II trial ACNS0126 offered concomitant oral temozolomide (TMZ) with RT followed by post-RT adjuvant TMZ (using the 5-day regimen) [36] to newly diagnosed children with HGG [20]. Temozolomide crosses the blood–brain barrier

(BBB) and has good oral bioavailability. Results of this study showed an overall 3-year EFS of 11 % and OS of 22 % (3-year EFS of 13 % for AA and 7 % for GBM) [20].

Unfortunately, the use of temozolomide in children has not improved outcomes for pediatric HGG, especially when accounting for improvements in neuroimaging, surgical technique, and delivery of RT. Apart from considering the fact that children who were enrolled in ACNS0126 were given TMZ the evening before daily RT when compared to 2 h or less on the day of RT (as administered on the adult EORTC/NCIC CTG trial), the most likely reason for the lack of a favorable impact of TMZ on survival in pHGG is due to the innate biological differences between pediatric and adult HGG. However, due to the favorable toxicity profile and the ability to add to this chemotherapy backbone in current and future studies, temozolomide-containing regimens are in common use at diagnosis. The completed phase II study ACNS0423 added adjuvant lomustine (CCNU) to TMZ following chemoradiation with TMZ; results are pending publication.

Other current clinical trials for newly diagnosed patients are incorporating *antiangiogenesis* strategies concurrent with and/or adjuvant to RT, such as bevacizumab, a recombinant humanized monoclonal antibody to the vascular endothelial growth factor A (VEGF-A). The current COG randomized phase II/III study ACNS0822 assigns patients to receive either temozolomide (TMZ), bevacizumab, or the HDAC inhibitor vorinostat (SAHA) as radiosensitizers with RT followed by TMZ and bevacizumab. A multi-cooperative group (ITCC/SIOP-E, Australian CCTG) randomized phase II study is comparing bevacizumab concurrent with TMZ and RT followed by TMZ and bevacizumab to chemoradiation with TMZ followed by adjuvant TMZ.

High-dose myeloablative chemotherapy with autologous hematopoietic stem cell rescue (ASCR) has resulted in survival for selected groups of patients (those with minimal or no residual disease prior to consolidation with myeloablative chemotherapy). The majority of reports are limited to small numbers of patients either newly diagnosed [37] or with recurrent disease [38]. However, overall long-term survival rates remain poor with significant long-term morbidity and mortality from the treatment regimen, and this therapeutic approach is not currently recommended for newly diagnosed patients.

Treatment of Infants with HGG

Although HGG is rare in this age group, infants (children younger than 3 years) have a better outcome than older children. In order to avoid the long-term devastating side effects of RT to the developing brain, clinical trials have been designed to either delay or totally avoid RT. There is a subset of patients younger than 3 years of age who have improved outcomes with chemotherapy alone [39–41]. Whenever possible, RT should be omitted or delayed in the treatment of children <3 years with HGG.

Local Therapies

One of the major limitations of HGG treatment is the successful and efficient delivery of effective therapies. The blood–brain barrier (BBB), although disrupted in some types of tumors (AA, cortical GBM), is largely intact (midline HGGs: thalamic GBM, DIPG) and plays an active role in restricting the delivery of systemically administered conventional and biological therapies. This leads to decreased effective concentration of the therapeutic agents in the tumor. In order to overcome this limitation, several alternative drug delivery strategies have been tried including: osmotic disruption of the BBB, use of lipophilic drugs, inhibition of membrane pumps such as p-glycoprotein, and intra-arterial and intrathecal chemotherapy; however, these treatment approaches have met with limited success. Novel controlled release systems which circumvent the BBB include direct intra-tumoral injection through an indwelling catheter or implantable chemotherapy-impregnated biodegradable wafers for which the best studied (in adults) includes BCNU. Convection-enhanced delivery

Table 10.3 Molecular targets in pediatric high-grade glioma

Target	Agent	Recurrent/relapsed	Median PFS (mo.)	PFS-6 (%)	Reference
VEGF	Bevacizumab (with irinotecan)	Recurrent/relapsed	4.5	42	[44]
EGFR	Erlotinib	Recurrent/relapsed	1.5	34	[45, 46]
	Gefitinib	Recurrent/relapsed	NR	15 (1-year PFS)	[47]
	Nimotuzumab	Recurrent/relapsed	1.8	NR	[48, 49]
PDGFR	Imatinib	Recurrent/relapsed	NR	18	[50, 51]
mTOR	Temsirolimus	Recurrent/relapsed	1.9	NR	[52]
αV-integrin	Cilengitide	Recurrent/relapsed	1.0	NR	[43]

EGFR epidermal growth factor receptor, *mTOR* mammalian target of rapamycin, *NR* not reported, *PDGFR* platelet-derived growth factor, *VEGF* vascular endothelial growth factor

Adapted from Jones C, Perryman L, Hargrave D. Paediatric and adult malignant glioma: close relatives or distant cousins? Nat Rev Clin Oncol 2012; 9: 400–413. With permission from Nature Publishing Group

(CED) using external or implantable subcutaneous pumps allows intra-tumoral injection of novel therapeutic agents (chemotherapy, cytotoxic cytokines, and radio-immunotherapeutic agents) and is in early stages of clinical development in adults and children.

Novel Therapeutic Approaches: Targeted Therapies and Immunotherapy

The increased understanding of the biology and the pathways involved in HGGs has led to development of novel targeted therapies [32]. Broadly, these can be divided into small molecule receptor tyrosine kinase inhibitors (RTKI) versus EGFR, VEGFR, IGF1R, etc.; specific signaling pathway inhibitors (PI3K/AKT/mTOR, Ras/Raf/MEK, and CDK pathways); chromatin-remodeling/post-translational histone modification pathway inhibitors; antiangiogenic therapies; radiosensitizers; and immunotherapies [42]. Recent encouraging results in glioma immunotherapy in adults and children including EGFRvIII and dendritic cell-based tumor vaccines have led to a number of clinical trials in various stages of clinical trial development [42].

Recurrent HGGs

Relapse or progression of disease is very common in pediatric HGG and mortality approaches 100 % in these cases. The tumor recurrence can be local (at or adjacent to the site of the primary tumor) or disseminated (especially in nonresponsive tumors). Treatment options for relapsed HGG are limited and depend on factors such as the patient's age, performance status, response to initial therapy, time since original diagnosis, and whether tumor recurrence is local or diffuse. Limited therapeutic options include repeat resection, re-irradiation, and systemic chemotherapy. A large number of single-agent phase I/II trials have been conducted in children with recurrent HGG, but the majority of agents tested have revealed minimal or no activity (range of response rates: 0–23 %) (Table 10.3). The Pediatric Preclinical Testing Program, along with the Pediatric Brain Tumor Consortium (PBTC, USA), COG, and other cooperative groups, is developing a preclinical pipeline prior to testing these new agents in early phase clinical trials in children. Targeted therapies such as bevacizumab as single agents or in combination with cytotoxic chemotherapy have been used with some success in adults but have been disappointing in children. Recently completed phase II studies combining O6-benzylguanine O6BG with temozolomide [53] and the anti-integrin agent cilengitide (ACNS0621) [43] for recurrent disease have not provided sufficient response data to proceed to phase III studies. Patients with no or minimal residual disease following re-resection of a recurrent tumor may benefit from myeloablative chemotherapy with ASCR; however, this approach remains experimental.

Outcome

The overall clinical outcome for children with HGG is poor, with only ~30 % of the patients surviving within 3 years of diagnosis. Yet, children have a more favorable prognosis than adults where a 5-year OS using chemoradiation strategies is approaching 10 % [54]. Age at diagnosis, histologic grade, and extent of surgical resection all have an important bearing on the survival outcomes. Children younger than 3 years of age have improved outcomes when compared to older children. Patients with AA (grade III) have a more favorable prognosis than those with GBM (grade IV) emphasizing the importance of central neuropathological review. Children who undergo a GTR have a better 5-year PFS when compared to children who have an STR or a biopsy. Biological characteristics including the absence of TP53, lack of MGMT expression, and the presence of IDH1 mutations and wild-type H3.3 have all been identified as good prognostic factors with improved overall survival. Postsurgical adjuvant therapy (chemotherapy, RT) increases survival rate when compared to surgery alone.

Long-term survivors of children with HGG usually have profound therapy-induced

sequelae [55]. Functional neurological deficits are usually seen in patients with large cortical tumors in the eloquent areas of the brain. Some of the devastating therapy (chemotherapy and cranio-spinal RT) induced side effects include severe neurocognitive deficits, endocrinopathies, sterility, growth failure, and the risk of second malignancies (including meningioma) [55, 56].

Summary and Future Directions

Pediatric HGGs are not the same as adult malignant gliomas. Recent integrated genomic studies have identified six different biological subgroups of GBM across all ages. The clinical and biological data clearly show that GBM in adults and children have significant differences in their underlying biology (Table 10.2) [57]. Even within a given tumor type, there is a distinct molecular heterogeneity that occurs between different ages and brain location. Chromatin remodeling defects are central to the pathogenesis of pediatric and young adult HGG. Historically, treatment protocols for pediatric HGG have been derived from adult therapies and have had poor outcomes. Future molecularly driven classifications and treatment strategies should take into account distinct biological differences including genetic drivers and, in the pediatric setting, identify relevant therapeutic targets and design appropriate preclinical model systems to test these targets. Positive findings from such model systems when incorporated into biology-based trials will hopefully facilitate rapid translation of therapeutic breakthroughs into the clinic.

Acknowledgments Dr. Issai Vanan is the Father Peter J Mckenna St. Baldrick's Cancer Research Scholar, supported by the St. Baldrick's Foundation, USA. Dr. Eisenstat holds the Muriel and Ada Hole Kids with Cancer Society Chair in Pediatric Oncology, University of Alberta.

References

1. Louis DN, Ohgaki H, Wiestler OD, Cavenee WK, Burger PC, Jouvet A, et al. The 2007 WHO classification of tumours of the central nervous system. Acta Neuropathol. 2007;114(2):97–109.
2. Dolecek TA, Propp JM, Stroup NE, Kruchko C. CBTRUS Statistical Report: primary brain and central nervous system tumors diagnosed in the United States in 2005–2009. Neuro Oncol. 2012;14:v1–49.
3. Kaderali Z, Lamberti-Pasculli M, Rutka JT. The changing epidemiology of paediatric brain tumours: a review from the hospital for sick children. Childs Nerv Syst. 2009;25(7):787–93.
4. Kyritsis AP, Bondy ML, Rao JS, Sioka C. Inherited predisposition to glioma. Neuro Oncol. 2010;12(1):104–13.
5. Benesch M, Wagner S, Berthold F, Wolff JE. Primary dissemination of high-grade gliomas in children: experiences from four studies of the Pediatric Oncology and Hematology Society of the German Language Group (GPOH). J Neurooncol. 2005;72(2):179–83.
6. Wilne SH, Dineen RA, Dommett RM, Chu TP, Walker DA. Identifying brain tumours in children and young adults. BMJ. 2013;347:f5844.
7. Peet AC, Arvanitis TN, Leach MO, Waldman AD. Functional imaging in adult and paediatric brain tumors. Nat Rev Clin Oncol. 2012;9(12):700–11.

8. Wen PY, MacDonald DR, Reardon DA, Cloughesy TF, Sorensen AG, Galanis E, et al. Updated response assessment criteria for high-grade gliomas: response assessment in Neuro-Oncology Working Group. J Clin Oncol. 2010;28:1963–72.

9. Warren KE, Poussaint TY, Vezina G, Hargrave D, Packer RJ, Goldman S, et al. Challenges with defining response to antitumor agents in pediatric neuro-oncology: a report from the response assessment in pediatric neuro-oncology (RAPNO) working group. Pediatr Blood Cancer. 2013;60(9):1397–401.

10. Fouladi M, Hunt DL, Pollack IF, Dueckers G, Burger PC, Becker LE, et al. Outcome of children with centrally reviewed low-grade gliomas treated with chemotherapy with or without radiotherapy on Children's Cancer Group high-grade glioma study CCG-945. Cancer. 2003;98(6):1243–52.

11. Pollack IF, Boyett JM, Yates AJ, Burger PC, Gilles FH, Davis RL, Finlay JL, Children's Cancer Group. The influence of central review on outcome associations in childhood malignant gliomas: results from the CCG-945 experience. Neuro Oncol. 2003;5(3):197–207.

12. Gilles FH, Tavaré CJ, Becker LE, Burger PC, Yates AJ, Pollack IF, Finlay JL. Pathologist interobserver variability of histologic features in childhood brain tumors: results from the CCG-945 study. Pediatr Dev Pathol. 2008;11(2):108–17.

13. Parsons DW, Jones S, Zhang X, Lin JC, Leary RJ, Angenendt P, et al. An integrated genomic analysis of human glioblastoma multiforme. Science. 2008;321(5897):1807–12.

14. Noushmehr H, Weisenberger DJ, Diefes K, Phillips HS, Pujara K, Berman BP, et al. Identification of a CpG island methylator phenotype that defines a distinct subgroup of glioma. Cancer Cell. 2010;17(5):510–22.

15. Paugh BS, Zhu X, Qu C, Endersby R, Diaz AK, Zhang J, et al. Novel oncogenic PDGFRA mutations in pediatric high-grade gliomas. Cancer Res. 2013;73(20):6219–29.

16. Phillips JJ, Aranda D, Ellison DW, Judkins AR, Croul SE, Brat DJ, et al. PDGFRA amplification is common in pediatric and adult high-grade astrocytomas and identifies a poor prognostic group in IDH1 mutant glioblastoma. Brain Pathol. 2013;23(5):565–73.

17. Pollack IF, Hamilton RL, James CD, Finkelstein SD, Burnham J, Yates AJ, Children's Oncology Group, et al. Rarity of PTEN deletions and EGFR amplification in malignant gliomas of childhood: results from the Children's Cancer Group 945 cohort. J Neurosurg. 2006;105(5 Suppl):418–24.

18. Bax DA, Gaspar N, Little SE, Marshall L, Perryman L, Regairaz M, et al. EGFRvIII deletion mutations in pediatric high-grade glioma and response to targeted therapy in pediatric glioma cell lines. Clin Cancer Res. 2009;15(18):5753–61.

19. Pollack IF, Hamilton RL, Sobol RW, Burnham J, Yates AJ, Holmes EJ, et al. O6-methylguanine-DNA methyltransferase expression strongly correlates with outcome in childhood malignant gliomas: results from the CCG-945 Cohort. J Clin Oncol. 2006;24(21):3431–7.

20. Cohen KJ, Pollack IF, Zhou T, Buxton A, Holmes EJ, Burger PC, et al. Temozolomide in the treatment of high-grade gliomas in children: a report from the Children's Oncology Group. Neuro Oncol. 2011;13(3):317–23.

21. Schlosser S, Wagner S, Mühlisch J, Hasselblatt M, Gerss J, Wolff JE, Frühwald MC. MGMT as a potential stratification marker in relapsed high-grade glioma of children: the HIT-GBM experience. Pediatr Blood Cancer. 2010;54(2):228–37.

22. Hegi ME, Diserens AC, Gorlia T, Hamou MF, de Tribolet N, Weller M, et al. MGMT gene silencing and benefit from temozolomide in glioblastoma. N Engl J Med. 2005;352(10):997–1003.

23. Schwartzentruber J, Korshunov A, Liu XY, Jones DT, Pfaff E, Jacob K, et al. Driver mutations in histone H3.3 and chromatin remodelling genes in paediatric glioblastoma. Nature. 2012;482(7384):226–31.

24. Sturm D, Witt H, Hovestadt H, Khuong-Quang DA, Jones DTW, Konermann C, et al. Hotspot mutations in H3F3A and IDH1 define distinct epigenetic and biological subgroups of glioblastoma. Cancer Cell. 2012;22:425–37.

25. Chan KM, Fang D, Gan H, Hashizume R, Yu C, Schroeder M, et al. The histone H3.3K27M mutation in pediatric glioma reprograms H3K27 methylation and gene expression. Genes Dev. 2013;27(9):985–90.

26. Fontebasso AM, Liu XY, Sturm D, Jabado N. Chromatin remodeling defects in pediatric and young adult glioblastoma: a tale of a variant histone 3 tail. Brain Pathol. 2013;23(2):210–6.

27. Paugh BS, Qu C, Jones C, Liu Z, Adamowicz-Brice M, Zhang J, et al. Integrated molecular genetic profiling of pediatric high-grade gliomas reveals key differences with the adult disease. J Clin Oncol. 2010;28(18):3061–8.

28. Bjerke L, Mackay A, Nandhabalan M, Burford A, Jury A, Popov S, et al. Histone H3.3 mutations drive pediatric glioblastoma through upregulation of MYCN. Cancer Discov 2013; Epub ahead of print.

29. Rheinbay E, Louis DN, Bernstein BE, Suvà ML. A telltail sign of chromatin: histone mutations drive pediatric glioblastoma. Cancer Cell. 2012;21(3):329–31.

30. Fontebasso AM, Schwartzentruber J, Khuong-Quang DA, Liu XY, Sturm D, Korshunov A, et al. Mutations in SETD2 and genes affecting histone H3K36 methylation target hemispheric high-grade gliomas. Acta Neuropathol. 2013;125(5):659–69.

31. Dasgupta T, Haas-Kogan DA. The combination of novel targeted molecular agents and radiation in the treatment of pediatric gliomas. Front Oncol. 2013;3:110.

32. Jones C, Perryman L, Hargrave D. Paediatric and adult malignant glioma: close relatives or distant cousins? Nat Rev Clin Oncol. 2012;9:400–13.

33. Wisoff JH, Boyett JM, Berger MS, Brant C, Li H, Yates AJ, et al. Current neurosurgical management

and the impact of the extent of resection in the treatment of malignant gliomas of childhood: a report of the Children's Cancer Group trial no. CCG-945. J Neurosurg. 1998;89(1):52–9.

34. Sposto R, Ertel IJ, Jenkin RD, Boesel CP, Venes JL, Ortega JA, et al. The effectiveness of chemotherapy for treatment of high grade astrocytoma in children: results of a randomized trial. A report from the Childrens Cancer Study Group. J Neurooncol. 1989;7(2):165–77.

35. Finlay JL, Boyett JM, Yates AJ, Wisoff JH, Milstein JM, Geyer JR, et al. Randomized phase III trial in childhood high-grade astrocytoma comparing vincristine, lomustine, and prednisone with the eight-drugs-in-1-day regimen. Childrens Cancer Group. J Clin Oncol. 1995;13(1):112–23.

36. Stupp R, Mason WP, van den Bent MJ, Weller M, Fisher B, Taphoorn MJ, European Organisation for Research and Treatment of Cancer Brain Tumor and Radiotherapy Groups, National Cancer Institute of Canada Clinical Trials Group, et al. Radiotherapy plus concomitant and adjuvant temozolomide for glioblastoma. N Engl J Med. 2005;352(10):987–96.

37. Massimino M, Gandola L, Luksch R, Spreafico F, Riva D, Solero C, et al. Sequential chemotherapy, high-dose thiotepa, circulating progenitor cell rescue, and radiotherapy for childhood high-grade glioma. Neuro Oncol. 2005;7(1):41–8.

38. Finlay JL, Dhall G, Boyett JM, Dunkel IJ, Gardner SL, Goldman S, Children's Cancer Group, et al. Myeloablative chemotherapy with autologous bone marrow rescue in children and adolescents with recurrent malignant astrocytoma: outcome compared with conventional chemotherapy: a report from the Children's Oncology Group. Pediatr Blood Cancer. 2008;51(6):806–11.

39. Geyer JR, Finlay JL, Boyett JM, Wisoff J, Yates A, Mao L, Packer RJ. Survival of infants with malignant astrocytomas. A Report from the Childrens Cancer Group. Cancer. 1995;75(4):1045–50.

40. Duffner PK, Krischer JP, Burger PC, Cohen ME, Backstrom JW, Horowitz ME, et al. Treatment of infants with malignant gliomas: the Pediatric Oncology Group experience. J Neurooncol. 1996;28(2–3):245–56.

41. Dufour C, Grill J, Lellouch-Tubiana A, Puget S, Chastagner P, Frappaz D, et al. High-grade glioma in children under 5 years of age: a chemotherapy only approach with the BBSFOP protocol. Eur J Cancer. 2006;42(17):2939–45.

42. Tanaka S, Louis DN, Curry TW, Batchelor TT, Dietrich J. Diagnostic and therapeutic avenues for glioblastoma: no longer a dead end? Nat Rev Clin Oncol. 2013;10(1):14–26.

43. MacDonald TJ, Vezina G, Stewart CF, Turner D, Pierson CR, Chen L, et al. Phase II study of cilengitide in the treatment of refractory or relapsed high-grade gliomas in children: a report from the Children's Oncology Group. Neuro Oncol. 2013;15(10):1438–44.

44. Gururangan S, Chi SN, Young Poussaint T, Onar-Thomas A, Gilbertson RJ, Vajapeyam S, et al. Lack of efficacy of bevacizumab plus irinotecan in children with recurrent malignant glioma and diffuse brainstem glioma: a Pediatric Brain Tumor Consortium study. J Clin Oncol. 2010;28(18):3069–75.

45. Geoerger B, Hargrave D, Thomas F, Ndiaye A, Frappaz D, Andreiuolo F, et al. ITCC (Innovative Therapies for Children with Cancer) European Consortium Innovative Therapies for Children with Cancer pediatric phase I study of erlotinib in brainstem glioma and relapsing/refractory brain tumors. Neuro Oncol. 2011;13(1):109–18.

46. Broniscer A, Baker SJ, Stewart CF, Merchant TE, Laningham FH, Schaiquevich P, et al. Phase I and pharmacokinetic studies of erlotinib administered concurrently with radiotherapy for children, adolescents, and young adults with high-grade glioma. Clin Cancer Res. 2009;15(2):701–7.

47. Geyer JR, Stewart CF, Kocak M, Broniscer A, Phillips P, Douglas JG, et al. A phase I and biology study of gefitinib and radiation in children with newly diagnosed brain stem gliomas or supratentorial malignant gliomas. Eur J Cancer. 2010;46(18):3287–93.

48. Massimino M, Bode U, Biassoni V, Fleischhack G. Nimotuzumab for pediatric diffuse intrinsic pontine gliomas. Expert Opin Biol Ther. 2011;11(2):247–56.

49. Lam C, Bouffet E, Bartels U. Nimotuzumab in pediatric glioma. Future Oncol. 2009;5(9):1349–61.

50. Pollack IF, Jakacki RI, Blaney SM, Hancock ML, Kieran MW, Phillips P, et al. Phase I trial of imatinib in children with newly diagnosed brainstem and recurrent malignant gliomas: a Pediatric Brain Tumor Consortium report. Neuro Oncol. 2007;9(2):145–60.

51. Baruchel S, Sharp JR, Bartels U, Hukin J, Odame I, Portwine C, et al. A Canadian paediatric brain tumour consortium (CPBTC) phase II molecularly targeted study of imatinib in recurrent and refractory paediatric central nervous system tumours. Eur J Cancer. 2009;45(13):2352–9.

52. Geoerger B, Kieran MW, Grupp S, Perek D, Clancy J, Krygowski M, et al. Phase II trial of temsirolimus in children with high-grade glioma, neuroblastoma and rhabdomyosarcoma. Eur J Cancer. 2012; 48(2):253–62.

53. Warren KE, Gururangan S, Geyer JR, McLendon RE, Poussaint TY, Wallace D, et al. A phase II study of O6-benzylguanine and temozolomide in pediatric patients with recurrent or progressive high-grade gliomas and brainstem gliomas: a Pediatric Brain Tumor Consortium study. J Neurooncol. 2012;106(3):643–9.

54. Stupp R, Hegi ME, Mason WP, van den Bent MJ, Taphoorn MJ, Janzer RC, European Organisation for Research and Treatment of Cancer Brain Tumour and Radiation Oncology Groups, National Cancer Institute

of Canada Clinical Trials Group. Effects of radiotherapy with concomitant and adjuvant temozolomide versus radiotherapy alone on survival in glioblastoma in a randomised phase III study: 5-year analysis of the EORTC-NCIC trial. Lancet Oncol. 2009;10(5):459–66.

55. Merchant TE, Pollack IF, Loeffler JS. Brain tumors across the age spectrum: biology, therapy and late effects. Semin Radiat Oncol. 2010;20(1):58–66.

56. Sands SA, Zhou T, O'Neil SH, Patel SK, Allen J, McGuire Cullen P, et al. Long-term follow-up of children treated for high-grade gliomas: children's oncology group L991 final study report. J Clin Oncol. 2012;30(9):943–9.

57. Fontebasso AM, Bechet D, Jabado N. Molecular biomarkers in pediatric glial tumors: a needed wind of change. Curr Opin Oncol. 2013;25(6):665–73.

Diffuse Intrinsic Pontine Glioma

11

Magimairajan Issai Vanan, Vivek Mehta,
and David D. Eisenstat

Introduction

The brainstem (derived from the embryonic mesencephalon) includes three neuroanatomic regions: the midbrain, the pons, and the medulla oblongata. Tumors of the brainstem comprise at least 10 % of all central nervous system (CNS) tumors in children ages 0–19 years in the USA; the majority of these tumors are gliomas [1]. Prior to modern imaging techniques, all brainstem gliomas were regarded as a single pathological entity, and the prognosis was considered uniformly poor. Various imaging modalities have been used to classify brainstem tumors based on the growth pattern and amenability to surgical resection. Diffuse intrinsic pontine gliomas (DIPG) are the most common brainstem tumors

M.I. Vanan, M.D., M.P.H., F.A.A.P.
Departments of Pediatrics and Child Health,
Oncology and Cell Biology, Cancer Care Manitoba,
Manitoba Institute of Cell Biology, University of
Manitoba, Winnipeg, MB, Canada

V. Mehta, M.D., M.Sc.
Division of Neurosurgery, Department of Surgery,
Stollery Children's Hospital/University of Alberta,
Edmonton, AB, Canada

D.D. Eisenstat, M.D., M.A., F.R.C.P.C. (✉)
Departments of Pediatrics, Medical Genetics and
Oncology, Stollery Children's Hospital, University
of Alberta, Edmonton Clinic Health Academy,
Edmonton, AB, Canada
e-mail: eisensta@ualberta.ca

in children, are most often WHO grade IV, and account for greater than 80 % of brainstem gliomas in this age group. The widespread infiltration of this tumor and predominantly high-grade features, coupled with its critical location and inoperability, has led to a uniformly poor outcome in children with DIPG.

Epidemiology

DIPG occurs in all age groups but is most commonly diagnosed in children between the ages of 5 and 10 years. There is equal predilection for both sexes (M:F = 1:1), and the prognosis is significantly worse than that of other brainstem tumors. Because of their infiltrative nature and brainstem localization, DIPGs are not amenable to surgical resection. Over the years, many classification schemes have been proposed for brainstem tumors (Table 11.1), and most of them utilized the best neuroimaging modalities available at the time of classification [4]. The earliest classifications relied on computed axial tomography (CT) and surgical observations; however, the more recent schemes include magnetic resonance imaging (MRI). All these systems categorize the tumor by the pattern of growth (diffuse or focal) or imaging characteristics. In the broadest sense, these tumors are divided into two groups, either focal or diffuse. The more complex schemes subdivide these tumors by location within the brainstem (midbrain, pons, or medulla), growth pattern

Table 11.1 Brainstem tumor classification systems

Reference	Classification system	
Epstein [2]	Intrinsic	Diffuse
		Focal
		Cervicomedullary
	Exophytic	Anterolateral
		Posterolateral
	Disseminated	Positive CSF cytology
		Positive myelography
Choux et al. [3]	Type I	Diffuse
	Type II	Intrinsic, focal
	Type III	Exophytic, focal
	Type IV	Cervicomedullary

(intrinsic or exophytic), direction and extent of tumor growth, the presence or absence of contrast enhancement, and the presence of hemorrhage or hydrocephalus. In one of the most recent classifications proposed by Choux et.al, based on both CT and MRI characteristics, brainstem tumors are divided into four types [4]. DIPGs are classified as type I tumors (not to be confused with WHO grade I). These lesions appear hypointense on CT with non-delineated borders and do not significantly enhance on T1-weighted MRI sequences with gadolinium as the contrast reagent. DIPGs are characterized by diffuse infiltration and swelling of the brainstem (Fig. 11.1).

Clinical Features

The clinical features of patients with brainstem tumors vary with respect to tumor location and the nature/pattern of growth of these tumors. Patients with DIPG have a short latency (usually less than 2–3 months) between the onset of clinical symptoms and diagnosis. The classic triad of symptoms includes *cerebellar signs* (e.g., ataxia, dysmetria, dysarthria), *long-tract signs* (e.g., increased tone, hyperreflexia, clonus, Babinski sign, motor deficit, etc.), and isolated or multiple *cranial nerve palsies* (unilateral or bilateral), more commonly 6th and 7th nerve palsies. Patients with diffuse brainstem tumors associated with neurofibromatosis type 1(NF1) usually have tumor that may mimic DIPG on imaging.

However, in the context of NF1, these are low-grade gliomas (LGG, WHO grades I–II) that can be asymptomatic or diagnosed in the context of an insidious history of isolated cranial nerve palsy or motor deficit. Careful clinical examination for the stigmata of NF-1 and family history should help in the identification of these lesions that usually do not require any active treatment. In DIPG, signs and symptoms of increased intracranial pressure (due to obstructive hydrocephalus from expansion of the pons) are seen in less than 10 % of children. Various other nonspecific symptoms present either at the time of diagnosis or at the time of progression include sensory abnormalities, behavioral changes (night terrors, pathologic laughter, and separation anxiety), urinary problems, declining school performance, respiratory symptoms including sleep apneas, etc.

Diagnostic Evaluation

Neuroimaging

The two most commonly used neuroimaging modalities for diagnosing DIPG are CT and MRI. DIPGs appear hypodense on CT with a nonspecific pattern of enhancement and comprise almost 80 % of all pontine tumors. Invasion into the adjacent midbrain and medulla is common, but they rarely affect the fourth ventricle (in 10 % of cases). The diagnosis of DIPG is mostly based on characteristic MRI findings in the presence of typical clinical features (Fig. 11.1) [4]. The classic MRI findings include the appearance of a diffusely expansile pontine mass with or without encirclement of the basilar artery. Most diffuse brainstem tumors appear to be hypointense on T1-weighted MR images and hyperintense on T2-weighted images. Prominent peritumoral edema is commonly seen. The ventral pons may appear swollen and infiltrated. There is variable contrast enhancement ranging from homogeneous rim enhancement to patchy enhancement to the complete absence of enhancement.

Other MR-based imaging technologies can play a very important role in the management of DIPG, especially in monitoring of response to

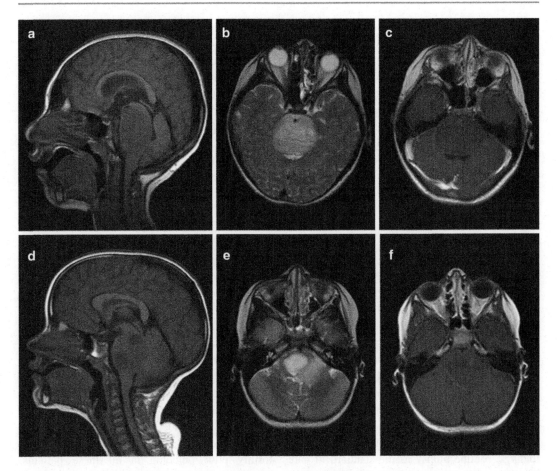

Fig. 11.1 (a–c) **A** 7-year-old male with DIPG. (a) Sagittal T1 with gadolinium, (b) axial T2, and (c) axial T1 with gadolinium. (d–f) **A** 6-year-old female with DIPG. (a) Sagittal T1 with gadolinium, (b) axial T2, and (c) axial T1 with gadolinium. Both tumors demonstrate minimal contrast enhancement

therapy. Response assessment during or post che-motherapy/targeted therapy by MRI is done using the Response Assessment in Neuro-Oncology (RANO) criteria [5] with decreased tumor size, decreased steroid use, and improved neurologic symptoms indicative of response. These criteria were developed primarily for contrast-enhancing tumors like supratentorial GBM in adults (WHO grade IV), and DIPGs frequently do not enhance or they may exhibit variable patterns of enhance-ment. Conventional MRI instructs us regarding tumor structure and location and cannot reliably differentiate therapy-related phenomena such as efficacy, pseudo-progression, or pseudo-response. Hipp et al. [6] used multiparametric imaging in a prospective study to evaluate out-come of children with DIPG. In their study,

increased perfusion (as determined using DSC MRI) at any single time point was associated with shorter survival (RR=4.91), and increasing perfusion over time was a poor prognostic factor. In other studies using MR spectroscopy (MRS) in DIPG, the choline:N-acetylaspartate ratio (CHO:NAA) has been shown to be prognostic, with those patients having a CHO:NAA ratio higher than the median of 2.1 demonstrating a greater risk of early mortality compared to patients with CHO:NAA ≤2.1. Changes in this ratio during follow-up had an impact on progno-sis; increase in the CHO:NAA ratio was inversely associated with survival, while a decreasing CHO:NAA ratio was associated with a longer life expectancy. Neuroimaging using MRS can also be used in DIPG to evaluate the pyramidal tracts when combined with diffusion tensor (DT) tractography to differentiate between benign and malignant lesions (such as brainstem LGG associated with NF-1) and selection of a tumor site for biopsy to differentiate from nonneoplastic processes including neurodegenerative conditions (Alexander disease, ADEM/acute demyelinating encephalomyelitis, central pontine myelinolysis), infections (paracoccidioidomycosis), etc.

Pathology

Role of Biopsy

Historically, prior to CT and MRI, stereotactic brainstem biopsies were performed on a regular basis for histological confirmation of the diagnosis. Due to the heterogeneity of these tumors, the significant morbidity potentially associated with the biopsies, the minimal alteration of the treatment plan based on biopsy results, the prevalence of poor candidates for biopsy at the time of presentation (i.e., those with focal neurological deficits, increased ICP), and the widespread availability of MRI with characteristic radiologic findings, routine biopsy as the standard of care was discontinued in the early 1990s [7].

However, compared to the majority of centers in North America, routine biopsy of children with suspected DIPG has been performed in Europe in the last decade (UK and France). In two of the largest series of brainstem tumor biopsies in children [8, 9], no mortality was reported and transient reversible morbidity (cranial nerve palsy, worsening hemiparesis) lasting only a few days were reported in less than 10 % of patients. More recently, Grill et al. reported on 20 newly diagnosed DIPG patients who had a stereotactic biopsy [10] and new multidisciplinary consensus statements have been developed to gliomas, including DIPG [11]. In summary, the authors conclude that brainstem biopsy is relatively safe in experienced hands using modern neurosurgical techniques. The rationale behind this paradigm shift is that stereotactic biopsies may enable to perform prognostic genomic testing on small

tissue samples (such as H3.3 mutations with increased or decreased survival) and allow identification of potentially druggable targets. With the availability of small molecule inhibitors to these targets, it may be possible to develop new clinical approaches. However, this approach still remains experimental, and pilot studies in Europe and North America are ongoing to confirm the safety of stereotactic biopsies in the context of multicenter trials and their potential for influencing therapy.

Histopathology

The histologic appearance of diffuse intrinsic pontine gliomas is similar to that of other high-grade astrocytomas in other locations (grades III–IV). Classic features including an increased mitotic index, cellular anaplasia, areas of tumor necrosis, and hemorrhage with increased angiogenesis are most often seen. Pretreatment biopsy samples correlate well histologically with autopsy samples. The utility of differentiating between WHO grade III and IV histology in the pons is probably not relevant due to the uniformly poor outcome in all these patients. Biopsies when indicated (atypical radiologic features, exophytic tumors, long clinical latency) are obtained from areas of tumors easily accessible to the neurosurgeon, and due to tumor heterogeneity might not be truly representative (i.e., showing features of lower-grade tumor such as grade II). It has been shown that tumor grade by histology is not predictive of prognosis in typical DIPG. DIPG predominantly spread by contiguity extending rostrally into the brainstem and caudally into the cerebellar peduncles and the medulla. Leptomeningeal dissemination is seen in 10–20 % of the cases at the time of diagnosis. However, this number increases to 50–60 % in patients with recurrent or progressive DIPG or at the time of autopsy. For this reason, some authors consider that baseline MRI of both the brain and spine at diagnosis followed by periodic surveillance of the spine during therapy should be performed.

Molecular Genetics and Tumor Biology

A number of recent comprehensive studies have established that DIPGs can be considered a separate biologic entity when compared to adult and the majority of pediatric supratentorial GBMs at the genetic and epigenetic levels. The recently proposed integrated genomic classification categorizes the majority of DIPG into the histone variant H3.3 K27 group (midline infratentorial tumors with the H3.3 K27M mutation).

Recurrent somatic driver mutations in the H3F3A gene that affect its coded protein, the replication-independent histone 3 variant (H3.3), lead to an amino acid substitution at a key residue, namely, lysine (K) 27. This K27M mutation is seen in over 70 % of DIPG cases [12]. The K27M mutations are also seen in 10–20 % of the supratentorial midline HGGs. This mutation is seen in both pretreatment biopsy samples and autopsy material indicating that it is present at diagnosis and not induced by therapy. DIPG can be classified into *wild type* and *mutated* based on the K27M-H3.3 mutation with distinct clinical, genetic, and prognostic features [12]. Tumors with a wild-type (wt) H3.3 at the K27 residue often have atypical clinical presentation (long latency of symptoms, atypical MRI findings) and show high-grade histology on biopsy samples with a few long-term survivors when compared to the H3.3 K27M mutated DIPGs. Also specific focal chromosome number gains involving the ASAP2 (2p25.1) and MYCN (2p24.3) genes may be seen in K27 wild-type tumors [12]. The H3.3 K27M-mutated DIPGs have worse overall survival when compared to wild-type tumors, and this association is independent of patient age and histological diagnosis [12]. These mutated tumors have glial differentiation on histology and are exclusively associated with gain or amplification of PDGFRA (4q12, seen in 40 % of cases) and MYC/PVT1 (8q24). In one study, TP53 mutations were seen in 77 % of DIPG tumors and were associated with both wild-type and mutated H3.3 tumors [12]. ATRX mutations are infrequent in DIPGs (9 %) when compared to supratentorial pediatric HGGs (29 %) and are seen in mutated K27M-H3.3 tumors in children of an older age group [12]. In another study, mutations involving the replication-dependent histone 3 variant (H3.1) that lead to the same amino acid substitution (H3.1 K27M) were seen in 9 % of the patients with DIPG [13]. A summary of the DIPG classification based on the H3.3 mutation status is given in Table 11.2.

Table 11.2 Integrated genomic classification of DIPG

		H3.3 or H3.1 (K27M mutant)	H3.3 or H3.1 (wild type)
Clinical features			
	Age in years (mean)	8.1	4.6
	Atypical clinical features (longer duration of symptoms, atypical radiology)	–	+
	Overall survival	< 1 year	4–5 years; some long-term survivors
Genomic features			
	Copy number Abnormalities (gains/amplifications)	1. PDGFRA (4q12) 2. MYC/PVT1 (8q24)	1. ASAP2 (2p25) 2. MYCN (2p24)
	TP53 mutation	++ (~80 %)	++ (~80 %)
	ATRX	+ (older children)	–
Potential therapeutic targets/agents			
		Histone modifying agents + RTK Inhibitors	

Based on data from Refs. [12, 15]

When compared to pediatric high-grade gliomas (pHGG), DIPGs show a higher frequency of chromosomal imbalance with gains of chromosomes 2, 8q, and 9q. Losses of chromosomes 16q, 17p, and 20p occur more frequently in DIPG when compared to adult HGG [14]. Receptor tyrosine kinases (RTKs) appear to be upregulated at the genomic or expression level (or both) in the majority of pediatric DIPGs. The most common recurrent focal gain in pediatric DIPG encompasses PDGFRA, with amplification in at least 30 % of DIPGs, and an even larger number showing overexpression at the RNA and protein levels. EGFR gain does not appear to be a frequent event in pediatric DIPG. Multiple dual amplifications of other RTKs like MET, IGF1R, and ERBB4 alone or in combination with PDGFRA are also reported in DIPG. These discoveries, along with reported oncogenic PI3K pathway mutations in PI3KCA, support new treatment approaches targeting this pathway [10, 14–16].

Cell of Origin and Animal Models

There are several unique features of DIPG, which suggest that these tumors are related to dysregulation of a normal postnatal neurodevelopmental process (reviewed in [14]): distinct age of incidence (5–10 years of age), specific anatomical site, and unique biological features (H3.3 K27M mutations, RTK and cell cycle regulatory pathways which play a role in normal brainstem embryogenesis). Monje et al. identified a neural precursor-like cell population in the human ventral pons that is linked (both anatomically and temporally) to the incidence of DIPG [17]. During normal growth and development of the brain, these pontine precursor-like cells (PPC) are spatiotemporally restricted to the ventral brainstem, and the density of the PPC varies during different time periods (present during infancy, decreases by 2 years of age, and increases again during middle childhood). Using mouse models, the authors showed that the signaling by the Hedgehog pathway is increased and contributes to PPC proliferation. This time period in the mouse corresponds to the middle childhood period in humans when DIPG occurs. However, aberrant Hedgehog signaling alone did not result in DIPG in this mouse model, indicating the need for additional genetic mutations (PDGFRA, MYC/PVT1, TP53, etc.) [17].

Mouse Models for Preclinical Testing

Two broad categories of mouse models are available for preclinical testing in DIPG. A genetically engineered mouse model (GEMM) using the avian retroviral RCAS/tv-a system (overexpression of PDGFRA with simultaneous loss of Ink4a-ARF in periventricular cells lining the fourth ventricle and the aqueduct of Sylvius) results in a high-grade glioma histologically similar to human DIPG in immunocompetent mice with high penetrance/short latency and similar invasive features [18]. The direct implantation models use xenografts (primary tumor cells or brain tumor initiating cells/BTICs) derived from patient samples and orthotopically implant modified human glioma cells into the pons. The tumors formed are strikingly similar to human DIPG and are monitored for growth and treatment response using bioluminescence imaging and other small animal imaging techniques [19, 20].

Therapy

DIPG is almost invariably fatal with a mean overall survival of 9–12 months from the time of diagnosis. Radiation therapy prolongs survival by a mean of 3–6 months, but is still considered aggressive palliative therapy. A number of adjuvant therapies such as radiation sensitizers, differentiation agents, and cytotoxic drugs have been studied, but none of them have had any significant impact on the outcomes for these patients.

In the context of typical DIPG, there is no role for surgical resection. However, as we understand more about the biology of these tumors and biologic-based therapies become available, we may require tissue at diagnosis in order to personalize therapy, and routine biopsies may become the standard of care in the future [21].

Radiation Therapy

The current standard of care for children with newly diagnosed DIPG includes fractionated focal radiation therapy (RT) to the tumor along with 1–2 cm margins (54–60Gy, 1.8–2 Gy fractions over a period of 6 weeks). Supportive care in the form of corticosteroids is used to treat the peritumoral edema. To date, RT is the only form of treatment that appears to have a transient benefit in DIPG. Lower doses of RT (<50Gy) have shown a worse outcome, and higher doses using hyperfractionated RT (66–78 Gy) do not appear to provide a survival advantage when compared to standard fractionation protocols. Pilot studies using hypofractionation have reported results that are similar to those observed with normal fractionation. However, the advantage of this technique is to reduce the total duration of treatment (13–18 fractions instead of 30–33). Following completion of radiation, there is clinical progression of disease in almost all cases with radiologic evidence of local recurrence within 3–6 months. However, it is not exceptional to observe evidence of leptomeningeal dissemination at recurrence.

Although RT appears beneficial, radiation sensitizers have not improved outcomes to date. The use of concurrent RT with radiosensitizers including platinum compounds (carboplatin), topoisomerase inhibitors (etoposide, trofosfamide, topotecan), and other agents (metronomic temozolomide, etanidazole) has not been successful. The current Children's Oncology Group (COG) study for DIPG (ACNS0927) is a phase I/II study evaluating vorinostat (SAHA, an HDAC inhibitor) as radiosensitizer used concurrently (with RT) and as maintenance therapy [21].

In the absence of effective neoadjuvant or adjuvant chemotherapy, some institutions are providing palliative re-irradiation with/without concurrent chemotherapy to a dose of 18–20 Gy given over 9–10 fractions (1.8–2.0 Gy/fraction). Preferred candidates may be those children who have experienced durable responses to prior radiation without evidence of clinical/radiological progression off therapy [22]. However, further studies involving larger patient cohorts are required before including re-irradiation as a standard of care for patients with DIPG in the setting of disease progression.

Chemotherapy

Different chemotherapeutic strategies including neoadjuvant (pre-RT) multi-agent chemotherapy, concurrent chemotherapy with RT (both fractionated and hyperfractionated protocols), and adjuvant chemotherapy have not shown improved survival when compared to RT alone (reviewed in [23]). In particular, the current standard of care for adult GBM, RT with concurrent and adjuvant temozolomide, did not improve outcomes for DIPG [24, 25].

Local Therapies

One of the major limitations of DIPG treatment is the successful and efficient delivery of effective therapies. The blood–brain barrier (BBB) is largely intact in DIPG and plays an active role in restricting the delivery of systemically administered conventional and biological therapies. This leads to decreased effective concentration of the therapeutic agents in the tumor. In order to overcome this limitation, several alternative drug delivery strategies have been tried including: osmotic disruption of the BBB, use of lipophilic drugs, inhibition of membrane pumps, intra-arterial and intrathecal chemotherapy, etc., but have met with limited success. Convection-enhanced delivery (CED), using external or implantable subcutaneous pumps, allows intratumoral injection of novel therapeutic agents (chemotherapy, cytotoxic interleukins, radioimmunotherapeutic agents), and there are ongoing phase I/II clinical trials in DIPG.

Targeted Therapies

Recent understanding of the biology of DIPG using autopsy as well as biopsy samples has led to identification of several novel therapeutic

Table 11.3 Molecular Targets in DIPG

Target	Agent	Newly diagnosed or recurrent/relapsed	Median PFS (month)	PFS-6 (%)	Reference
VEGF	Bevacizumab	Recurrent/relapsed	2.5	10	[26]
VEGFR/EGFR	Vandetanib	Newly diagnosed with RT	NR	88	[27]
EGFR	Erlotinib	Newly diagnosed with RT	8	90	[26]
	Gefitinib	Newly diagnosed with RT	7.4	88	[28]
	Nimotuzumab	Newly diagnosed with RT	5.5	NR	[29]
PDGFR	Imatinib	Newly diagnosed with RT	NR	70	[30]
mTOR	Temsirolimus	Recurrent/Relapsed	2.5	NR	[31]
Farnesyltransferase	Tipifarnib	Newly diagnosed with RT	NR	44	[32]

Adapted from Jones C, Perryman L, Hargrave D. Paediatric and adult malignant glioma: close relatives or distant cousins. Nat Rev Clin Oncol 2012; 9:400–413. With permission from Nature Publishing Group

targets and small molecule inhibitors (Table 11.3). Some of the contemporary clinical trials using targeted therapies in DIPG are summarized in a recent review [14]. Immunotherapy using dendritic cell vaccines in DIPG is limited by the availability of tissue to generate tumor-associated antigens.

Outcome/Prognosis

The prognosis of patients with DIPG is extremely poor and is almost always fatal. However, there are some favorable prognostic factors seen in a minority of patients. Some of the clinically favorable prognostic factors include: (a) young age at presentation (<3 years), (b) prolonged latency between onset of symptoms and diagnosis (>6 months), and (c) absence of cranial nerve palsies or long-tract involvement at presentation. The H3.3 K27M-mutated DIPGs have a worse overall survival when compared to wild-type H3.3 tumors, and this association is independent of patient age and histological diagnosis.

Future Directions

Currently, there is no effective treatment for DIPG. Recent advances in the genetics and biology of HGGs have identified DIPG as a distinct group of tumors from the majority of pediatric HGG. Defects in chromatin remodeling

(via H3.3/H3.1 K27M somatic mutations as a primary event with one or more secondary hits including TP53, PDGFRA, MYC/PVT1) leading to age- and brain-location-specific defects in chromatin structure are fundamental in the pathogenesis of DIPG tumors. Further understanding of the defects downstream of the H3.3/H3.1 K27M mutation [33] along with development of relevant animal models with these mutations will help in therapeutic advances against this deadly tumor. Future clinical trials should be based on molecular classification of tumor tissue obtained from biopsy, as this will help in better treatment stratification and more specific targeted therapies.

Acknowledgments Dr. Issai Vanan is the Father Peter J. Mckenna St. Baldrick's Cancer Research Scholar, supported by the St. Baldrick's Foundation, USA. Dr. Eisenstat holds the Muriel and Ada Hole Kids with Cancer Society Chair in Pediatric Oncology, University of Alberta.

References

1. Dolecek TA, Propp JM, Stroup NE, Kruchko C. CBTRUS Statistical Report: primary brain and central nervous system tumors diagnosed in the United States in 2005–2009. Neuro Oncol. 2012;14 Suppl 5:v1–49.
2. Epstein F. A staging system for brainstem gliomas. Cancer. 1985;56:1804–6.
3. Choux M, Lena G, Do L. Brainstem tumors. In: Choux M, Di Rocco C, Hockley A, editors. Pediatric neurosurgery. New York: Churchill Livingstone; 2000. p. 471–91.

4. Recinos PF, Sciubba DM, Jallo GI. Brainstem tumors: where are we today? Pediatr Neurosurg. 2007;43: 192–201.

5. Wen PY, Macdonald DR, Reardon DA, Cloughesy TF, Sorensen AG, Galanis E, et al. Updated response assessment criteria for high-grade gliomas: response assessment in Neuro-Oncology Working Group. J Clin Oncol. 2010;28:1963–72.

6. Hipp S, Steffen-Smith E, Hammoud D, Shih J, Bent R, Warren K. Predicting outcome of children with diffuse intrinsic pontine gliomas using multi-parametric imaging. Neuro Oncol. 2011;13:904–9.

7. Albright A, Packer R, Zimmerman R, Rorke L, Boyett J, Hammond G. Magnetic resonance scans should replace biopsies for the diagnosis of diffuse brainstem gliomas: a report from the Children's Cancer Group. Neurosurgery. 1993;33:1026–9.

8. Cartmill M, Punt J. Diffuse brain stem glioma. A review of stereotactic biopsies. Childs Nerv Syst. 1999;15:235–7.

9. Roujeau T, Machado G, Garnett MR, Miquel C, Puget S, Geoerger B, et al. Stereotactic biopsy of diffuse pontine lesions in children. J Neurosurg. 2007;107 Suppl 1:1–4.

10. Grill J, Puget S, Andreiulo F, Philippe C, MacConaill L, Kieran MW. Critical oncogenic mutations in newly diagnosed pediatric diffuse intrinsic pontine glioma. Pediatr Blood Cancer. 2012;58:489–91.

11. Walker DA, Liu J, Kieran M, Jabado N, Picton S, Packer R, et al. A multi-disciplinary consensus statement concerning surgical approaches to low-grade, high-grade astrocytomas and diffuse intrinsic pontine gliomas in childhood (CPN Paris 2011) using the Delphi method. Neuro Oncol. 2013;15:462–8.

12. Khuong-Quang DA, Buczkowicz P, Rakopoulos P, Liu XY, Fontebasso AM, Bouffet E, et al. K27M mutation in histone H3.3 defines clinically and biologically distinct subgroups of pediatric diffuse intrinsic pontine gliomas. Acta Neuropathol. 2012;124: 439–47.

13. Wu G, Broniscer A, McEachron TA, Lu C, Paugh BS, Becksfort J, et al. Somatic histone H3 alterations in pediatric diffuse intrinsic pontine gliomas and non-brainstem glioblastomas. Nat Genet. 2012;44:251–3.

14. Jones C, Perryman L, Hargrave D. Paediatric and adult malignant glioma: close relatives or distant cousins. Nat Rev Clin Oncol. 2012;9:400–13.

15. Paugh BS, Qu C, Jones C, Liu Z, Adamowicz-Brice M, Zhang J, Bax DA, et al. Integrated molecular genetic profiling of pediatric high-grade gliomas reveals key differences with the adult disease. J Clin Oncol. 2010;28:3061–8.

16. Puget S, Philippe C, Bax DA, Job B, Varlet P, Junier MP, et al. Mesenchymal transition and PDGFRA amplification/mutation are key distinct oncogenic events in pediatric diffuse intrinsic pontine gliomas. PLoS One. 2012;7:e30313.

17. Monje M, Mitra SS, Freret ME, Raveh TB, Kim J, Masek M, et al. Hedgehog-responsive candidate cell of origin for diffuse intrinsic pontine glioma. Proc Natl Acad Sci U S A. 2011;108:4453–8.

18. Becher OJ, Hambardzumyan D, Walker TR, Helmy K, Nazarian J, Albrecht S, et al. Preclinical evaluation of radiation and perifosine in a genetically and histologically accurate model of brainstem glioma. Cancer Res. 2010;70:2548–57.

19. Caretti V, Zondervan I, Meijer DH, Idema S, Vos W, Hamans B, et al. Monitoring of tumor growth and post-irradiation recurrence in a diffuse intrinsic pontine glioma mouse model. Brain Pathol. 2011;21: 441–51.

20. Aoki Y, Hashizume R, Ozawa T, Banerjee A, Prados M, James DC, et al. An experimental xenograft mouse model of diffuse pontine glioma designed for therapeutic testing. J Neurooncol. 2012;108:29–35.

21. Gajjar A, Packer RJ, Foreman NK, Cohen K, Haas-Kogan D, Merchant TE. Children's Oncology Group's 2013 blueprint for research: central nervous system tumors. Pediatr Blood Cancer. 2013;60:1022–6.

22. Fontanilla HP, Pinnix CC, Ketonen LM, Woo SY, Vats TS, Rytting ME, et al. Palliative reirradiation for progressive diffuse intrinsic pontine glioma. Am J Clin Oncol. 2012;35:51–7.

23. Jansen MHA, van Vuurden DG, Vandertop WP, Kaspers GJL. Diffuse intrinsic pontine gliomas: a systematic update on clinical trials and biology. Cancer Treat Rev. 2012;38:27–35.

24. Cohen KJ, Heideman RL, Zhou T, Holmes EJ, Lavey RS, Bouffet E, Pollack IF. Temozolomide in the treatment of children with newly diagnosed diffuse intrinsic pontine gliomas : a report from the Children's Oncology Group. Neuro Oncol. 2011;13:410–6.

25. Chassot A, Canale S, Varlet P, Puget S, Rougeau T, Negretti L, et al. Radiotherapy with concurrent and adjuvant temozolomide in children with newly diagnosed diffuse intrinsic pontine glioma. J Neurooncol. 2012;106:399–407.

26. Geoerger B, Hargrave D, Thomas F, Ndiaye A, Frappaz D, Andreiulo F, et al. Innovative Therapies for Children with Cancer pediatric phase I study of erlotinib in brainstem glioma and relapsing/refractory brain tumors. Neuro Oncol. 2011;13:109–18.

27. Broniscer A, Baker JN, Tagen M, Onar-Thomas A, Gilbertson RJ, Davidoff AM, et al. Phase I study of vandetanib during and after radiotherapy in children with diffuse intrinsic pontine glioma. J Clin Oncol. 2010;28:4762–8.

28. Pollack IF, Stewart CF, Kocak M, Poussaint TY, Broniscer A, Banerjee A, et al. A phase II study of gefitinib and irradiation in children with newly diagnosed brainstem gliomas: a report from the Pediatric Brain Tumor Consortium. Neuro Oncol. 2011;13: 290–7.

29. Massimino M, Bode U, Biassoni V, Fleischhack G. Nimotuzumab for pediatric diffuse intrinsic pontine gliomas. Expert Opin Biol Ther. 2011;11:247–56.

30. Geoerger B, Kieran MW, Grupp S, Perek D, Clancy J, Krygowski M, et al. Phase II trial of temsirolimus in

children with high-grade glioma, neuroblastoma and rhabdomyosarcoma. Eur J Cancer. 2012;48:253–62.

31. Pollack IF, Jakacki RI, Blaney SM, Hancock ML, Kieran MW, Phillips P, et al. Phase I trial of imatinib in children with newly diagnosed brainstem and recurrent malignant gliomas: a Pediatric Brain Tumor Consortium report. Neuro Oncol. 2007;9: 145–60.

32. Haas-Kogan DA, Banerjee A, Kocak M, Prados MD, Geyer JR, Fouladi M, et al. Phase I trial of tipifarnib in children with newly diagnosed intrinsic diffuse brainstem glioma. Neuro Oncol. 2008;10:341–7.

33. Lewis PW, Müller MM, Koletsky MS, Cordero F, Lin S, Banaszynski LA, et al. Inhibition of PRC2 activity by a gain-of-function H3 mutation found in pediatric glioblastoma. Science. 2013;340:857–61.

Embryonal Brain Tumors

12

Tiffany Sin Yu Chan, Xin Wang, Tara Spence,
Michael D. Taylor, and Annie Huang

Introduction

Medulloblastoma (MB) and central nervous system primitive neuroectodermal tumor (CNS-PNET) are primary grade 4 embryonal brain tumors that require multimodal therapies. Although MB and CNS-PNETs are treated with similar approaches and treatment regimens, they represent biologically different diseases. Recent studies have revealed molecular subgroups for both MB and CNS-PNET which correlate with distinct clinicopathologic features and treatment response. This chapter will summarize current clinical understanding of MB and CNS-PNET in the context of recent molecular studies and postulate on the direction of future therapeutic approaches for these diseases.

T.S.Y. Chan, B.Sc.
Department of Cell Biology/Arthur and Sonia Labatt
Brain Tumour Research Centre, The Hospital for Sick
Children, Toronto, ON, Canada

X. Wang, B.H.Sc. (Hon). • M.D. Taylor, M.D.
Department of Developmental and Stem Cell Biology,
The Hospital for Sick Children, Toronto, ON, Canada

T. Spence, M.Sc. • A. Huang, M.D., Ph.D. (✉)
Department of Cell Biology, The Hospital for Sick
Children, Toronto, ON, Canada
e-mail: annie.huang@sickkids.ca

Medulloblastoma

Epidemiology

Medulloblastoma is the most common malignant brain tumor in childhood, representing up to 25 % of all pediatric brain tumors. First described by Bailey and Cushing in 1925, MB arises from the cerebellum and is classified as a World Health Organization (WHO) grade 4 tumor. MB predominantly arises in children, with peak incidence between the ages of 3–4 and 8–9. The annual incidence has been estimated at 1 in every 200,000 children under the age of 15 [1]. Consistent with the classification of an embryonal tumor, MB is rarely seen in adults; 70 % of patients present before the age of 20. There is a modest male preponderance in a ratio of 1.4:1 [2]. A small proportion of MBs (<5 %) have inherited disorders with germline mutations, these include: Gorlin's syndrome (also called as nevoid basal cell carcinoma syndrome) associated with patched-1 (*PTCH1*) gene mutations, Turcot syndrome associated with mutations in the adenomatous polyposis coli (*APC*) gene, and Li-Fraumeni syndrome caused by TP53 mutations [1]. These familial cancer syndromes provided some of the first clues about biological pathways that underlie MB pathogenesis.

K. Scheinemann and E. Bouffet (eds.), *Pediatric Neuro-oncology*,
DOI 10.1007/978-1-4939-1541-5_12, © Springer Science+Business Media New York 2015

Clinical Presentation

Patients with MB frequently present with signs and symptoms related to hydrocephalus secondary to fourth ventricular obstruction, with predominant symptoms of vomiting, headache, and nausea. Due to the localizing posterior fossa mass, ataxia, dysmetria, and diplopia secondary to sixth nerve palsy are often accompanying symptoms. The most common symptoms, especially in younger children, are nonspecific and include morning headaches with vomiting, irritability, and lethargy – subtle clinical signs that can present diagnostic challenges [3].

The differential diagnosis for MB includes a range of tumors with a predilection for the cerebellum. These include pilocytic astrocytoma, ependymoma, and other rarer embryonal tumors including atypical teratoid/rhabdoid tumors (ATRT) and ETANTR/EMTR (embryonal neoplasm with abundant neuropil and true rosettes). It can be difficult to distinguish these tumor entities by clinical symptoms alone; however, patients with pilocytic astrocytoma or ependymoma tend to have a longer duration of symptoms.

Imaging Findings

The initial diagnosis of MB is usually made on non-contrast computed tomography (CT) followed by magnetic resonance imaging (MRI) with contrast which is the preferred modality, and later confirmed with histopathology [4]. The classical CT finding is a hyper-attenuating midline mass that markedly enhances with contrast medium. Foraminal extension of tumor and a predominantly cystic mass with a mural nodule would, respectively, favor ependymoma and pilocytic astrocytoma over MB (Fig. 12.1). The presence of leptomeningeal or nodular metastases would favor a diagnosis of MB or another related embryonal tumor such as ATRT. It is important to note that both CT and MRI characteristic of MB may overlap with that of other tumor types; hence, surgical histopathology is needed for definitive tumor diagnosis. Spinal MRI is part of standard preoperative investigations for posterior fossa tumors and can demonstrate evidence of nodular or leptomeningeal dissemination. Attention should be paid to kidney abnormalities when spinal MRI scan is performed as the presence of metastatic lesions at this level would favor ATRT rather than MB.

Histopathology

Microscopically, MB is often referred to as a "small round blue cell tumor," given the characteristics of densely packed cells with prominent nuclei surrounded by scant cytoplasm under H&E staining. The WHO classification of tumors of the central nervous system identifies five major histological variants in MB: classic, desmoplastic, large cell, anaplastic, and medulloblastoma with extensive nodularity (MBEN) [5]. Large cell and anaplastic variants have been correlated with poorer patient outcomes, while the best survival has been reported in patients with desmoplastic or MBEN histology; however, prognostic correlations may be influenced by age and other clinical features. Furthermore, as histologic categorization may be influenced by tumor heterogeneity, patient prognostication based on histopathological findings alone may not be accurate. The histologic differential diagnosis for MB includes atypical teratoid/rhabdoid tumor (ATRT) and rare embryonal tumors such as ETANTR [6]. Both entities which arise predominantly in younger children should be part of the differential work-up in all young patients with suspected MB. As characteristic rhabdoid cells may be present in variable amounts in ATRTs, immunostaining for the IN1/SNF gene product, which is nearly universally absent in ATRT but retained in MB tumors, should be included in the diagnostic work-up. Most but not all ETANTR exhibit classic histologic features of ependymoblastic rosettes and neuronal differentiation on a neuropil background and can be differentiated from MB by strong immuno-positivity for LIN28 and/or genomic amplification of the C19MC locus on 19q13.42 [7, 8].

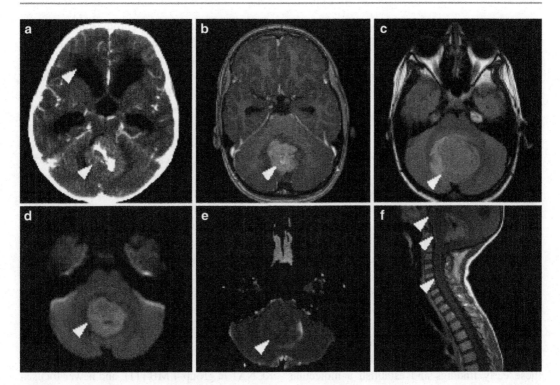

Fig. 12.1 CT and MR imaging of medulloblastoma.(**a**) Axial contrast-enhanced CT showing a hyperdense mass compressing the 4th ventricle (*white arrow*). Note the hydrocephalus with accompanying trans-ependymal flow (*white arrow*). (**b**) Axial T1 gadolinium-enhanced MRI and (**c**) axial FLAIR showing an enhancing mass in the midline cerebellum. (**d**) Axial T1 and (**e**) accompanying axial diffusion coefficient map showing restricted diffusion. (**f**) Sagittal T1 gadolinium-enhanced MRI through the midline spine showing laminar leptomeningeal enhancement along the dorsal and ventral aspects of the spinal cord and ventral brainstem indicative of metastatic dissemination (arrows)

Current MB Staging and Risk Stratification

Traditionally, MB patients are assigned into different treatment risk groups according to clinical features, which include age, the extent of resection, and the presence of metastasis at time of diagnosis. High-risk patients are defined as those <3 years of age, with more than 1.5 cm postsurgical residual tumor or evidence of metastasis at presentation [3]. Up to one third of MB patients present with leptomeningeal metastasis to the brain and/or spine, which may be detected on a preoperative MRI scan of the brain and spine. Postoperative MR imaging of the brain should be performed as soon as possible after surgery to avoid postoperative artifactual imaging changes to assess tumor residual. Staging is completed with cytological examination of the cerebrospinal fluid (CSF) for evidence of microscopic dissemination. Patients with nonmetastatic disease and no significant postoperative residual tumor, who are greater than 36 months of age, are stratified as standard risk.

Currently, all MB patients receive risk-adapted multimodality protocols based on clinical risk stratification schema. However, it is now increasingly clear that stratification based on clinical assessment alone is inadequate. It has been argued that current staging system fails to detect the true extent of disease and results in frequent over-/undertreatment of patients. Devastating acute and long-term treatment sequelae in survivors are major concerns for MB patients treated with intensive chemoradiotherapeutic treatment. Conversely, even with aggressive therapies, up to 30 % of MB patients will succumb to their disease. The lack of reliable clinical predictors of MB outcome has prompted substantial studies to identify biological predictors of clinical phenotype in MB.

Molecular Features of MB

MB was first linked to abnormalities in the Wingless (WNT) and Sonic Hedgehog (SHH) developmental signaling pathways based on observed association of MB with Turcot syndrome and Gorlin's syndrome, and demonstration of alterations, respectively, in the APC and PTCH genes in some MB [9]. Early small cohort studies also suggested that specific genetic alterations, notably, MYCC gene amplification and CTNNB1 mutations, had prognostic correlations in MB (reviewed in ref [10]). Recent global gene expression and copy number studies of substantial cohorts of MB have helped to consolidate these early findings and establish a molecular classification system for MB that correlates with clinical phenotypes and patient outcomes. Specifically several global gene expression profiling studies of substantial MB cohorts have now demonstrated that MB is comprised of four molecular variants termed WNT, Sonic Hedgehog (SHH), and group 3 and group 4 subtypes which are associated with distinct developmental pathway signatures and/or cytogenetic abnormalities. The 4 MB subgroups also correlate with distinct tumor histology, patient demographics, and survival [10]. The WNT subgroup exhibits the best prognosis of any subgroup (greater than 95 % survival) and typically occurs in older children and exhibit classic histology. SHH MB represents an intermediate prognosis subgroup with overall survival ranging from 60 to 80 % and is predominantly seen in infants and young adults; MB with desmoplastic histology is almost exclusively restricted to this subgroup. Group 3 and 4 tumors which are not associated with any specific developmental signatures have the worst overall survival. MYCC gene amplification was observed only in group 3 tumors which also display frequently anaplastic histology, while group 4 tumors commonly (>30 %) exhibited isochromo-

some 17q (i17q, loss of chromosome 17p and gain of 17q). Characteristics of these subgroup variants are summarized in Fig. 12.2 [10]. These findings have helped to significantly advance our understanding of MB molecular biology and provided valuable diagnostic and prognostic tools that are currently in consideration for use in upfront risk stratification of patients in clinical trials across North America and Europe. A significant challenge is the development of robust diagnostic assays that can be used in clinical trials to reliably distinguish MB subgroups with high sensitivity and specificity. Currently, most consistent results to subtype MB have been reported with the use of nuclear CTNNB1 immuno-positivity and monosomy 6 which identifies WNT MB and MYCC amplifications which identifies group 3 MB; however, assays to reliably identify SHH and group 4 MB are lacking. Promising assays for MB subgrouping which include immunostains for SFRP1 in SHH, NPR3 in group 3, and KCNA1 in group 4 MB [11], and newer focused transcriptional and methylation assays remain to be validated.

The availability of tools to segregate molecular subtypes of MB will profoundly alter the design of MB clinical trials [11]. In addition to enhanced risk stratification for current conventional treatment regimens, molecular subtyping of MB will enable concerted investigations of novel therapy tailored to subgroup-specific biology. The inclusion of molecular analyses with traditional histo-clinical examination will be the standard of care in establishing the diagnosis and treatment stratification of MB in the near future.

Therapeutic Approaches

Multimodal approach of maximal safe surgical resection, radiotherapy to the primary tumor site and craniospinal axis, and systemic adjuvant chemotherapy are the current standard of care. Patients with MB often present with significant obstructive hydrocephalus, and thus management of increased intracranial pressure is commonly the priority. Patients may be managed with corticosteroids to alleviate tumor edema or require CSF

Molecular Subgroups of Medulloblastoma

CONSENSUS	WNT	SHH		Group 4
Cho (2010)	C6	C3	C1/C5	C2/C4
Northcott (2010)	WNT	SHH	Group C	Group D
Kool (2008)	A	B	E	C/D
Thompson (2006)	B	C, D	E, A	A, C

DEMOGRAPHICS

Age Group: infant, child, adult

Gender: ♀ ♂

	WNT	SHH	Group C	Group 4
Age Group				
Gender	♂♂:♀♀	♂♂:♀♀	♂♂:♀	♂♂:♀

CLINICAL FEATURES

	WNT	SHH	Group C	Group 4
Histology	classic, rarely LCA	desmoplastic/nodular, classic, LCA	classic, LCA	classic, LCA
Metastasis	rarely M+	uncommonly M+	very frequently M+	frequently M+
Prognosis	very good	infants good, others intermediate	poor	intermediate

GENETICS

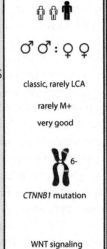 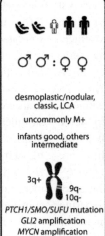 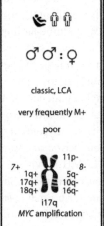 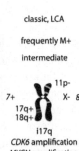

WNT	SHH	Group C	Group 4
6-	3q+ / 9q- / 10q-	7+ / 1q+ / 17q+ / 18q+ / 11p- / 5q- / 10q- / 16q- / 8-	7+ / 17q+ / 18q+ / 11p- / X- / 8-
CTNNB1 mutation	PTCH1/SMO/SUFU mutation GLI2 amplification MYCN amplification	i17q MYC amplification	i17q CDK6 amplification MYCN amplification

GENE EXPRESSION

WNT	SHH	Group C	Group 4
WNT signaling	SHH signaling	Photoreceptor/GABAergic	Neuronal/Glutamergic
MYC +	MYCN +	MYC +++	minimal MYC / MYCN

Fig. 12.2 Genetic, demographic, and clinicopathological features of the four molecular subgroups of medulloblastoma

diversion prior to surgery. With current treatment strategies, an anticipated 5-year overall survival (OS) has reached up to 80 % for patients with localized disease. However, metastatic and recurrent MBs still result in a significant mortality.

Surgery and Radiotherapy

Maximal safe resection of the posterior fossa mass is a key component and goal for patients with MB. With modern surgical techniques, gross total resection can be achieved in a majority of patients. As residual disease is associated with poorer outcome, immediate reoperation or second look surgery after adjuvant chemo- or radiotherapy may be considered.

Radiotherapy remains a critical part of the multimodal approach and is delivered early,

within a month postsurgery, as delayed radiation results in poorer outcome [12]. The goal of radiotherapy is to control for both residual microscopic tumor in the primary site and to treat or prevent leptomeningeal disease along the craniospinal axis. Due to the severe toxic effects of irradiation to the developing nervous system, craniospinal radiation is often avoided or delayed in patients under the age of 3. Children with both average- and high-risk MB patients receive the same dose of local tumor bed irradiation of 5,400–5,580 cGy, but receive risk-adapted craniospinal irradiation. Children without tumor residual or metastasis received a 2,340 cGy craniospinal irradiation, while high-risk patients receive at least 3,600 cGy to the neuraxis [13]. Further reduction of craniospinal irradiation to 1,800 cGy for average-risk patients is currently being investigated in a phase III randomized control study by the North American Children's Oncology Trial Group (COG).

In European and North American trials, the standard of care for MB involves postsurgical radiation followed typically by adjuvant cisplatin-based or high-dose chemotherapy. With such regimens, a 5-year survival for average-risk MB patients has reached 75–85 %; however, survival of high-risk patients is significantly poorer with a 5-year OS of 30–65 %. Significant improvement in survival has been achieved with chemoradiotherapy combination regimens; however, high-dose craniospinal radiotherapy continues to be associated with a high incidence of treatment-related complications. In addition to cognitive impairment, ototoxicity, thyroid dysfunction, growth failure, and endocrine abnormalities are significant sequelae in MB survivors. Intensity-modulated and proton-based radiation therapies represent promising newer normal tissue-sparing radiotherapeutic approaches. In addition to the use of conventional concomitant chemotherapy, development of novel radiosensitizers would be an important step toward minimizing radiation-associated toxicity.

Chemotherapy

Adjuvant chemotherapy plays an important role in the management of both average- and high-risk MB patients and has been used with the intent to permit reduction in radiation doses for older children or to avoid or delay radiation in younger children.

Radiation-sparing approaches for younger children with MB have been varied both in terms of chemotherapeutic regimens and inclusion of age range. In addition, some groups have used focal radiation up-front. Global trial groups have used three general approaches in children <3–5 years of age with MB to achieve a 5-year OS ranging between 50 and 70 %. These regimens have generally differed in the use of methotrexate, intraventricular treatment, and use of high-dose chemotherapy for consolidation. While the SFOP [14] group has used chemotherapy-based regimens without methotrexate, the UKCCSG/SIOP

[15] and the German trial group protocol [13] employed a methotrexate-based chemotherapy backbone with intraventricular methotrexate treatment in the German experience. The Head Start consortium, which pioneered the use of high-dose chemotherapy, currently employs a methotrexate-based induction regimen with a single high-dose/stem cell rescue as consolidation [16], while treatment in the COG protocol is consolidated with 3 cycles of high-dose therapy and stem cell rescue [17]. As favorable outcomes with desmoplastic MB in young children have been seen across different infant MB studies, planned trials are examining desmoplasia as a criterion for stratification. An ongoing COG high-risk infant MB/CNS-PNET protocol is examining the benefits of methotrexate during induction in high-dose chemotherapy-based regimens, while the relative merits of single versus three stem cell rescue in consolidation remain to be investigated.

Treatment approaches to older children with MB have been more consistent. With the exception of a stem cell-based protocol from St. Jude's, most trial groups have employed a conventional chemotherapy-based regimen with similar drugs. For average-risk patients, over the age of 3, both the COG and SIOP trial groups have employed a chemotherapy-based regimens with CCNU, VCR, and cisplatin, followed by reduced dose 2,340 cGy craniospinal irradiation and reported similar 5-year EFS, respectively, of 81 % [18] and 77 % [19]. In the St. Jude Medulloblastoma-96 protocol where standard-dose craniospinal in radiation is followed by four cycles of cyclophosphamide-based, dose-intensive chemotherapy, 5-year OS of 85 % has been reported [20], suggesting that dose intensification may benefit some average-risk patients.

Overall survival of patients with high-risk disease, specifically those presenting with metastasis, has been less favorable with 60–65 % long-term survival observed across chemotherapy and high-dose-based regimens. However, improved results have been reported by the Milan strategy in which patients received postoperative methotrexate, etoposide, cyclophosphamide, and carboplatin in a 2-month schedule, followed by hyperfractionated accelerated radiotherapy (HART). This regimen resulted in a 5-year OS of

73 %. COG also reported better survival in a phase I/II trial for high-risk MB in which patients received 15–30 doses of carboplatin along vincristine as radiosensitizers, followed by cisplatin-based maintenance chemotherapy. This study reported the highest overall survival at 82 % in high-risk MB patients who received 6 months of maintenance chemotherapy with cyclophosphamide thus suggesting a role for biologic-based maintenance chemotherapy in MB therapy [21].

Due to the increased incidence of secondary malignancies from irradiation and chemotherapy, periodic surveillance with brain and spine MRIs for disease recurrence, as well as secondary malignancies, is performed. In addition, regular neuropsychological and medical surveillance for end-organ toxicity is indicated for MB survivors. Recurrent disease, which occurs in approximately 25 % of patients with MB, remains a significant clinical challenge. Most relapses tend to occur within the first 3 years post-diagnosis, and long-term survival in this population remains very poor, with no clear effective rescue regimens reported. Limited successes have been reported with high-dose chemotherapy/autologous stem cell rescue regimens in older children with recurrent MB [22]. Higher salvage rates have been reported in younger children, who have not received prior irradiation, with radiation-based rescue protocols [23].

Molecular Therapeutic Targets

Basic research has led to tremendous gains in biological knowledge regarding MB. Specifically, the establishment of molecular subgroups for MB and the development of multiple group specific animal models are poised to transform future clinical trials and treatments for MB patients. It is expected that in the near future, patients will be stratified and treated based on the biological subgroup-specific makeup of their disease, which will hopefully lead to improved outcomes with less adverse effects. One main goal is to reduce morbidity of current treatment regimens in children with favorable biology disease. Specifically reducing chemotherapy and craniospinal irradiation for the

Table 12.1 Examples of preclinical pharmaceutical agents for targeted therapeutics in medulloblastoma

Drug name	Mode of action	Stage	Reference
GDC-0449	Smo inhibitor	Phase I	[24, 25]
LDE225	Smo inhibitor	Phase II	[26]
Lapatinib	ERBB2 inhibitor	Phase II	[27]
PHA665752	MET inhibitor	Preclinical	[28]
Tipifarnib	Farnesyltransferase inhibitor	Preclinical	[29]
IPI-926	Smo inhibitor	Preclinical	[30]

favorable WNT subgroup could be one tangible approach that will minimize treatment toxicity.

To date, multiple pharmacological inhibitors for SHH-driven MB subgroups have been designed and have shown promising antitumor effects in SHH MB mouse models, and some are currently under clinical trials (Table 12.1). Promising preclinical studies, however, have not correlated with sustained disease response due to development of drug resistance with monotherapies [25]. These observations suggest that a combination of targeted therapies with conventional chemotherapy regimens may be required for optimal efficacy. Additionally, the use of several biologic agents that target signaling cross talk between SHH signaling and other key molecular pathways, such as AKT, Notch, TGF-β(beta), may also offer novel approaches to tailored therapy [31]. The feasibility of employing combination signaling therapies has been assessed in MB preclinical models. For instance, retinoic acid, which induces apoptosis together with histone deacetylase inhibitors, exhibits synergistic effects in xenograft and transgenic models [32]. Furthermore, a combination of LDE225 with PI3K inhibitors also markedly delays development of resistance thus suggesting the importance and promise of multiple pathway inhibition for sustained tumor response [26].

Recent studies implicate the PI3K/AKT pathway, an effector and downstream target of MYCN/C, respectively, in SHH and group 3 MB biology. Thus, PI3K/AKT inhibitors also represent attractive new drug approaches for these patients [33]. Indeed small molecule inhibitors of PI3K/AKT have been demonstrated to suppress MB tumorigenesis in in vitro cell culture conditions [34], as well as in MYC-driven mouse models [33]. As MYC overexpression confers aggressive and metastatic behavior in MB [35], there has been considerable interest in directly targeting MYC or altering MYC downstream effects. Intriguingly, recent studies in myeloma and lymphoma models have shown the effective use of BET bromo-domain inhibitors to suppress MYC expression [36]. More interestingly, recent focus on screening synthetic lethal targets for MYC-driven cancer also identified potential new targets such as the core SUMOylation machinery and eukaryotic initiation factor complex assembly that are required to support MYC oncogenic state [36], for therapeutic opportunities. It is anticipated that with further dissection of MB subgroups and development of more precise subtype models that treatment of MB will approach a truly tailored approach with regimens that incorporate a spectrum of biologic agents that will improve patient outcomes with minimal sequelae.

Central Nervous System Primitive Neuroectodermal Tumor/ Pineoblastoma

Epidemiology

Central nervous system primitive neuroectodermal tumors (CNS-PNETs) encompass a collection of embryonal tumors which are poorly differentiated with varying degrees of neuronal, astrocytic, or ependymal differentiation. They represent ~2.5 % of all childhood brain tumors [5] and are predominantly hemispheric in location but can also arise in multiple other CNS locations including the posterior fossa. In the most recent WHO classification system, CNS-PNETs are subcategorized based on location and histology and include CNS-PNET-NOS or supratentorial-PNET which are hemispheric tumors without any distinctive histologic features that overlap with tumors previously labeled as SPNET. Other categories identified by specific histologic features include CNS-neuroblastoma, CNS-ganglioneuroblastoma, medulloepithelioma, and ependymoblastoma. Cerebral neuroblastomas

and ganglioneuroblastoma, respectively, display only neuronal differentiation or with the presence of ganglion cells. Medulloepitheliomas are rare and diagnosed based on the presence of features resembling embryonic neural tube formation, while ependymoblastoma are characterized by distinct multilayered "ependymoblastic" rosettes; however, accuracy and specificity of this subclassification is under debate [5], and ependymoblastomas has been proposed to overlap with the recently described aggressive ETANTR/EMTR histologic entity [6]. These observations highlight the significant challenge in histological classification of CNS-PNET, particularly for subtypes which exhibit closely related variant histology. Emerging data suggest these may also represent closely related biological and molecular entities. CNS-PNETs diagnosis and classification have been challenging and remain in flux. Notably, pineal region PNET has been considered and treated as SPNET in clinical trials; however, their biologic relatedness to tumors currently classified under the CNS-PNET umbrella remains unclear. A full understanding of the molecular spectrum of this broad category of CNS-PNET and their relationship to tumors restricted to the pineal region is critical for development of more specific diagnostics and therapeutics.

Clinical/Imaging Findings

Clinical presentation of CNS-PNETs varies and can include a broad range of symptoms related to tumor location; however, signs and symptoms of increased intracranial pressure are most common. CNS-PNETs located in the cerebral hemispheres usually present as heterogeneously enhancing large, deep-seated lesions that may contain areas of calcification and may be difficult to distinguish from other malignant hemispheric lesions.

Molecular Features of CNS-PNETs

Although CNS-PNETs may share close histologic resemblance with MB, cumulative studies of small tumor cohorts show they lack genomic features commonly found in MB including isochromosome 17q and MYCC amplification, reviewed in [37]. Li et al. [8] first studied a substantial cohort of 40 hemispheric CNS-PNET using global gene expression and copy number profiling and reported the discovery of a novel oncogenic miRNA cluster that was amplified in 25 % of CNS-PNETs. They demonstrated that tumors with C19MC amplification were frequently CNS-PNETs with variant histologic features and included tumors labeled as ETANTRs, CNS-PNETs with ependymal differentiation, medulloepithelioma, and ependymoblastoma. In a subsequent study, Korshunov et al. [38] confirmed that the C19MC amplicon identified CNS-PNETs variants with histologic features of rosette formation that they called EMTR. In a more recent study, Picard et al. conducted global profiling and immunohistochemical analyses on 142 CNS-PNETs arising in the cerebral hemisphere and demonstrated that the C19MC-amplified tumors (called group 1) also expressed high levels of LIN28, a pluripotency marker [7]. Notably, C19MC amplification/LIN28-positive CNS-PNETs are not restricted to the cerebral hemispheres, indicating C19MC/LIN28 identifies a single molecular disease that may exhibit disparate histologies and location. Thus, C19MC amplification and LIN28 expression represent powerful molecular tools to identify and define the true incidence of group 1 CNS-PNETs, which may not be as uncommon as previously anticipated.

Picard et al. [7] also identified two other molecular classes of CNS-PNETs with oligoneural (group 2) and mesenchymal (group 3) gene expression signatures in their global study. Group 2 CNS-PNETs characterized by an oligoneural gene signature, arose most frequently in older children, and were predominantly localized (15 % were metastatic). The group 3 mesenchymal subgroup, which were identified by the lack of both LIN28 and OLIG2 expression, were found across age groups and had the highest incidence (65 %) of metastases [7]. Thus, OLIG2 expression may serve as an important marker to identify CNS-PNETs with low risk of metastasis. To date no specific histologic features which correlate with group 2 and 3 CNS-PNETs signatures

have been identified. Interestingly, a recent study suggested that a specific mutation of the H3.3 gene (H3.3G34R), which is seen in about 25 % of glioblastoma, is also found in subset of CNS-PNETs [39]. These findings highlight long-standing challenges with histologic diagnosis of CNS-PNET and suggest that molecular features of some tumors diagnosed as CNS-PNETs and GBMs may overlap. Together with the identification of candidate immuno-markers for CNS-PNETs, these studies will now enable better categorization of the spectrum of undifferentiated malignant neuroepithelial tumors arising in the cerebrum.

Although certain copy number features were more commonly seen in group 2 versus group 3 tumors, no cytogenetic alterations exclusive to group 2 and 3 tumors were observed. N-Myc amplification and deletion of CDKN2A/B tumor suppressor locus (Chr9p21.3) which have been previously reported were observed in a proportion of group 2 and 3 tumors [40]. Future larger-scale studies will enable more comprehensive analysis of the clinical implications of these genetic lesions in CNS-PNETs.

Therapeutic Approaches for CNS-PNETs

Similar to MB, maximal safe surgery is also recommended for CNS-PNETs; however, due to the deep-seated nature of these tumors, safe complete tumor resection is often difficult to achieve. Currently, postsurgical therapy for CNS-PNET is similar to that for high-risk medulloblastoma [41, 42] with delivery of higher dose craniospinal irradiation in older children. However, survival rates of CNS-PNET are significantly poorer, with overall survival rates reported at <50 % regardless of therapy received [17, 41]. Determinants of treatment failures in CNS-PNETs are not clear; however, limited data from a number of small studies suggest that an extent of resection and treatment with irradiation are important prognostic factors [43]. Notably, predominant local failures reported in retrospective studies of CNS-PNETs together with pilot studies of risk-adapted radiation

[44, 45] suggest that a proportion of older children with hemispheric CNS-PNETs may be cured with reduced dose or volume of irradiation. As group 2 OLIG2+ CNS-PNETs are predominantly localized, OLIG2 may represent a promising marker for treatment stratification of CNS-PNETs.

Poorest outcomes have been observed in infants with CNS-PNET and may reflect omission or reduction of radiotherapy as radiotherapy has been identified as a significant predictor of progression-free and overall survival [42, 44]. However, it may also reflect the distinct biology of CNS-PNETs arising in younger children. Data to date suggest a particularly aggressive course for the ETANTR/EMTR tumors which comprise group 1 CNS-PNETs. Gene expression signatures suggest activation of SHH and noncanonical WNT pathways in C19MC/LIN28+ group 1 tumors [7]; thus SHH pathway inhibitors, such as GDC-0449 or LDE225, represent promising novel therapeutics that warrants further investigation in this disease. Significantly, recent studies demonstrate that LIN28 activates the insulin-PI3K-mTOR pathway in these tumors and treatment with mTOR inhibitors abrogates growth of an ETANTR/EMTR cell line [46]. These studies suggest that drugs targeting the insulin-mTOR signaling warrant further evaluation in this disease.

Pineoblastoma

Pineoblastomas are grade 4 tumors arising in the pineal region that have traditionally been included as "supratentorial PNETs" in clinical trials, as they histologically resemble small round blue cell embryonal tumors that arise in other regions of the CNS. They comprise 40 % of tumors arising within the pineal parenchyma [5]. The differential diagnosis for pineoblastomas includes germ cell tumors and low-grade glial tumors that arise in the region of the tectal plate/pineal gland as well as benign pineal tumors and other nonmalignant masses. Radiologic features of an enhancing poorly circumscribed pineal mass would favor a malignant tumor diagnosis such as germ cell tumor or pineoblastoma. Histopathologic features

of pineoblastoma predominantly resemble that of primitive pineal or retinal tissues. Only a small number of pineoblastomas have been examined at the molecular level [40, 47]; thus a comprehensive molecular picture has yet to emerge. Notably tumors with molecular features of ETANTR/EMTR have also been reported in the pineal region, suggesting that a proportion of tumor diagnosed as pineoblastomas in younger children may be C19MC/LIN28 group 1 CNS-PNETs.

Demographically pineoblastomas are most frequently found in younger children and may be associated with heritable RB1 alterations and present concurrently with retinoblastoma [48]. Thus, ophthalmological examination of young children presenting with pineoblastoma is recommended to rule out "trilateral" retinoblastoma. Children can present with hydrocephalus due to third ventricular obstruction as well as ocular signs of a pineal mass.

Younger children with pineoblastoma frequently present with or recur with metastatic disease thus making treatment pineoblastoma highly challenging [49]. Metastatic disease at diagnosis and young age has been identified as negative prognosticators and is likely to be age-related treatment approaches. Notably, although Fangusaro et al. [50] reported worse outcomes for pineoblastoma than hemispheric CNS-PNET treated in the Head Start protocol, outcomes for pineoblastomas in older children treated with chemoradiotherapy protocols have been reported to be significantly better than hemispheric CNS-PNETs [51, 52]. Whether these discrepant observations reflect age-related differences in pineoblastoma biology remains to be studied.

Prospects and Future Directions

Since the first publication on gene expression signatures of embryonal tumors [53], molecular studies of MB and rarer embryonal tumors, such as CNS-PNETs, have rapidly advanced. Discovery of clinically relevant molecular subclasses of MB and CNS-PNETs has highlighted the molecular heterogeneity of these tumors and provided new diagnostic and prognostic tools.

With new molecular tools in hand, we are poised to quickly enter an era of trials where molecular information will significantly enhance clinical predictors for risk stratification and patient outcomes. Additionally these studies have uncovered novel targetable genes and pathways that necessitate the development of biology-based therapeutic trials for evaluation. For both MB and CNS-PNETs, the rapid pace of these significant achievements has only been possible with the establishment of large collaborative consortia which have provided the power to delineate molecular subgroups in relatively rare diseases. Similar global efforts will be necessary in clinical trials to enable robust translation of biological discoveries to precision in patient care. Additionally, continued global effort will be necessary to provide further refinement in molecular classification, particularly for rarer types of embryonal brain tumors such as CNS-PNETs and pineoblastoma.

References

1. Packer RJ, et al. Medulloblastoma and primitive neuroectodermal tumors. Handb Clin Neurol. 2012;105: 529–48.
2. McKean-Cowdin R, et al. Trends in childhood brain tumor incidence, 1973-2009. J Neurooncol. 2013;115(2):153–60.
3. Packer RJ, Vezina G. Management of and prognosis with medulloblastoma: therapy at a crossroads. Arch Neurol. 2008;65(11):1419–24.
4. Tortori-Donati P, et al. Medulloblastoma in children: CT and MRI findings. Neuroradiology. 1996;38(4): 352–9.
5. Louis DN, International Agency for Research on Cancer. WHO classification of tumours of the central nervous system, World Health Organization classification of tumours. 4th ed. Lyon: International Agency for Research on Cancer; 2007.
6. Gessi M, et al. Embryonal tumors with abundant neuropil and true rosettes: a distinctive CNS primitive neuroectodermal tumor. Am J Surg Pathol. 2009; 33(2):211–7.
7. Picard D, et al. Markers of survival and metastatic potential in childhood CNS primitive neuroectodermal brain tumours: an integrative genomic analysis. Lancet Oncol. 2012;13(8):838–48.
8. Li M, et al. Frequent amplification of a chr19q13.41 microRNA polycistron in aggressive primitive neuroectodermal brain tumors. Cancer Cell. 2009;16(6): 533–46.
9. Oliver TG, Wechsler-Reya RJ. Getting at the root and stem of brain tumors. Neuron. 2004;42(6):885–8.
10. Taylor MD, et al. Molecular subgroups of medulloblastoma: the current consensus. Acta Neuropathol. 2012;123(4):465–72.
11. Northcott PA, et al. The clinical implications of medulloblastoma subgroups. Nat Rev Neurol. 2012; 8(6):340–51.
12. Rieken S, et al. Outcome and prognostic factors of radiation therapy for medulloblastoma. Int J Radiat Oncol Biol Phys. 2011;81(3):e7–13.
13. Rutkowski S, et al. Treatment of early childhood medulloblastoma by postoperative chemotherapy alone. N Engl J Med. 2005;352(10):978–86.
14. Grill J, et al. Treatment of medulloblastoma with postoperative chemotherapy alone: an SFOP prospective trial in young children. Lancet Oncol. 2005;6(8): 573–80.
15. Grundy RG, et al. Primary postoperative chemotherapy without radiotherapy for treatment of brain tumours other than ependymoma in children under 3 years: results of the first UKCCSG/SIOP CNS 9204 trial. Eur J Cancer. 2010;46(1):120–33.
16. Fangusaro J, et al. Intensive chemotherapy followed by consolidative myeloablative chemotherapy with autologous hematopoietic cell rescue (AuHCR) in young children with newly diagnosed supratentorial primitive neuroectodermal tumors (sPNETs): report of the Head Start I and II experience. Pediatr Blood Cancer. 2008;50(2):312–8.
17. Geyer JR, et al. Multiagent chemotherapy and deferred radiotherapy in infants with malignant brain tumors: a report from the Children's Cancer Group. J Clin Oncol. 2005;23(30):7621–31.
18. Packer RJ, et al. Phase III study of craniospinal radiation therapy followed by adjuvant chemotherapy for newly diagnosed average-risk medulloblastoma. J Clin Oncol. 2006;24(25):4202–8.
19. Lannering B, et al. Hyperfractionated versus conventional radiotherapy followed by chemotherapy in standard-risk medulloblastoma: results from the randomized multicenter HIT-SIOP PNET 4 trial. J Clin Oncol. 2012;30(26):3187–93.
20. Gajjar A, et al. Risk-adapted craniospinal radiotherapy followed by high-dose chemotherapy and stem-cell rescue in children with newly diagnosed medulloblastoma (St Jude Medulloblastoma-96): long-term results from a prospective, multicentre trial. Lancet Oncol. 2006;7(10):813–20.
21. Jakacki RI, et al. Outcome of children with metastatic medulloblastoma treated with carboplatin during craniospinal radiotherapy: a Children's Oncology Group Phase I/II study. J Clin Oncol. 2012;30(21):2648–53.
22. Pizer B, et al. Treatment of recurrent central nervous system primitive neuroectodermal tumours in children and adolescents: results of a Children's Cancer and Leukaemia Group study. Eur J Cancer. 2011; 47(9):1389–97.
23. Donahue B, et al. Radiation therapy quality in CCG/ POG intergroup 9961: implications for craniospinal

irradiation and the posterior fossa boost in future medulloblastoma trials. Front Oncol. 2012;2:185.

24. LoRusso PM, et al. Phase I trial of hedgehog pathway inhibitor vismodegib (GDC-0449) in patients with refractory, locally advanced or metastatic solid tumors. Clin Cancer Res. 2011;17(8):2502–11.

25. Rudin CM, et al. Treatment of medulloblastoma with hedgehog pathway inhibitor GDC-0449. N Engl J Med. 2009;361(12):1173–8.

26. Buonamici S, et al. Interfering with resistance to smoothened antagonists by inhibition of the PI3K pathway in medulloblastoma. Sci Transl Med. 2010;2(51):51.

27. Fouladi M, et al. A molecular biology and phase II trial of lapatinib in children with refractory CNS malignancies: a pediatric brain tumor consortium study. J Neurooncol. 2013;114(2):173–9.

28. Kongkham PN, et al. Inhibition of the MET Receptor Tyrosine Kinase as a Novel Therapeutic Strategy in Medulloblastoma. Transl Oncol. 2010;3(6):336–43.

29. Fouladi M, et al. A phase II study of the farnesyl transferase inhibitor, tipifarnib, in children with recurrent or progressive high-grade glioma, medulloblastoma/primitive neuroectodermal tumor, or brainstem glioma: a Children's Oncology Group study. Cancer. 2007;110(11):2535–41.

30. Lee MJ, et al. Hedgehog pathway inhibitor saridegib (IPI-926) increases lifespan in a mouse medulloblastoma model. Proc Natl Acad Sci U S A. 2012;109(20): 7859–64.

31. de Bont JM, et al. Biological background of pediatric medulloblastoma and ependymoma: a review from a translational research perspective. Neuro Oncol. 2008;10(6):1040–60.

32. Spiller SE, et al. Response of preclinical medulloblastoma models to combination therapy with 13-cis retinoic acid and suberoylanilide hydroxamic acid (SAHA). J Neurooncol. 2008;87(2):133–41.

33. Pei Y, et al. An animal model of MYC-driven medulloblastoma. Cancer Cell. 2012;21(2):155–67.

34. Baryawno N, et al. Small-molecule inhibitors of phosphatidylinositol 3-kinase/Akt signaling inhibit Wnt/beta-catenin pathway cross-talk and suppress medulloblastoma growth. Cancer Res. 2010;70(1):266–76.

35. Zhou L, et al. Silencing of thrombospondin-1 is critical for myc-induced metastatic phenotypes in medulloblastoma. Cancer Res. 2010;70(20):8199–210.

36. Prochownik EV, Vogt PK. Therapeutic Targeting of Myc. Genes Cancer. 2010;1(6):650–9.

37. Li MH, et al. Molecular genetics of supratentorial primitive neuroectodermal tumors and pineoblastoma. Neurosurg Focus. 2005;19(5):E3.

38. Korshunov A, et al. Focal genomic amplification at 19q13.42 comprises a powerful diagnostic marker for embryonal tumors with ependymoblastic rosettes. Acta Neuropathol. 2010;120(2):253–60.

39. Gessi M, et al. H3.3 G34R mutations in pediatric primitive neuroectodermal tumors of central nervous system (CNS-PNET) and pediatric glioblastomas: possible diagnostic and therapeutic implications? J Neurooncol. 2013;112(1):67–72.

40. Miller S, et al. Genome-wide molecular characterization of central nervous system primitive neuroectodermal tumor and pineoblastoma. Neuro Oncol. 2011;13(8):866–79.

41. Reddy AT, et al. Outcome for children with supratentorial primitive neuroectodermal tumors treated with surgery, radiation, and chemotherapy. Cancer. 2000;88(9): 2189–93.

42. Timmermann B, et al. Role of radiotherapy in supratentorial primitive neuroectodermal tumor in young children: results of the German HIT-SKK87 and HIT-SKK92 trials. J Clin Oncol. 2006;24(10):1554–60.

43. McBride SM, Daganzo SM, Banerjee A, Gupta N, Lamborn KR, Prados MD, Berger MS, Wara WM, Haas-Kogan DA. Radiation is an important component of multimodality therapy for pediatric non-pineal supratentorial primitive neuroectodermal tumors. Int J Radiat Oncol Biol Phys. 2008;72(5):1319–23.

44. Johnston DL, et al. Supratentorial primitive neuroectodermal tumors: a Canadian pediatric brain tumor consortium report. J Neurooncol. 2008;86(1):101–8.

45. Massimino M, et al. Evolving of therapeutic strategies for CNS-PNET. Pediatr Blood Cancer. 2013;60(12): 2031–5.

46. Spence T, et al. A novel C19MC amplified cell line links Lin28/let-7 to mTOR signaling in Embryonal Tumor with Multilayered Rosettes. J Neurooncol. 2014;16(1):62–71.

47. Fevre-Montange M, et al. Microarray analysis reveals differential gene expression patterns in tumors of the pineal region. J Neuropathol Exp Neurol. 2006;65(7): 675–84.

48. Antoneli CB, et al. Trilateral retinoblastoma. Pediatr Blood Cancer. 2007;48(3):306–10.

49. Duffner PK, et al. Lack of efficacy of postoperative chemotherapy and delayed radiation in very young children with pineoblastoma. Pediatric Oncology Group. Med Pediatr Oncol. 1995;25(1):38–44.

50. Fangusaro JR, et al. Brainstem primitive neuroectodermal tumors (bstPNET): results of treatment with intensive induction chemotherapy followed by consolidative chemotherapy with autologous hematopoietic cell rescue. Pediatr Blood Cancer. 2008;50(3): 715–7.

51. Jakacki RI, et al. Survival and prognostic factors following radiation and/or chemotherapy for primitive neuroectodermal tumors of the pineal region in infants and children: a report of the Childrens Cancer Group. J Clin Oncol. 1995;13(6):1377–83.

52. Cohen BH, et al. Prognostic factors and treatment results for supratentorial primitive neuroectodermal tumors in children using radiation and chemotherapy: a Childrens Cancer Group randomized trial. J Clin Oncol. 1995;13(7):1687–96.

53. Pomeroy SL, et al. Prediction of central nervous system embryonal tumour outcome based on gene expression. Nature. 2002;415(6870):436–42.

Ependymoma

13

Juliette Hukin, John-Paul Kilday, and Uri Tabori

Epidemiology

Ependymomas are the third most common brain tumours in the paediatric population compromising 5–10 % of all newly diagnosed childhood brain tumours. Ependymoma represents the second most common malignant brain tumour in childhood. Most childhood intracranial ependymomas arise from the posterior fossa and approximately 25–38 % are of supratentorial origin [1]. Ten to thirteen percent of childhood ependymomas arise from the spinal cord; it is the most common intramedullary spinal cord tumour in childhood. Sixty percent of childhood ependymoma is diagnosed under the age of 5 years; the majority in this age group arises from the posterior fossa and tends to behave more aggressively. In contrast spinal ependymoma is the most common location over all age groups and represents more than 75 % of adult cases of ependymoma. There is predominance in males 0.23:0.17 and in Caucasians 0.21 per 100,000 patient years vs. an incidence of 0.13 per 100,000 patient years in African Americans [1]. Neurofibromatosis (NF) type 2, a familial autosomal dominant condition, predisposes to spinal ependymoma.

J. Hukin, M.B.B.S., F.R.C.P.C. (✉)
Division of Neurology and Oncology,
British Columbia Children's Hospital, Vancouver,
BC, Canada
e-mail: jhukin@cw.bc.ca

J.-P. Kilday, M.B.Ch.B., M.R.C.P.C.H., Ph.D.
Pediatric Brain Tumor Program, Department of
Hematology/Oncology, Hospital for Sick Children,
Toronto, ON, Canada

U. Tabori, M.D.
Department of Hematology/Oncology, The Hospital
for Sick Children/Institute of Medical Sciences,
University of Toronto/The Arthur and Sonia Labatt
Brain Tumour Research Centre, Toronto, ON, Canada

Location and Presenting Symptoms

Posterior fossa ependymomas arise from the floor of the fourth ventricle, the lateral recess (40 %) and the roof of the fourth ventricle (10 %). Seventy-five percent of supratentorial ependymomas arise from the parenchyma; the remainder arise from the lateral ventricle or rarely the third ventricle. The parenchymal ependymoma is thought to arise from the rests of ependymal cells retained in parenchyma during development. They do often arise near the ventricle and may extend into the ventricle. Spinal ependymomas arise from the cauda equina and the central canal of the spinal cord.

K. Scheinemann and E. Bouffet (eds.), *Pediatric Neuro-oncology*,
DOI 10.1007/978-1-4939-1541-5_13, © Springer Science+Business Media New York 2015

Leptomeningeal disease is described in 5–10 % of ependymomas. Five-year event-free survival of those with microscopic dissemination identified on CSF cytology is similar to those with macroscopic disease, magnetic resonance imaging (MRI) positive +/– CSF: approximately 27 %.

Presenting symptoms depend on location and age. Infants present with accelerated head growth, full fontanelle, irritability, vomiting, regression, head tilt with or without neurological deficit, e.g. hemiparesis, cranial nerve deficit and ataxia. Older children often present with headache, vomiting, papilloedema, ataxia and cranial nerve deficit. The spinal cord tumours present more insidiously with progressive back pain over a few months, worse after sleeping or waking the child in the night. The children with cauda equina or conus lesions develop saddle anaesthesia, constipation and urinary retention or overflow incontinence. Those with lesions higher up in the cord present more commonly with scoliosis with or without suspended sensory loss and motor deficits.

Imaging Findings

Standard of care for imaging these tumours to delineate precisely the anatomy of tumour location, the best surgical approach and the extent of the disease is by MRI plus gadolinium of the brain and spine. However 50 % of tumours show calcification, which is most easily visualised on CT. CT however is being used less frequently due to the ionising radiation exposure it entails. MRI T1 with and without contrast, T2, diffusion weighted images are usually performed; some centres also evaluate MRI perfusion and spectroscopy.

Posterior fossa ependymoma: typically signal intensity on T2 weighted images is similar to grey matter throughout most of the lesion, but there may be heterogeneity. On T1 the tumour demonstrates low signal intensity and predominantly solid enhancement. The lesion may extend through the foramen of Luschka into the cerebellopontine angle (15 %) and/or through the foramen of Magendie (60 %) onto the posterior aspect of the cervical cord and may encase blood vessels and lower cranial nerves (Fig. 13.1).

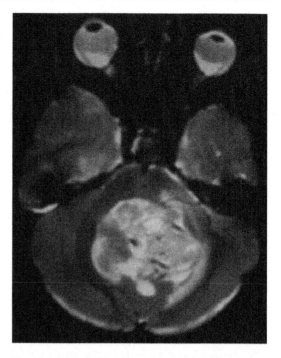

Fig. 13.1 This MRI shows a very large posterior fossa ependymoma filling the fourth ventricle and extending into the left cerebellopontine angle through the foramen of Luschka (Reprinted from Teo C, Nakaji P, Symons P, et al. Ependymoma. Child's Nervous System 2003; 19(5–6): 270–285. With permission from Springer Verlag)

Supratentorial tumours tend to be more heterogeneous, with cystic, calcified and haemorrhagic components. They usually have avidly enhancing areas interspersed with nonenhancing regions (Figs. 13.2 and 13.3).

Pathology

Histological classification of ependymomas is most frequently defined using the World Health Organization (WHO) grading scheme for CNS tumours [2]. According to this system, ependymomas can be divided into four pathological subgroups: subependymoma and myxopapillary ependymoma (both WHO grade I), classic (grade II) and anaplastic (grade III). Within the classic subgroup are four morphological variants: cellular, papillary, clear cell and tanycytic tumours (Table 13.1).

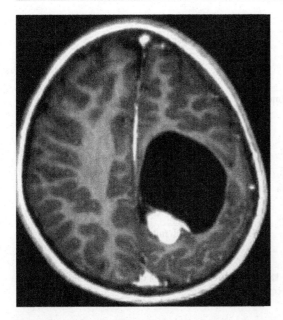

Fig. 13.2 Supratentorial ependymoma. The location makes these tumours more readily resectable. This patient did not have adjuvant therapy and has enjoyed 4 years of recurrence-free survival (Reprinted from Teo C, Nakaji P, Symons P, et al. Ependymoma. Child's Nervous System 2003; 19(5–6): 270–285. With permission from Springer Verlag)

Subependymomas are benign nodules usually found in the intracranial ventricles of adults. Similarly, myxopapillary ependymomas are rarely seen in children and tend to arise almost exclusively in the spine, at the level of the cauda equina. Paediatric intracranial ependymomas are typically of a classic or anaplastic histology. Hallmark microscopic features of classic ependymomas include either perivascular pseudorosettes, formed by the radial arrangement of tumour cells around a blood vessel (perivascular), or true rosettes where the cells circumferentially surround a central lumen or canal [3]. Positive cytoplasmic staining for glial fibrillary acid protein (GFAP) and vimentin is a frequent immunohistochemical finding. Anaplastic ependymomas are additionally differentiated by displaying numerous mitotic figures, substantial necrosis, an increased cellular nucleus/cytoplasmic ratio and microvascular proliferation. Assigning a specific WHO grade to a given tumour remains subjective, lacking uniformity, and is often difficult as ependymomas frequently demonstrate marked intratumoral heterogeneity. This is emphasised by the reported

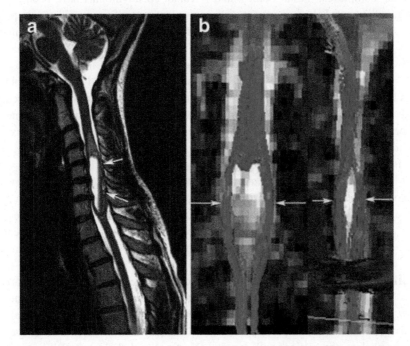

Fig. 13.3 Ependymoma: there is a tumour in the lower cervical spinal cord (**a**) with displacement of the fibres visible on the tractogram (**b**) (Reprinted from Vargas MI, Delavelle J, Jlassi H, et al. Clinical applications of diffusion tensor tractography of the spinal cord. Neuroradiology 2008; 50(1): 25–29. With permission from Springer Verlag)

Table 13.1 Current WHO classifications of ependymomas

WHO grading system	Subgroups	Histopathology
I	Subependymoma	Isomorphic nuclei embedded in a dense fibrillary matrix of glial cell processes with frequent microcystic change
	Myxopapillary ependymoma	Mitoses rare or absent
		GFAP-expressing cuboidal to elongated tumour cells arranged in a papillary manner around vascular stromal cores
II (classic)	Cellular ependymoma	Monomorphic nuclear morphology
	Papillary ependymoma	Mitoses rare or absent
	Clear cell ependymoma	Perivascular pseudorosettes and ependymal rosettes
	Tanycytic ependymoma	
III (anaplastic)		High mitotic activity. Palisading necrosis. Microvascular proliferation. Perivascular pseudorosettes

[Reprinted from Louis DN, Ohgaki H, Wiestler OD, et al. The 2007 WHO classification of tumours of the central nervous system. Acta Neuropathol 2007;114:97–109. With permission from Springer Verlag]

incidence of anaplastic ependymoma, varying from 7 to 89 % of cohorts analysed.

Electron microscopy may be used to confirm the histological identification of ependymoma; characteristic features include cilia, microvilli, long junctional complexes, basal bodies and intracytoplasmic filaments [4].

Biology

Recent times have witnessed an increase in studies aiming to improve our understanding of the nature and origins of molecular genetic abnormalities found in ependymoma. What is becoming apparent is that ependymoma is a biologically diverse and complex entity which, akin to medulloblastoma, appears to be comprised of biologically and functionally distinct molecular subclasses.

Predisposition Syndromes

The majority of paediatric ependymomas arise spontaneously without a known predisposition syndrome. Nevertheless, associations with certain conditions have been reported. For instance, neurofibromatosis type 2 is an autosomal dominant condition caused by a germline mutation in the *NF2/Merlin* gene (22q12.2). This disorder is particularly associated with the formation of vestibular schwannomas, although spinal ependymomas can be a relatively common finding [5]. Intracranial ependymomas have been described as a rare feature of Turcot syndrome type 2 [6]. This familial disorder is caused by inherited mutations of the *APC* gene (5q22.2) and is characterised by the development of intestinal polyps, yet is more commonly associated with medulloblastoma formation. Familial ependymomas occurring in the absence of such inherited syndromes have also been described, although these are extremely rare.

Cell of Origin

The morphological similarity between neoplastic ependymoma cells and normal ependymal cells lining the CNS ventricular system made the latter a presumed cell of origin for this tumour. However, recent stem cell characterisation studies have suggested that tumour initiation may actually arise in primitive radial glial cells (RGCs), which demonstrate both stem (CD133+/ Nestin+) *and* glial (Rc2+/Blbp+) immunophenotypes. These RGCs have been shown in vitro to self-renew, and differentiate, whilst also forming ependymomas when transplanted into immuno-compromised mice, making them attractive candidates [7, 8]. If this concept proves correct, it may lead to a shift in therapy by targeting these ependymoma-initiating cells in addition to reducing tumour bulk.

Molecular Subgroups

Earlier biological studies have shown distinct molecular differences between spinal, supratentorial and posterior fossa ependymomas, suggesting tumour location may be an important driving factor for these lesions [7]. Whilst the precise number remains uncertain, up to nine molecular subclasses of ependymoma from these three sites have now been suggested according to a combination of intrinsic chromosomal abnormalities and characteristic 'driving' gene mutations (such as *NOTCH1* or *EPHB2* amplification). For instance, at least two molecularly distinct subclasses of posterior fossa ependymoma have been confirmed, each associated with a specific patient age group and clinical outcome [9]. Likewise, supratentorial tumours can be divided into two groups according the expression of genes controlling neuronal differentiation [10].

There is also evidence from chromosome imbalance work that childhood and adult ependymomas are biologically distinct, irrespective of tumour location, with gain of chromosomes 1q, 7 and 9 and loss of chromosomes 22, 3 and 9p being frequent in paediatric tumours [11]. Moreover, a 'balanced' genomic profile, without chromosomal gain or loss, has been reported in up to 58 % of paediatric ependymomas, particularly those under 3 years of age. This contrasts with adult ependymomas where a balanced genome is found in less than 10 % of cases [11].

Prognostic Factors

Due to the relatively poor survival outcomes of ependymoma when compared with other paediatric CNS tumours, there remains great interest in determining prognostic factors for this tumour group in order to risk stratify patients and tailor therapy appropriately. Several clinical, pathological and biological correlates of outcome have been assessed, primarily using data from retrospective cohort studies.

Clinicopathological Factors

Surgical Resection

The degree of tumour removal, particularly a gross total resection (GTR), appears the most favourable and consistent clinical prognostic factor reported from retrospective case series, with 5-year survival rates being reported as high as 80 %, compared to 22–47 % for cases of incomplete resection [11–13]. However, literature suggests that for approximately one-third of childhood intracranial ependymomas, GTR is not achieved. This is particularly the case for infratentorial tumours extending to involve the lower cranial nerves and associated vasculature, where aggressive resection can be associated with substantial morbidity.

Tumour Location

There is insufficient evidence that intracranial location impacts on patient prognosis, independent of that explained by surgical accessibility and the ease of achieving a GTR. There is data, albeit limited, to suggest complete resection for certain supratentorial ependymomas can be curative [14]. Indeed, the North American Children's Oncology Group (COG) currently recommends only a post-operative observation strategy for grade II supratentorial tumours where GTR has been achieved.

Age

Historically, a younger age at diagnosis has frequently been associated with shorter patient survival. Possible explanations for this include an age-related difference in underlying tumour biology, or the practice of delaying or avoiding adjuvant radiotherapy to the developing central nervous system. However, whilst the majority of studies reveal an association with age, this is not consistent as some studies report no prognostic difference between contrasting paediatric age groups [15].

WHO Grade

A distinct difference in survival outcomes between anaplastic and classical ependymomas, according to the WHO grading system, remains unproven. This probably reflects the difficulty of applying such a classification scheme in clinical practice due to intratumoural heterogeneity, inter-observer variability and the inability to uniformly define anaplasia. Whilst some studies have observed an adverse prognosis for anaplastic ependymomas, other studies have refuted this. Unfortunately, alternative classification schemes have also failed to prove either reproducible or prognostic [16].

Biological Factors

Molecular Subgroups

As stated, advances in tumour molecular analysis (high-throughput gene expression and genomic arrays, tissue microarray analysis by immunohistochemistry and fluorescence in situ hybridisation, etc.) have enabled new biological subgroups of ependymoma to be identified. For instance, gene expression profiling of posterior fossa ependymomas has delineated at least two distinct prognostic groups [9, 17]. One such set of tumours (termed 'Group A' or '1') were often located laterally in the cerebellopontine angle, frequently demonstrated overexpression of genes including *laminin-alpha 2* (*LAMA2*), or genes involved in mesenchymal/extracellular matrix development such as *Tenascin-C* (*TNC*), and were associated with a younger patient age, recurrence and metastasis. The contrasting group of ependymomas ('Group B' or '2') were primarily located centrally, found predominantly in adolescents or adults and were less invasive. Consequently, the progression-free survival (PFS) and overall survival (OS) rates for Group A/1 ependymomas were significantly poorer than for Group 2/B tumours. Likewise, biological prognostic subgroups of supratentorial ependymomas have been identified according to the expression of genes implicated in neuronal differentiation such as *NFL70*, where overexpression independently conferred an improved PFS [10].

Chromosomal Imbalances

Gain of chromosome 1q is the most common chromosomal imbalance observed in paediatric ependymomas, when compared to adult tumours [11]. Nevertheless, it is only observed in approximately 20 % of cases [18]. Several retrospective genomic studies performed in both North America and Europe, including analyses of uniformly treated clinical trial cohorts, have confirmed an adverse prognostic role for 1q gain, being associated with a worse patient PFS and OS. Studies have also proposed incorporating 1q gain into future patient risk group stratifications in order to tailor therapy more appropriately [19]. The precise mechanism of 1q gain and why, in turn, this seems to impart a worse outcome for patients remains unclear.

Gain of another chromosomal region, 9q33-34, has been shown to occur relatively frequently at recurrence, in addition to being associated with an adverse prognosis in paediatric ependymoma. This region encompasses the loci of genes thought to be implicated in ependymoma pathogenesis such as *NOTCH1* and *TNC* [18].

Individual Molecular Markers

Several biological markers have been proposed as correlates of adverse outcome in paediatric ependymoma from retrospective case series of paediatric ependymoma. These include overexpression of human telomerase reverse transcriptase (hTERT) [20] and its nuclear chaperone Nucleolin [21], the extracellular matrix proteins TNC and LAMA2 [9, 22], p53 [23], EGFR [24, 25], the transcription factor EVI-1 [26] and the stem cell marker Nestin [27].

However, all of these putative prognostic candidates have not been completely validated, either by generating reproducible findings in different retrospective cohorts or indeed in a prospective clinical trial setting. Until this is undertaken, definitive conclusions regarding their effectiveness as prognostic markers in paediatric ependymoma should be considered with caution.

Evidence has shown, however, that ependymoma can no longer be considered a single biological entity. Indeed, as suggested by Grill and colleagues, due to the biological complexity and diversity of paediatric ependymoma, future prognostic predictions may require a set of several biomarkers which have relevance for a particular molecular subset of the tumour, as is currently the case for medulloblastomas [18].

Treatment

Surgery is the main initial treatment modality but curative as single modality therapy when complete removal is possible with acceptable functional outcome only in the minority of childhood ependymoma. This mainly applies for tumours arising from the spinal cord. Following reports of potential cure of supratentorial ependymoma with resection alone [14], COG has been evaluating the possibility of observation only in supratentorial WHO grade 2 ependymoma following a complete resection; the results of this clinical trial are awaited.

Posterior fossa tumours represent the majority of cases in childhood; a GTR is aimed for, sometimes sacrificing cranial nerve function, as the extent of resection is recognised to have an impact on cure rate. There is always careful consideration of long-term surgical morbidity vs. improving cure rate with the extent of resection. Most centres would not consider that the requirement of lifelong tracheostomy or G-tube is an acceptable intentional morbidity of surgery. Unfortunately these tumours may be wrapped around major blood vessels in the posterior fossa as well as infiltrating lower cranial nerves thus making it impossible to perform a total resection. Intraoperative brainstem monitoring, sensory- and motor-evoked potentials should be considered where the tumour likely involves cranial nerve, brainstem or spinal cord, to minimise postsurgical morbidity. In addition intracranial ependymomas can be very vascular, particularly the large tumours of young children, requiring a second stage surgical resection either up front or following some chemotherapy [28].

Spinal cord tumours are generally WHO grade 1 and can be observed even in the absence of a complete resection, with the aim to reresect at the time of progression or recurrence and consideration of involved field post-operative radiation at that time.

There is a small risk of recurrence with metastases; however, this is rare with spinal ependymoma. Occasionally multiple primaries of the spinal cord occur; this should raise the suspicion of neurofibromatosis type 2.

Radiation therapy to the involved field has been standard for WHO grade 2 and grade 3 tumours following resection, and provides a survival advantage [29]. Conformal, stereotactic and proton beam radiation are presently being used to the tumour bed to provide more precise radiation and less long-term morbidity. Radiation is being reconsidered in children as young as 12 months of age, as it is proposed that the long-term cognitive decline in the young is significantly less dramatic and more acceptable with focal radiation as opposed to craniospinal radiation, particularly with more precise techniques [30]. Long-term prospective multi-institutional studies especially in children < 5 years of age at the time of the radiation have yet to confirm satisfactory long-term morbidity. Molecular signatures of ependymoma may in the future help us identify which intracranial ependymomas will behave less aggressively and may either not need radiation or may not need a GTR to be cured; type B posterior fossa ependymoma has an excellent prognosis [9]. In general it is deemed only necessary to radiate the craniospinal axis if there is evidence of dissemination at diagnosis, as failure in patients with localised disease is at the primary site in 90 % of patients.

The role of chemotherapy in treating ependymomas is not clear. It can induce a partial or complete response in some patients and it may be helpful in facilitating second-look surgery.

It has been used to delay radiotherapy in infant protocols with disappointing results for the most part but effective in some patients obviating the need for radiation [31–33]. It is presently being evaluated in residual and anaplastic disease following resection and radiation in the open COG protocol for those who are 12 months of age or older.

Chemotherapy after resection and radiation for those with residual intracranial ependymoma post resection was proposed by Needle in 1997 and consisted of a regime of carboplatin, vincristine, ifosfamide and etoposide delivered for four cycles [34]. The 5-year PFS was 74 %, superior to radiation alone following surgery. Chemotherapy after surgery but before radiation has been evaluated by Garvin to manage residual disease after surgery. Vincristine, cisplatin and cyclophosphamide were delivered in four cycles with each lasting 21 days. Of 35 patients evaluable for response, 40 % had a complete response, 17 % a partial response and 14 % progressed through chemotherapy. The pre-irradiation chemotherapy group demonstrated EFS comparable to those with no residual who were treated post resection with radiation alone. However benefit from chemotherapy was restricted to patients who had had more than 90 % of the tumour resected [28].

Attempts have been made to delay or avoid radiation in infants due to concern regarding long-term morbidity following brain radiation particularly of children under 3 years of age. The Baby Pediatric Oncology Group protocol consisting of 28-day cycles of chemotherapy is used for children younger than 36 months to delay radiation until the child reaches that age. The chemotherapy consisted of vincristine, cyclophosphamide alternating with cisplatin and etoposide. Those less than 24 months of age at diagnosis had a significantly worse outcome 12 % 5-year PFS vs. 55 % 5-year PFS in those 24–36 months of age at diagnosis; this is presumed to be due to more prolonged delay in radiation [32]; however, potential confounding factors include younger age with more aggressive tumour biology and lesions less amenable to a meaningful resection. Grundy reports the UK/SIOP experience of alternating cycles of myelosuppressive and non-myelosuppressive chemotherapy, with a 5-year cumulative incidence of freedom from radiotherapy of 42 % in infants with non-metastatic ependymoma at diagnosis. The median time to progression was 1.6 years and 80 % had local recurrences [31]. Head Start 1 and 2 chemotherapy including IV methotrexate in induction for five metastatic ependymomas [33] provided 80 % overall survival; however, radiation-free survival in the whole ependymoma group ($n=29$) was only 8 %; those without dissemination did not receive methotrexate with this protocol.

Venkatramani reports a more favourable outcome in supratentorial ependymoma: 86 % 3 year event-free survival following treatment with the Head Start 3 regimen [35].

Recurrent Ependymoma

Recurrent ependymoma is still a challenge which occurs in up to half the cases depending on the above prognostic factors. Recurrent ependymoma has a unique pattern which is different than other malignant paediatric brain tumours such as medulloblastoma and ATRT and can be exploited for therapeutic use. Most of tumour recurrences are local and complete surgical resection can be achieved. Upon successive relapse, tumours tend to metastasise. Pathologically, tumours tend to change to higher grade with successive recurrences [36].

Treatment and Outcome of Recurrent Ependymoma

In most series, recurrent ependymoma still has dismal outcome. However, the course may be indolent and protracted enabling the study of multiple approaches. Surgical resection is often feasible in local recurrence and in selected cases of well-demarcated nodules. Although not curative, this can result in prolonged tumour-free survival. Due to its indolent course, multiple chemotherapeutic regimens and combinations were tested with or without novel agents. These results have not resulted in significant tumour control or change in outcome.

Radiation therapy for children who were not irradiated upfront has resulted in cure for a significant proportion of patients [31] and should be considered, especially with aggressive surgery when appropriate. Reirradiation has been shown to be both feasible and safe and improve outcome [36–38]. Radiosurgery has shown some positive results in selected cases but larger series do not reveal improved outcome and recurrence outside the radiation field is common.

Conformal reirradiation to a total cumulative dose of more than 100 Gy to local recurrence is associated with high rates of local tumour control and lack of radiation necrosis if performed more than a year from initial radiation therapy. Craniospinal radiation, with surgery of primary and metastatic disease, has shown prolonged PFS in several series [36, 38, 39]. Although improved overall survival has been shown using this approach, larger prospective studies are required to determine the curative potential of this approach.

Novel therapies have shown frustrating unsatisfactory results so far. Nevertheless, rational therapies stemming from biological studies have shown some encouraging results. In a drug screen based on molecular characterisation of supratentorial ependymoma, 5FU has shown efficacy in vitro and in vivo and this regimen is being tested in a phase II clinical trial [40]. Better understanding of the events which characterise recurrent ependymomas may lead to additional rational targeted therapies which may improve outcome to these patients.

Long-Term Outcome and Summary

The long-term cure and outcome of patients is improving with advances in neurosurgical techniques allowing a meaningful resection whilst minimising secondary neurological deficits. Also imperative to better long-term outcome includes the ability to provide precise radiation to the majority of patients without craniospinal disease minimising long-term cognitive and functional impairment. Increased availability of neuroimaging will potentially allow earlier detection and thus possibly decrease morbidity associated with metastasis, large vascular tumours, attachment to cranial nerves and around major blood vessels and hydrocephalus, all features contributing to long-term morbidity in survivors. The role of chemotherapy although limited at this time is helpful in some cases and may play a larger role in the future for specific more aggressive subtypes. Advances in molecular biology may assist in the future, regarding stratification of therapy and novel therapies for the most challenging tumours.

References

1. McGuire CS, Sainani KL, Fisher PG. Incidence patterns for ependymoma: a surveillance, epidemiology, and end results study. J Neurosurg. 2009;110:725–9.
2. Louis DN, Ohgaki H, Wiestler OD, et al. The 2007 WHO classification of tumours of the central nervous system. Acta Neuropathol. 2007;114:97–109.
3. Goldwein JW, Leahy JM, Packer RJ, et al. Intracranial ependymomas in children. Int J Radiat Oncol Biol Phys. 1990;19:1497–502.
4. Rosenblum MK. Ependymal tumors: a review of their diagnostic surgical pathology. Pediatr Neurosurg. 1998;28:160–5.
5. Evans DG. Neurofibromatosis type 2 (NF2): a clinical and molecular review. Orphanet J Rare Dis. 2009;4:16.
6. Onilude OE, Lusher ME, Lindsey JC, Pearson AD, Ellison DW, Clifford SC. APC and CTNNB1 mutations are rare in sporadic ependymomas. Cancer Genet Cytogenet. 2006;168:158–61.
7. Taylor MD, Poppleton H, Fuller C, et al. Radial glia cells are candidate stem cells of ependymoma. Cancer Cell. 2005;8:323–35.
8. Johnson RA, Wright KD, Poppleton H, et al. Cross-species genomics matches driver mutations and cell compartments to model ependymoma. Nature. 2010; 466:632–6.
9. Witt H, Mack SC, Ryzhova M, et al. Delineation of two clinically and molecularly distinct subgroups of posterior fossa ependymoma. Cancer Cell. 2011; 20:143–57.
10. Andreiuolo F, Puget S, Peyre M, et al. Neuronal differentiation distinguishes supratentorial and infratentorial childhood ependymomas. Neuro Oncol. 2010; 12(11):1126–34.
11. Kilday JP, Rahman R, Dyer S, et al. Pediatric ependymoma: biological perspectives. Mol Cancer Res. 2009; 7:765–86.
12. Bouffet E, Perilongo G, Canete A, Massimino M. Intracranial ependymomas in children: a critical review of prognostic factors and a plea for cooperation. Med Pediatr Oncol. 1998;30:319–29; discussion 29–31.
13. Merchant TE, Li C, Xiong X, Kun LE, Boop FA, Sanford RA. Conformal radiotherapy after surgery for paediatric ependymoma: a prospective study. Lancet Oncol. 2009;10:258–66.
14. Hukin J, Epstein F, Lefton D, Allen J. Treatment of intracranial ependymoma by surgery alone. Pediatr Neurosurg. 1998;29:40–5.
15. Robertson PL, Zeltzer PM, Boyett JM, et al. Survival and prognostic factors following radiation therapy and chemotherapy for ependymomas in children: a report of the Children's Cancer Group. J Neurosurg. 1998;88:695–703.
16. Ellison DW, Kocak M, Figarella-Branger D, et al. Histopathological grading of pediatric ependymoma: reproducibility and clinical relevance in European trial cohorts. J Negat Results Biomed. 2011;10:7.

17. Wani K, Armstrong TS, Vera-Bolanos E, et al. A prognostic gene expression signature in infratentorial ependymoma. Acta Neuropathol. 2012;123:727–38.

18. Andreiuolo F, Ferreira C, Puget S, Grill J. Current and evolving knowledge of prognostic factors for pediatric ependymomas. Future Oncol. 2013;9:183–91.

19. Godfraind C, Kaczmarska JM, Kocak M, et al. Distinct disease-risk groups in pediatric supratentorial and posterior fossa ependymomas. Acta Neuropathol. 2012;124:247–57.

20. Tabori U, Wong V, Ma J, et al. Telomere maintenance and dysfunction predict recurrence in paediatric ependymoma. Br J Cancer. 2008;99:1129–35.

21. Ridley L, Rahman R, Brundler MA, et al. Multifactorial analysis of predictors of outcome in pediatric intracranial ependymoma. Neuro Oncol. 2008;10:675–89.

22. Puget S, Grill J, Valent A, et al. Candidate genes on chromosome 9q33-34 involved in the progression of childhood ependymomas. J Clin Oncol. 2009;27: 1884–92.

23. Korshunov A, Golanov A, Timirgaz V. Immunohisto-chemical markers for prognosis of ependymal neoplasms. J Neurooncol. 2002;58:255–70.

24. Gilbertson RJ, Bentley L, Hernan R, et al. ERBB receptor signaling promotes ependymoma cell proliferation and represents a potential novel therapeutic target for this disease. Clin Cancer Res. 2002;8: 3054–64.

25. Senetta R, Miracco C, Lanzafame S, et al. Epidermal growth factor receptor and caveolin-1 coexpression identifies adult supratentorial ependymomas with rapid unfavorable outcomes. Neuro Oncol. 2011;13:176–83.

26. Koos B, Bender S, Witt H, et al. The transcription factor evi-1 is overexpressed, promotes proliferation, and is prognostically unfavorable in infratentorial ependymomas. Clin Cancer Res. 2011;17:3631–7.

27. Milde T, Hielscher T, Witt H, et al. Nestin expression identifies ependymoma patients with poor outcome. Brain Pathol. 2012;22:848–60.

28. Garvin Jr JH, Selch MT, Holmes E, Berger MS, Finlay JL, Flannery A, Goldwein JW, Packer RJ, Rorke-Adams LB, Shiminski-Maher T, Sposto R, Stanley P, Tannous R, Pollack IF, Children's Oncology Group. Phase II study of pre-irradiation chemotherapy for childhood intracranial ependymoma. Children's Cancer Group protocol 9942: a report from the Children's Oncology Group. Pediatr Blood Cancer. 2012;59: 1183–9.

29. Koshy M, Rich S, Merchant TE, Mahmood U, Regine WF, Kwok Y. Post-operative radiation improves survival in children younger than 3 years with intracranial ependymoma. J Neurooncol. 2011;105: 583–90.

30. Landau E, Boop FA, Conklin HM, Wu S, Xiong X, Merchant TE. Supratentorial ependymoma: disease control, complications, and functional outcomes after irradiation. Int J Radiat Oncol Biol Phys. 2013; 85:193–9.

31. Grundy RG, Wilne SA, Weston CL, et al. Primary postoperative chemotherapy without radiotherapy for intracranial ependymoma in children: the UKCCSG/SIOP prospective study. Lancet Oncol. 2007;8: 696–705.

32. Duffner PK, Krischer JP, Sanford RA, et al. Prognostic factors in infants and very young children with intracranial ependymomas. Pediatr Neurosurg. 1998;28: 215–22.

33. Zacharoulis S, Levy A, Chi SN, et al. Outcome for young children newly diagnosed with ependymoma, treated with intensive induction chemotherapy followed by myeloablative chemotherapy and autologous stem cell rescue. Pediatr Blood Cancer. 2007; 49:34–40.

34. Needle MN, Goldwein JW, Grass J, et al. Adjuvant chemotherapy for the treatment of intracranial ependymoma of childhood. Cancer. 1997;80:341–7.

35. Venkatramani R, Ji L, Lasky J, et al. Outcome of infants and young children with newly diagnosed ependymoma treated on the "Head Start" III prospective clinical trial. J Neurooncol. 2013;113:285–91.

36. Bouffet E, Hawkins CE, Ballourah W, et al. Survival benefit for pediatric patients with recurrent ependymoma treated with reirradiation. Int J Radiat Oncol Biol Phys. 2012;83:1541–8.

37. Liu AK, Foreman NK, Gaspar LE, Trinidad E, Handler MH. Maximally safe resection followed by hypofractionated re-irradiation for locally recurrent ependymoma in children. Pediatr Blood Cancer. 2009;52:804–7.

38. Merchant TE, Boop FA, Kun LE, Sanford RA. A retrospective study of surgery and reirradiation for recurrent ependymoma. Int J Radiat Oncol Biol Phys. 2008;71:87–97.

39. Messahel B, Ashley S, Saran F, et al. Relapsed intracranial ependymoma in children in the UK: patterns of relapse, survival and therapeutic outcome. Eur J Cancer. 2009;45:1815–23.

40. Atkinson JM, Shelat AA, Carcaboso AM, et al. An integrated in vitro and in vivo high-throughput screen identifies treatment leads for ependymoma. Cancer Cell. 2011;20:384–99.

Central Nervous System Germ Cell Tumors (CNS-GCT)

14

Ute Bartels and Ash Singhal

Introduction

CNS GCTs are a heterogeneous group of tumors consisting of germinoma and non-germinomatous germ cell tumors (NGGCTs). NGGCTs include embryonal carcinoma, yolk sac tumors (or endodermal sinus tumors), choriocarcinoma, mature and immature teratoma, and teratoma with malignant transformation, as well as mixed pathology NGGCT. The terminology of "non-germinomatous germ cell tumors" has been repeatedly questioned as the term does not capture the variety of tumors properly. Many NGGCTs (so termed if the pathology includes at least one NGGCT subtype) are mixed in nature and may even entail components of germinoma. Hence some authors advocate substituting the term "mixed malignant germ cell tumors" (MMGCT) in place of "NGGCT" [1]. The authors of this chapter will continue to use the terms germinoma and NGGCT as there is not yet consensus around this new terminology. This chapter aims to capture the commonality and difference in the understanding of these tumors between the Western and Eastern world and the inherent challenges regarding adequate conclusions with respect to treatment and prognosis.

Epidemiology

Differences in incidence rates are observed according to gender and ethnicity. The mean annual incidence of CNS GCT is reported to be 1.06 per million children (0–18 years of age) in Canada [2]. In this study, the annual incidence of germinoma was approximately twice that of NGGCT. While other Western countries estimate similar incidence rates with CNS GCT accounting for up to 3.6 % of all pediatric intracranial CNS tumors [3], the rates are higher in Japan and the Far East accounting for up to 15.3 % of all pediatric intracranial CNS tumors [4, 5]. The reasons for variations in incidence remain elusive, but genetic predisposition or difference in viral infection rates according to ethnic background and/or geographical areas has been considered potential explanations. If the latter cause would apply, racial difference may disappear with second-generation immigrants from Asia to other continents. A retrospective Canadian epidemiological study suggested that this higher prevalence persisted in children of Asian descent; however, this trend did not reach statistical

U. Bartels, M.D. (✉)
Department of Hematology/Oncology,
The Hospital for Sick Children, Toronto, ON, Canada
e-mail: ute.bartels@sickkids.ca

A. Singhal, M.D., F.R.C.S. (C.)
Department of Pediatric Neurosurgery, University of British Columbia, BC Children's Hospital,
Vancouver, BC, Canada

K. Scheinemann and E. Bouffet (eds.), *Pediatric Neuro-oncology*,
DOI 10.1007/978-1-4939-1541-5_14, © Springer Science+Business Media New York 2015

significance due to the small sample size and missing information on ethnicity [2].

The peak incidence of CNS GCT is in the second decade of life and male gender is affected more often [3, 6, 7]. The male predominance is striking in GCT arising in the pineal area with a male-to-female ratio ranging up to 15:1, while girls are slightly more affected if GCTs arise in the suprasellar region [8, 9].

Pathology and Etiology of Germ Cell Tumors

CNS GCTs are the exact morphological homologues of extracranial and gonadal germ cell tumors. Each of the histological subtypes of GCT mimics elements of one or more of the three embryonic germ layers: endoderm, mesoderm, and ectoderm (Fig. 14.1). Uncertainty remains regarding the nature of the cell of origin.

Gonadotropins are considered to have a potential role in the etiology due to the midline location of GCTs, the neighborhood to diencephalic centers that regulate gonadotropins, and the increased prevalence in children of peripubertal age and in boys affected by Klinefelter syndrome (47, XXY) [10, 11]. Several case reports describe GCTs affecting siblings or children with NF-1 or Down syndrome [12–19] hypothesizing potential genetic links. The occurrence of extracranial germ cell tumors in patients years after successful treatment for CNS GCT may as well be suggestive of a possible genetic disposition [20, 21].

Germinoma

Germinomas account for approximately 60–70 % of intracranial germ cell tumors [5]. Most germinomas develop in the midline structures, namely the suprasellar and pineal regions [22]. Occurrences outside the midline and in the basal ganglia are rare [23, 24]. Progression-free survival (PFS) in germinomas is excellent with 5-year overall survival (OS) exceeding 90 % in retrospective and prospective series [6, 25, 26].

Clinical Presentation

The clinical presentation is determined by the location of the germinoma. Long-lasting histories up to years are not uncommon. Diabetes insipidus, a symptom of the vast majority of patients with suprasellar and bifocal germinoma, can remain clinically balanced and undiagnosed for a prolonged time period. Hence diligent history taking and review of polyuria and polydipsia is important. Symptoms of increased fluid intake, weight loss, and personality changes in an academic high achieving, peripubertal girl may

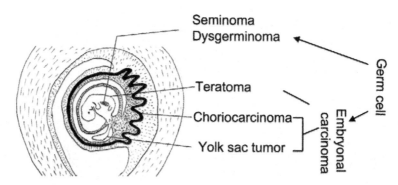

Fig. 14.1 Germinoma resembles the primordial germ cell tumor of the gonads. Teratoma mimics the fetus itself, yolk sac tumor resembles the yolk sac, choriocarcinoma is similar to trophoblast or placenta, and embryonal carcinoma is composed of immature embryonic tissues (Reprinted from [69])

mislead to an inappropriate diagnosis of an eating behavior disorder. New onset of diabetes insipidus should prompt diagnostic workup including brain magnetic resonance imaging (MRI). In case of documented pituitary stalk thickening, a careful clinical and imaging follow-up is recommended as about ~15–25 % of affected individuals may eventually develop germinoma [27, 28]. Other symptoms associated with suprasellar germinoma location are visual disturbances and endocrinopathies.

The most common symptoms of a pineal germinoma are symptoms of increased intracranial pressure due to obstruction of the aqueduct and Parinaud's syndrome. This syndrome is named for Henri Parinaud, French ophthalmologist (1844–1905), and its component of upward gaze palsy is most apparent at clinical presentation.

Basal ganglia germinoma accounts for 4–10 % of germinoma and is often characterized by insidious onset of symptoms over a long period of time (1–4.5 years). The presentation is generally different from midline germinoma and can include hemiparesis or choreoathetotic movements, personality changes, and ocular and speech disturbances.

Radiology

Classical imaging characteristics of suprasellar and pineal (or bifocal) germinoma are homogenous iso- or hypointense lesions on T1 weighted MRI and iso- or hyperintense on T2 weighted MRI (iso- or hyperdense on computed tomography—CT) with avid enhancement after contrast administration. Ventricular dissemination is not exceptional and usually characterized by linear or nodular enhancement along the ependymal ventricular lining. Basal ganglia germinoma may lack this avid enhancement and sometimes show no or little mass effect especially in the early stages of the disease. Ipsilateral cerebral and/or brainstem atrophy (Wallerian degeneration) is present in one third of patients with basal ganglia germinoma [29].

Tumor Markers

Intracranial germ cell tumors can secrete tumor markers in the bloodstream and/or in the cerebrospinal fluid (CSF). Most germinomas are marker negative and, in particular, they never secrete alpha-fetoprotein (AFP). However some germinomas may secrete human chorionic gonadotropin (hCG and hCGβ) either in serum or in the CSF due to the presence of syncytiotrophoblastic giant cells (STGCs). Retrospective and prospective analyses found elevated hCG levels in up to 40 % of germinoma patients [26, 30, 31]. The majority of cases have elevated hCG levels solely in CSF; however, the presence of both or elevated value in serum with normal value in CSF is described [31]. Sampling artifacts including the short half-life of hCG (1.5 days) may contribute to some variability in these findings.

There are conflicting data regarding the maximum level of hCG in germinoma and its prognostic significance. Moderate elevation of hCG in serum or CSF is considered diagnostic for germinoma, and a level below 50 IU/L is the threshold used in Europe and North America. The International Society of Pediatric Oncology (SIOP-CNS-GCT) study defines tumors exceeding hCG > 50 IU/L as malignant secreting NGGCT. By contrast, in Japan, biopsy-proven germinomas are all classified as germinoma irrespective of their level of hCG secretion [32].

Some authors have suggested a different prognosis for germinoma with elevated level of hCG. One study reported a 10-year survival advantage for patients with nonsecreting germinomas (90 %) compared to those with elevated hCG serum levels (60 %) [33]. However, most other studies did not find such differences in outcome [22, 30, 34, 35]. The current ongoing Children's Oncology Group germ cell tumor study increased the hCG threshold for eligibility into the germinoma treatment stratum, allowing patients to be enrolled as long as hCG level does not exceed 100 IU/L either in serum or CSF.

s-Kit in Germinoma

Immunohistochemical studies have shown that s-kit is highly expressed in germinoma cells. CSF studies have shown high levels of soluble-kit (s-kit) in patients with germinomas (with or without STGCs) compared to patients with NGGCTs [36]. s-Kit levels were also correlated with the clinical course of the disease, with higher s-kit concentration in samples obtained before treatment and in those collected at the time of tumor recurrence. These data suggest that CSF s-kit may represent a valuable tumor marker of germinomatous components.

Staging

As with malignant childhood brain tumors in general, MRI of the entire CNS (brain and spinal cord) at the time of initial diagnosis is essential for staging. If emergency surgery is deemed necessary for the patient (mostly for hydrocephalus management), then MRI of the spine—if not done prior to surgery—should be obtained within a 48–72 h window after the surgical intervention to avoid any artifact associated with the recent intervention. Tumor markers in serum and CSF are essential in midline lesions that are suspicious for GCT, and results will determine the need for biopsy, establish treatment strategy, and estimate prognosis. In addition, a lumbar CSF investigation for cytology prior to initiation of treatment is the gold standard; however, this may not always be feasible due to the presence of obstructive hydrocephalus and the associated life-threatening risk of brain herniation, particularly in the context of pineal germinomas. The CNS GCT SIOP trial allowed enrolment of patients if CSF cytology was undertaken either via ventricular route or lumbar puncture. Interestingly the Japanese working group dismisses CSF cytology because it is not taken into treatment considerations [37]. Data from prospective studies suggest [26, 38] that 15–20 % of germinoma patients have disseminated disease at diagnosis either on imaging (M+) or on CSF investigation (M1).

Treatment

Role of Radiation and Chemotherapy

Historically, craniospinal irradiation (CSI) has been the gold standard treatment for CNS germinoma [39–41]. Combined systemic chemotherapy with local irradiation has been introduced with the aim of reducing radiation doses and/or volume and herewith the incidence of late-onset sequelae while maintaining high cure rates [42, 43]. Focal radiation however resulted in increased number of ventricular relapses and subsequently whole-ventricular radiation (WVI) was utilized by the Japanese, French, and German working groups [26, 32, 38]. The relative contributions of chemotherapy and irradiation remain a topic of debate in the treatment of these highly curable CNS germinomas.

Radiation Therapy

The use of CSI dates from an era when staging was rarely performed and treatment was similar for non-metastatic and metastatic patients. Progressively, the relevance of CSI was questioned, particularly for patients with non-metastatic CNS germinoma. The low risk of isolated spinal relapse was initially suggested by Brada [44]. Rogers et al. conducted a meta-analysis of radiation therapy for germinoma patients and found a recurrence rate of 7.6 % after whole-brain or WVI and of 3.8 % after craniospinal radiation. No predilection for isolated spinal metastasis was found when CSI was omitted (2.9 % versus 1.2 %). The authors concluded that reduced-volume irradiation should replace CSI [25]. Ogawa's retrospective review of the Japanese experience concurs with a low risk of spinal relapse with an incidence of 4 % (2/56) for patients treated with CSI versus 3 % (2/70) for patients treated without spinal radiation [22]. Excellent PFS for localized germinomas with the use of either whole-brain or whole-ventricular irradiation is reported by several institutions [6, 41, 45–47].

There are studies suggesting that radiation dose can be reduced to less than 36 Gy WVI without pre-irradiation chemotherapy [48, 49]. However the use of radiation therapy alone has been associated with a risk of extra CNS relapses [40]. In addition the late effects of radiation with respect to neurocognitive and endocrine function and quality of life are well recognized. A retrospective study evaluating quality of life in germinoma long-term survivors ($n=52$) treated with radiation only identified significant issues: only 6 of 44 patients were married, 21 patients had no occupation, and 7 of 11 formerly employed patients had left their jobs [50]. In the hopes that reduced dose and volume of irradiation will diminish impact on neurocognitive function and quality of life in a meaningful way, neoadjuvant chemotherapy has been progressively introduced in the management of CNS germinoma.

Chemotherapy

Germinomas are highly sensitive to chemotherapy particularly to platinum compounds and cyclophosphamide [51, 52]. The largest chemotherapy-only experiences are reported in the First, Second, and Third International CNS Germ Cell Tumor Study. In the first study chemotherapy consisted of 4 cycles of carboplatin ($500 \, mg/m^2/day$, day 1 and 2), etoposide ($150 \, mg/m^2/day$, day 3), and bleomycin ($15 \, mg/m^2/day$, day 3). Patients with complete radiological and tumor marker response proceeded to 2 more identical cycles, whereas cyclophosphamide ($65 \, mg/kg$) was added to the 3-drug regimen for those with incomplete response. Twenty-two of 45 CNS germinoma patients relapsed, and even though most relapsed patients were salvageable with radiation therapy, the 2-year OS in this study was only 84 % [53]. Nineteen germinoma patients were enrolled in the second study using an intensified cisplatin and cyclophosphamide-based chemotherapy induction. Despite proof of effectiveness with a high rate of complete remission, the 5-year event-free survival (EFS) and OS rates were unsatisfactory at 47 ± 2.3 % and 68 ± 2.2 %, respectively. Moreover chemotherapy was asso-

ciated with unacceptable morbidity and mortality (four deaths), predominantly in patients with diabetes insipidus [54]. The third study included 25 patients and confirmed the inferior outcome of this strategy with a 6-year EFS of 45.6 % when avoiding radiation [55]. In conclusion current therapies cannot dismiss radiation without hampering the chances of EFS and OS.

Combined Chemo- and Radiation Therapy

Preirradiation chemotherapy with carboplatin, etoposide, and ifosfamide followed by focal irradiation (40 Gy) has been utilized in the SIOP-CNS-GCT-96 protocol for patients with non-metastatic germinomas. Physicians had the option to use this approach or alternatively CSI without chemotherapy. This prospective, multinational study included 190 patients with localized germinoma. The 5-year EFS and OS for patients treated with preirradiation chemotherapy ($n=65$) were 88 ± 0.4 % and 96 ± 0.3 %, respectively, whereas the 5-year EFS and OS of patients treated with craniospinal radiation ($n=125$) were 94 ± 0.2 % and 95 ± 0.2 %. While relapses (4/125) only occurred locally in the CSI group, 6 of 7 relapses occurred in the ventricular area in the chemotherapy/focal radiation treatment group [26]. As a consequence, the current open SIOP trial combines preirradiation chemotherapy with ventricular irradiation (24 Gy) with an additional boost of 16 Gy to the primary tumor bed in patients with localized disease. Metastatic germinoma patients will continue to be treated with CSI at doses outlined above as the 45 metastatic patients included in the aforementioned study showed an excellent 98 ± 0.2 % 5-year EFS and OS.

The risk of ventricular recurrence in patients treated with chemotherapy and focal radiation has also been well documented by the French and Japanese working groups. Alapetite et al. reported the SFOP (Societé Française d'Oncologie Pédiatrique) experience including 60 patients treated for CNS germinoma with a combination of carboplatin, etoposide, and ifosfamide followed by focal radiation (40 Gy). The 5-year EFS and OS were 84.2 % and 98.2 %, respectively. Ten of 60 patients relapsed at a median time of 32 (range: 10–121) months with the majority (n = 8) within the ventricular system [38]. The second trial of the Japanese GCT study group consisted of three cycles of carboplatin (450 mg/m²/day, day 1) and etoposide (150 mg/m²/day, day 1–3) chemotherapy followed by local irradiation (24 Gy). Five-year OS was 98 %. However 13 % of the patients (16/123) developed recurrence. In an interim analysis a high incidence of ventricular/locoregional relapses was reported [37]. As a consequence, current treatment in Japan, Europe, and North America combines chemotherapy with WVI. While the dose of WVI is 24 Gy in Europe and Japan, the current Children's Oncology Trial evaluates the efficacy of a reduced dose of 18 Gy WVI (plus boost to tumor bed to a total of 30 Gy) in chemotherapy-responsive germinoma patients with localized disease.

Choices of Chemotherapeutic Agents

Among the variety of chemotherapy regimens, no protocol has suggested better activity or improved outcome. Therefore, the main issue in the management of germinoma patients relates to the short- and long-term safety of the chemotherapy used. While substitution of cisplatin with carboplatin has raised concerns because of inferior outcome in extracranial nonseminomatous germ cell tumors [56], carboplatin regimens have shown similar efficacy when compared with cisplatin regimens in CNS germinoma [51, 53].

The vast majority of patients with suprasellar germinoma suffer from diabetes insipidus. Cisplatin- or ifosfamide-based chemotherapy requires hyperhydration, which significantly increases the risk for electrolyte imbalances and consequent complications such as seizures [57]. A combination of carboplatin and etoposide chemotherapy is currently employed by the Japanese and North American working groups. This offers the advantage of easier outpatient administration and reduced risk of hyperhydration-associated metabolic complications.

Role of Surgery

The Need for Biopsy and Second-Look Surgery

As a matter of principle, a biopsy is required in case of marker-negative lesions. The choice of the technique (stereotactic, endoscopic, open craniotomy) and the goal of surgery (tissue diagnosis versus tumor resection) are complex and largely determined by the anatomy of the lesion (size, accessibility through the ventricle, etc.) as well as the presence and extent of ventriculomegaly. If the tumor is felt to be a germinoma, the general goal of surgical intervention (apart from hydrocephalus management) is tissue diagnosis and not tumor resection.

Symptomatic obstructive hydrocephalus may necessitate an emergent intervention such as placement of an external ventricular drain (EVD) or an endoscopic third ventriculostomy (ETV). At the time of ETV, many groups favor attempted tumor biopsy, to confirm the histology (keeping in mind the risk of sampling error in mixed pathology tumors).

The need for tissue biopsy in patients with a bifocal lesion, considered metasynchronous and not metastatic, is debated. In the current SIOP and North American protocols, a biopsy is not required if the clinical presentation, imaging characteristics, and tumor marker profile (AFP negative, no or mild elevation of hCG) are consistent with a bifocal germinoma. With very rare exceptions, bifocal lesions associated with negative tumor markers are almost always pure germinoma [26, 38, 58]. The current North American GCT trial does not mandate a biopsy for suprasellar, pineal, or unifocal ventricular lesions (radiologically consistent with germinoma) if AFP is negative and the hCG is elevated to ≤50 IU/L. However, in this protocol, a biopsy is required for patients with hCG values above 50 IU/L to a maximum of 100 IU/L. The Japanese approach has been surgical removal of lesions whenever feasible and subsequent treatment is based on the final pathology result.

Germinoma are highly chemosensitive and response to treatment is often obvious within

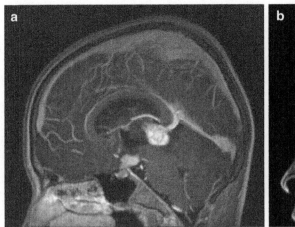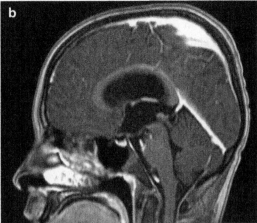

Fig. 14.2 Response to chemotherapy in a bifocal germinoma. Sagittal T1 weighted images after contrast. (**a**) At diagnosis. (**b**) After two cycles of chemotherapy with carboplatin/etoposide

days after the first cycle (Fig. 14.2). In our institutional experience an EVD can be removed within a week after the first chemotherapy cycle has been completed and before the patient becomes neutropenic. With this strategy VP shunts can most often be avoided. The presence of residual disease at the end of treatment is not predictive of worse outcome and patients with residual disease fare as well as those without [26]. Lack of chemotherapy responsiveness either in an hCG-positive or biopsy-proven germinoma raises concerns of a potential mixed GCT; hence, the current Children's Oncology Group GCT trial mandates second surgery at the end of chemotherapy in case of incomplete response when the residual suprasellar and pineal lesion are larger than 1 or 1.5 cm, respectively.

Prognosis

The overall survival in germinoma surpasses 90 % either with radiation alone or with combination of chemotherapy and radiation. Current treatment strategies include pre-radiation chemotherapy in order to reduce radiation dose and volume to minimize long-term sequelae. Current evidence suggests that extent of resection does not contribute to superior outcome but may add morbidity. Hence upfront surgery should be limited to a biopsy or avoided when possible [26, 59].

Non-germinomatous Germ Cell Tumors (NGGCTs)

NGGCTs (as the name implies) represent a group of pathologies distinct from germinoma and have substantially different diagnostic factors, pathological features, different surgical/chemotherapeutic/radiation therapy approaches, and different outcomes. As such, they should be considered entirely separately from germinomas. However, germinomas and NGCCT share a common location and clinical presentation, and this presents diagnostic challenges highlighted below.

Clinical Presentation

NGGCT, like germinoma, often presents with symptoms of hydrocephalus. These can include headaches, nausea, vomiting, blurred vision or diplopia, milestone regression, gait disturbance, and in more severe presentations, drowsiness or coma. Initial clinical findings can include significant findings in the ophthalmological examination, including papilledema, sixth nerve palsy, upgaze palsy, convergence nystagmus, retractory nystagmus, and papillary response abnormalities (light-near dissociation). Although these findings are generally termed "Parinaud's syndrome," Parinaud himself described only the upgaze palsy [60].

Endocrinopathies can frequently be present in NGGCT, with up to 90 % of patients having at least one endocrinopathy. These can include diabetes insipidus, growth retardation, and delayed or precocious puberty particularly in males with choriocarcinoma and teratomas [61]. Accordingly, endocrinology consultation and work-up is essential at presentation.

Radiology

While radiology can be helpful in the diagnosis of NGGCT, particularly with regard to staging and guiding initial management strategies, it is important to note that there are no absolute pathognomonic radiological features. CT is very helpful in determining the presence and location of calcification and hemorrhage. While calcification of the pineal is frequently a normal finding in older children and adults, the finding of a calcified pineal in a child under 6 years of age is cause for concern, and requires further work-up for CNS-GCT [62]. Germinomas as well as NGGCT can have central or peripheral calcification. More marked calcifications can be associated with teratoma. Hemorrhage can be associated with all CNS-GCT, but choriocarcinoma in particular is associated with hemorrhagic foci.

MRI is essential to characterizing the composition of the tumor. NGGCTs are generally more heterogeneous and enhance less avidly than germinoma. Teratomas have the propensity to show fat signal or cyst formation more frequently.

Tumor Markers

One unique characteristic that distinguishes many NGGCTs from germinoma is the expression of tumor markers. AFP is a glycoprotein that, when found in high levels in serum or CSF of children, can be indicative of an intracranial NGGCT. Likewise, beta-human chorionic gonadotropin (β-hCG) is also used as a tumor marker for intracranial NGGCTs, when found in serum and CSF in high concentrations. Normally, both

Table 14.1 Serum tumor marker

	AFP	β-hCG
Germinoma	–	–/(+)
Embryonal carcinoma	+/–	+/–
Yolk sac tumor	+++	–
Choriocarcinoma	–	+++
Immature teratoma	(+)/–	(+)/–
Mature teratoma	–	–

AFP and β-hCG are considered negative when found in very low concentrations in both the serum and CSF of children. Each subtype of NGGCT has its own general expression pattern of tumor markers. Choriocarcinomas tend to produce high levels of β-hCG (>100 IU/mL and often much higher, by an order of magnitude) but no AFP. In contrast, yolk sac tumors distinctively produce high levels of AFP and express no β-hCG. Embryonal cell carcinomas produce variable levels of both AFP and β-hCG in the serum and CSF. Immature teratomas inconsistently produce low concentrations of both AFP and β-hCG. Unlike their NGGCT brethren, mature teratomas produce no AFP and β-hCG in the serum and CSF (Table 14.1).

The consensus remains that the mere presence of AFP or β-hCG, in high concentration, is not diagnostically indicative of a particular NGGCT pathological subtype, but is predictive of a NGGCT present [61, 63].

Staging

As it applies to germinomas, complete CNS MRI is necessary either preoperatively or favorably within 48–72 h of surgical intervention to look for metastatic disease as well as synchronous lesions. Although there is some debate regarding the utility of CSF cytology (both in terms of the location sampled—lumbar versus ventricular—and in terms of the significance of the result), it remains the gold standard in most modern studies. As noted in the germinoma section, lumbar CSF sampling is not always deemed to be safe, based on concerns regarding herniation.

Treatment

Radiation

Unlike germinoma, NGGCTs are relatively non-responsive to radiation therapy alone, with reported 5-year survival statistics ranging from 20 to 40 % when standard radiation only was used [64]. Therapeutic strategies using chemotherapy in conjunction with radiation improved outcome significantly and as a consequence radiation therapy on its own should not be used to treat NGGCT [65]. Jackson et al. summarized the typical ranges for radiation dosage for the treatment of NGGCT in North America: between 30 and 36 Gy to the craniospinal axis, with a tumor boost of 20–54 Gy [66]. European treatment strategies combine chemotherapy with focal radiation to the tumor bed in non-metastatic NGGCT. Of note, mature teratoma generally lacks a response to all radiation types.

Chemotherapy

Like radiation therapy, chemotherapy alone has modest effectiveness in the treatment of NGGCT pathologies. Despite the sensitivity of NGGCT pathologies to chemotherapy, many advocate against chemotherapy-alone treatment regimens with exceptions for infants and very young children. Like germinoma, typically chemotherapeutic agents used to treat NGGCT are carboplatin or cisplatin, cyclophosphamide or ifosfamide, and etoposide [66]. One significant benefit of the use of chemotherapeutic agents in the treatment of NGGCTs is their ability to reduce the size and vascularity of the NGGCT before surgery [63]. The benefit on extent and safety of surgical resection after chemotherapy has been well recognized [67]. It bears note that mature teratomas lack response to chemotherapy.

Similar to germinoma treatment protocols, combined radiation therapy/chemotherapy is the recommended approach for treatment of NGGCT (Fig. 14.3). Multiple studies have, in aggregate, suggested 5-year overall survivals in the 70 % range utilizing combined chemotherapy and radiation [67]. European and North American protocols include a platinum agent, etoposide, and ifosfamide, followed by radiation. The optimal volume of radiation in NGGCT is still a matter of debate. While the SIOP protocol recommends focal radiation for non-metastatic NGGCT, the Children's Oncology Group has traditionally used craniospinal radiation at a dose of 36 Gy coupled with a tumor boost. The ongoing COG study is considering ventricular radiation with a boost to the tumor bed for NGGCT patients who achieve a complete response with chemotherapy. Despite the relative success of combination therapy in the treatment of many NGGCTs, teratomas (especially mature) generally lack a response to both chemotherapy and radiation therapy, and the therapy of choice is complete resection where feasible.

Surgical Management

In the urgent clinical situation, owing to hydrocephalus, the initial surgical management is CSF diversion (EVD or ETV) regardless of the provisional tumor type or markers. Serum and CSF tumor marker should be obtained whenever a GCT is part of the differential diagnosis. In cases where markers are positive and neuroimaging is consistent with NGGCT, chemotherapy can be initiated without a histopathological diagnosis. If the markers are negative, it is generally advisable to complete a biopsy (if technically feasible) at the time of ETV—this generally adds only a modest risk of tumor bleeding. However, biopsy of NGGCT, which can frequently have mixed pathologies, can be misleading owing to sampling error. For this reason (to afford maximal diagnostic tissue to provide pathological accuracy), as well as possible surgical restoration of normal CSF pathways, some authors justify the initial risks of surgery and advocate initial maximal tumor biopsy and reduction via craniotomy. This remains quite controversial in the pediatric neurosurgical literature [59]. Complete surgical resection is the treatment of choice for mature teratomas and benign immature teratomas.

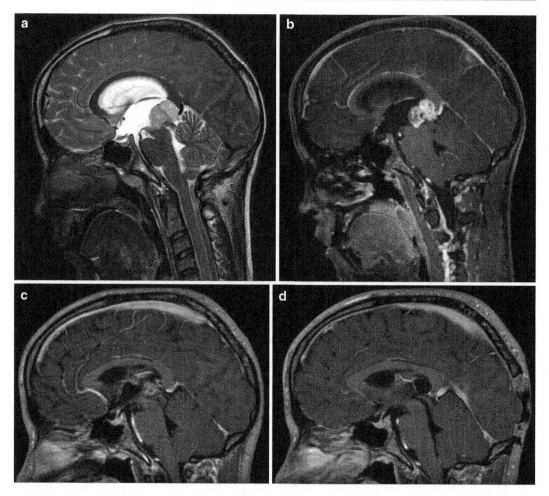

Fig. 14.3 Pineal NGGCT (yolk sac tumor/immature teratoma). Normalization of increased tumor markers (AFP, hCG) after two cycles of chemotherapy. (**a**) At diagnosis, sagittal T2. (**b**) At diagnosis, sagittal T1 + contrast. (**c**) Incomplete radiological response at the end of chemotherapy (total of six cycles of carboplatin, etoposide, ifosfamide). (**d**) Patient proceeded to surgery resulting in gross total resection followed by focal radiation therapy. Patient is well with no evidence of disease at 18-month follow-up

To monitor treatment response, serum and CSF tumor marker levels must be followed as well as serial imaging (MRI). In cases of radiological incomplete response/residual lesion after completion of chemotherapy and normalization of tumor markers, a surgical resection should be contemplated prior to radiation therapy. While the residual may represent a mature teratomatous component of a mixed NGGCT, a gross total resection of other viable tumor components prior to radiation improves OS [67].

There are multiple surgical approaches to pineal region NGGCT, including supratentorial, infratentorial, and transcallosal approaches via craniotomy. Each has relative merits and drawbacks, and the approach taken generally depends on the specific anatomy of the residual lesion.

Special note should be made regarding *growing teratomas*. For over 30 years, the literature has suggested that some NGGCTs radiographically enlarge—sometimes rapidly—during chemotherapy and/or radiation while serum tumor markers progressively improve, a condition referred to as "growing teratoma syndrome." This condition has recently been reported to occur in as many as 21 % of cases (11/52) of

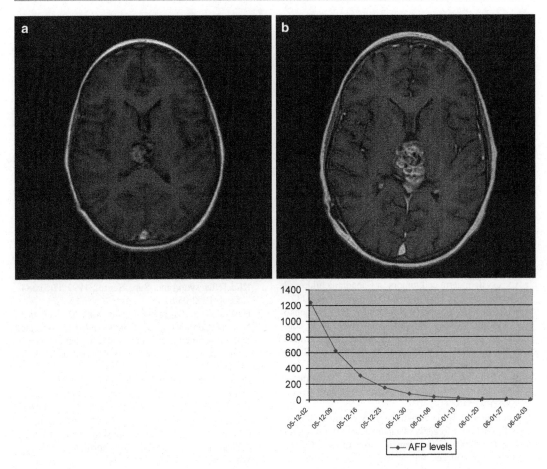

Fig. 14.4 Growing teratoma syndrome. Axial T1 weighted images after contrast. (**a**) At diagnosis. (**b**) Typical honeycomb shaped radiological progression while AFP normalized after two cycles of chemotherapy. Histological examination following complete resection showed mature teratoma

NGGCT, and the pathology was invariably mature teratoma [68]. As a consequence of the rapid growth and the lack of response of mature teratoma to adjuvant therapies, the management of growing teratoma must include surgical resection, and ideally gross total extirpation followed by radiation therapy (Fig. 14.4).

Conclusions and Future Directions

Ultimately, the recent history of CNS-GCT has been one of incremental improvement. The provision of care and treatment decision making, within the context of ongoing clinical trials, both has meant high quality care for that group of patients and has led to further improvements in care for the cohort of patients that have followed. Refinements in our collective understanding of CNS-GCT have meant improved surgical decision making (who to operate upon, which approaches to use, and how to minimize complications), improved selection of chemotherapeutic agents (from both an efficacy and safety point of view), and improved radiation treatments (what modality, what volume, what dose). Future patients will no doubt benefit from the lessons learned during the current era. Further refinements in surgical technology, pharmacological advances, and radiation technology will almost certainly make further meaningful improvements on survival rates and neurological and cognitive outcomes.

Other areas of focus, such as molecular targets, individual patient-tailored therapies, and radically different methods of disrupting tumor architecture or growth—such approaches are on the horizon and ever closer to impacting the care of children with CNS-GCT.

References

1. Finlay J, da Silva NS, Lavey R, Bouffet E, Kellie SJ, Shaw E, et al. The management of patients with primary central nervous system (CNS) germinoma: current controversies requiring resolution. Pediatr Blood Cancer. 2008;51(2):313–6.
2. Keene D, Johnston D, Strother D, Fryer C, Carret AS, Crooks B, et al. Epidemiological survey of central nervous system germ cell tumors in Canadian children. J Neurooncol. 2007;82(3):289–95. Epub 2006/11/23.
3. Dolecek TA, Propp JM, Stroup NE, Kruchko C. CBTRUS statistical report: primary brain and central nervous system tumors diagnosed in the United States in 2005-2009. Neuro Oncol. 2012;14 Suppl 5:v1–49.
4. Bouffet E, Matsutani M. Epidemiology of intracranial germ cell tumors (ICGCT) [Abstract]. Neuro Oncol. 2005;7(4):513–33.
5. Committee of Brain Tumor Registry of Japan. Report of Brain Tumor Registry of Japan (1969-1996). Neurol Med Chir. 2003;43(Supplement (11th edition)):1–111.
6. Borg M. Germ cell tumours of the central nervous system in children-controversies in radiotherapy. Med Pediatr Oncol. 2003;40(6):367–74.
7. Packer RJ, Cohen BH, Cooney K. Intracranial germ cell tumors. Oncologist. 2000;5(4):312–20.
8. Villano JL, Propp JM, Porter KR, Stewart AK, Valyi-Nagy T, Li X, et al. Malignant pineal germ-cell tumors: an analysis of cases from three tumor registries. Neuro Oncol. 2008;10(2):121–30. Epub 2008/02/22.
9. Villano JL, Virk IY, Ramirez V, Propp JM, Engelhard HH, McCarthy BJ. Descriptive epidemiology of central nervous system germ cell tumors: nonpineal analysis. Neuro Oncol. 2010;12(3):257–64. Epub 2010/02/20.
10. Prall JA, McGavran L, Greffe BS, Partington MD. Intracranial malignant germ cell tumor and the Klinefelter syndrome. Case report and review of the literature. Pediatr Neurosurg. 1995;23(4):219–24. Epub 1995/01/01.
11. Kaido T, Sasaoka Y, Hashimoto H, Taira K. De novo germinoma in the brain in association with Klinefelter's syndrome: case report and review of the literature. Surg Neurol. 2003;60(6):553–8; discussion 9. Epub 2003/12/13.
12. Aoyama I, Kondo A, Ogawa H, Ikai Y. Germinoma in siblings: case reports. Surg Neurol. 1994;41(4):313–7.
13. Wong TT, Ho DM, Chang TK, Yang DD, Lee LS. Familial neurofibromatosis 1 with germinoma involving the basal ganglion and thalamus. Childs Nerv Syst. 1995;11(8):456–8. Epub 1995/08/01.
14. Chik K, Li C, Shing MM, Leung T, Yuen PM. Intracranial germ cell tumors in children with and without Down syndrome. J Pediatr Hematol Oncol. 1999;21(2):149–51.
15. Fujita T, Yamada K, Saitoh H, Itoh S, Nakai O. Intracranial germinoma and Down's syndrome—case report. Neurol Med Chir (Tokyo). 1992;32(3):163–5.
16. Matsumura N, Kurimoto M, Endo S, Fukuda O, Takaku A. Intracranial germinoma associated with Down's syndrome. Report of 2 cases. Pediatr Neurosurg. 1998;29(4):199–202.
17. Tanabe M, Mizushima M, Anno Y, Kondou S, Dejima S, Hirao DJ, et al. Intracranial germinoma with Down's syndrome: a case report and review of the literature. Surg Neurol. 1997;47(1):28–31.
18. Hashimoto M, Hatasa M, Shinoda S, Masuzawa T. Medulla oblongata germinoma in association with Klinefelter syndrome. Surg Neurol. 1992;37(5):384–7. Epub 1992/05/01.
19. Hashimoto T, Sasagawa I, Ishigooka M, Kubota Y, Nakada T, Fujita T, et al. Down's syndrome associated with intracranial germinoma and testicular embryonal carcinoma. Urol Int. 1995;55(2):120–2. Epub 1995/01/01.
20. Flores NI, Krieger M, Dhall G, Finlay J. Second primary germ cell tumors in patients with prior primary central nervous system germ cell tumors: metachronous primaries or recurrent disease? 3rd international CNS germ cell tumour symposium, Corpus Christi College, Cambridge, 17th–20th April 2013. p. 73.
21. Watanabe T, Makiyama Y, Nishimoto H, Matsumoto M, Kikuchi A, Tsubokawa T. Metachronous ovarian dysgerminoma after a suprasellar germ-cell tumor treated by radiation therapy. Case report. J Neurosurg. 1995;83(1):149–53. Epub 1995/07/01.
22. Ogawa K, Shikama N, Toita T, Nakamura K, Uno T, Onishi H, et al. Long-term results of radiotherapy for intracranial germinoma: a multi-institutional retrospective review of 126 patients. Int J Radiat Oncol Biol Phys. 2004;58(3):705–13.
23. Villani A, Bouffet E, Blaser S, Millar BA, Hawkins C, Bartels U. Inherent diagnostic and treatment challenges in germinoma of the basal ganglia: a case report and review of the literature. J Neurooncol. 2008;88(3):309–14. Epub 2008/03/28.
24. Wong TT, Chen YW, Guo WY, Chang KP, Ho DM, Yen SH. Germinoma involving the basal ganglia in children. Childs Nerv Syst. 2008;24(1):71–8. Epub 2007/10/02.
25. Rogers SJ, Mosleh-Shirazi MA, Saran FH. Radiotherapy of localised intracranial germinoma: time to sever historical ties? Lancet Oncol. 2005;6(7):509–19.
26. Calaminus G, Kortmann R, Worch J, Nicholson JC, Alapetite C, Garre ML, et al. SIOP CNS GCT 96: final report of outcome of a prospective, multinational nonrandomized trial for children and adults with intracranial germinoma, comparing craniospinal

irradiation alone with chemotherapy followed by focal primary site irradiation for patients with localized disease. Neuro Oncol. 2013;15(6):788–96. Epub 2013/03/06.

27. Leger J, Velasquez A, Garel C, Hassan M, Czernichow P. Thickened pituitary stalk on magnetic resonance imaging in children with central diabetes insipidus. J Clin Endocrinol Metab. 1999;84(6):1954–60. Epub 1999/06/18.

28. Robison NJ, Prabhu SP, Sun P, Chi SN, Kieran MW, Manley PE, et al. Predictors of neoplastic disease in children with isolated pituitary stalk thickening. Pediatr Blood Cancer. 2013;60(10):1630–5. Epub 2013/05/15.

29. Ozelame RV, Shroff M, Wood B, Bouffet E, Bartels U, Drake JM, et al. Basal ganglia germinoma in children with associated ipsilateral cerebral and brain stem hemiatrophy. Pediatr Radiol. 2006;36(4):325–30.

30. Ogino H, Shibamoto Y, Takanaka T, Suzuki K, Ishihara S, Yamada T, et al. CNS germinoma with elevated serum human chorionic gonadotropin level: clinical characteristics and treatment outcome. Int J Radiat Oncol Biol Phys. 2005;62(3):803–8. Epub 2005/06/07.

31. Allen J, Chacko J, Donahue B, Dhall G, Kretschmar C, Jakacki R, et al. Diagnostic sensitivity of serum and lumbar CSF bHCG in newly diagnosed CNS germinoma. Pediatr Blood Cancer. 2012;59(7):1180–2. Epub 2012/02/04.

32. Matsutani M. Treatment of intracranial germ cell tumors: the second Phase II Study of Japanese GCT Study Group [abstract]. J Neurooncol. 2008;10(3):420.

33. Sawamura Y, Ikeda J, Shirato H, Tada M, Abe H. Germ cell tumours of the central nervous system: treatment consideration based on 111 cases and their long-term clinical outcomes. Eur J Cancer. 1998;34(1):104–10.

34. Fujimaki T, Matsutani M. HCG-procuding germinoma: Analysis of Japanese Pediatric Brain Tumor Study Group results [abstract]. Neuro-oncology. 2005;7(4):518.

35. Kim A, Ji L, Balmaceda C, Diez B, Kellie SJ, Dunkel IJ, et al. The prognostic value of tumor markers in newly diagnosed patients with primary central nervous system germ cell tumors. Pediatr Blood Cancer. 2008;51(6):768–73. Epub 2008/09/20.

36. Miyanohara O, Takeshima H, Kaji M, Hirano H, Sawamura Y, Kochi M, et al. Diagnostic significance of soluble c-kit in the cerebrospinal fluid of patients with germ cell tumors. J Neurosurg. 2002;97(1):177–83. Epub 2002/07/24.

37. Matsutani M. Oral presentation on CNS germinoma. Japanese pediatric brain tumor study group results. Second international symposium on central nervous system germ cell tumors November 18–21, 2005, Los Angeles, California; 2005.

38. Alapetite C, Brisse H, Patte C, Raquin MA, Gaboriaud G, Carrie C, et al. Pattern of relapse and outcome of non-metastatic germinoma

patients treated with chemotherapy and limited field radiation: the SFOP experience. Neuro Oncol. 2010;12(12):1318–25. Epub 2010/08/19.

39. Huh SJ, Shin KH, Kim IH, Ahn YC, Ha SW, Park CI. Radiotherapy of intracranial germinomas. Radiother Oncol. 1996;38(1):19–23.

40. Bamberg M, Kortmann RD, Calaminus G, Becker G, Meisner C, Harms D, et al. Radiation therapy for intracranial germinoma: results of the German cooperative prospective trials MAKEI 83/86/89. J Clin Oncol. 1999;17(8):2585–92.

41. Maity A, Shu HK, Janss A, Belasco JB, Rorke L, Phillips PC, et al. Craniospinal radiation in the treatment of biopsy-proven intracranial germinomas: twenty-five years' experience in a single center. Int J Radiat Oncol Biol Phys. 2004;58(4):1165–70.

42. Baranzelli MC, Patte C, Bouffet E, Couanet D, Habrand JL, Portas M, et al. Nonmetastatic intracranial germinoma: the experience of the French Society of Pediatric Oncology. Cancer. 1997;80(9):1792–7.

43. Fouladi M, Grant R, Baruchel S, Chan H, Malkin D, Weitzman S, et al. Comparison of survival outcomes in patients with intracranial germinomas treated with radiation alone versus reduced-dose radiation and chemotherapy. Childs Nerv Syst. 1998;14(10):596–601.

44. Brada M, Rajan B. Spinal seeding in cranial germinoma. Br J Cancer. 1990;61(2):339–40.

45. Tseng CK, Tsang NM, Wei KC, Jaing TH, Pai PC, Chang TC. Radiotherapy to primary CNS germinoma: how large an irradiated volume is justified for tumor control? J Neurooncol. 2003;62(3):343–8. Epub 2003/06/05.

46. Haas-Kogan DA, Missett BT, Wara WM, Donaldson SS, Lamborn KR, Prados MD, et al. Radiation therapy for intracranial germ cell tumors. Int J Radiat Oncol Biol Phys. 2003;56(2):511–8.

47. Roberge D, Kun LE, Freeman CR. Intracranial germinoma: on whole-ventricular irradiation. Pediatr Blood Cancer. 2005;44(4):358–62. Epub 2004/11/18.

48. Chen YW, Huang PI, Ho DM, Hu YW, Chang KP, Chiou SH, et al. Change in treatment strategy for intracranial germinoma: long-term follow-up experience at a single institute. Cancer. 2012;118(10):2752–62. Epub 2011/10/13.

49. Yen SH, Chen YW, Huang PI, Wong TT, Ho DM, Chang KP, et al. Optimal treatment for intracranial germinoma: can we lower radiation dose without chemotherapy? Int J Radiat Oncol Biol Phys. 2010;77(4):980–7. Epub 2009/10/30.

50. Sugiyama K, Yamasaki F, Kurisu K, Kenjo M. Quality of life of extremely long-time germinoma survivors mainly treated with radiotherapy. Prog Neurol Surg. 2009;23:130–9. Epub 2009/03/31.

51. Allen JC, DaRosso RC, Donahue B, Nirenberg A. A phase II trial of preirradiation carboplatin in newly diagnosed germinoma of the central nervous system. Cancer. 1994;74(3):940–4. Epub 1994/08/01.

52. Allen JC, Kim JH, Packer RJ. Neoadjuvant chemotherapy for newly diagnosed germ-cell tumors of the

central nervous system. J Neurosurg. 1987;67(1):65–70. Epub 1987/07/01.

53. Balmaceda C, Heller G, Rosenblum M, Diez B, Villablanca JG, Kellie S, et al. Chemotherapy without irradiation—a novel approach for newly diagnosed CNS germ cell tumors: results of an international cooperative trial. The First International Central Nervous System Germ Cell Tumor Study. J Clin Oncol. 1996;14(11):2908–15. Epub 1996/11/01.

54. Kellie SJ, Boyce H, Dunkel IJ, Diez B, Rosenblum M, Brualdi L, et al. Intensive cisplatin and cyclophosphamide-based chemotherapy without radiotherapy for intracranial germinomas: failure of a primary chemotherapy approach. Pediatr Blood Cancer. 2004;43(2):126–33.

55. da Silva NS, Cappellano AM, Diez B, Cavalheiro S, Gardner S, Wisoff J, et al. Primary chemotherapy for intracranial germ cell tumors: results of the third international CNS germ cell tumor study. Pediatr Blood Cancer. 2010;54(3):377–83. Epub 2010/01/12.

56. Horwich A, Sleijfer DT, Fossa SD, Kaye SB, Oliver RT, Cullen MH, et al. Randomized trial of bleomycin, etoposide, and cisplatin compared with bleomycin, etoposide, and carboplatin in good-prognosis metastatic nonseminomatous germ cell cancer: a Multiinstitutional Medical Research Council/European Organization for Research and Treatment of Cancer Trial. J Clin Oncol. 1997;15(5):1844–52. Epub 1997/05/01.

57. Afzal S, Wherrett D, Bartels U, Tabori U, Huang A, Stephens D, et al. Challenges and difficulties in management of patients with intracranial germ cell tumor having diabetes insipidus treated with cisplatin- and/or ifosfamide-based chemotherapy. Neuro Oncol. 2008;10(3):417.

58. Lafay-Cousin L, Millar BA, Mabbott D, Spiegler B, Drake J, Bartels U, et al. Limited-field radiation for bifocal germinoma. Int J Radiat Oncol Biol Phys. 2006;65(2):486–92.

59. Souweidane MM, Krieger MD, Weiner HL, Finlay JL. Surgical management of primary central nervous system germ cell tumors: proceedings from the sec-

ond international symposium on central nervous system germ cell tumors. J Neurosurg Pediatr. 2010;6(2):125–30. Epub 2010/08/03.

60. Echevarria ME, Fangusaro J, Goldman S. Pediatric central nervous system germ cell tumors: a review. Oncologist. 2008;13(6):690–9. Epub 2008/07/01.

61. Jorsal T, Rorth M. Intracranial germ cell tumours. A review with special reference to endocrine manifestations. Acta Oncol. 2012;51(1):3–9. Epub 2011/12/14.

62. Zimmerman RA, Bilaniuk LT. Age-related incidence of pineal calcification detected by computed tomography. Radiology. 1982;142(3):659–62. Epub 1982/03/01.

63. Kamoshima Y, Sawamura Y. Update on current standard treatments in central nervous system germ cell tumors. Curr Opin Neurol. 2010;23(6):571–5. Epub 2010/10/05.

64. Kretschmar C, Kleinberg L, Greenberg M, Burger P, Holmes E, Wharam M. Pre-radiation chemotherapy with response-based radiation therapy in children with central nervous system germ cell tumors: a report from the Children's Oncology Group. Pediatr Blood Cancer. 2007;48(3):285–91. Epub 2006/04/07.

65. Dhall G, Khatua S, Finlay JL. Pineal region tumors in children. Curr Opin Neurol. 2010;23(6):576–82. Epub 2010/11/03.

66. Jackson C, Jallo G, Lim M. Clinical outcomes after treatment of germ cell tumors. Neurosurg Clin N Am. 2011;22(3):385–94, viii. Epub 2011/08/02.

67. Murray MJ, Horan G, Lowis S, Nicholson JC. Highlights from the Third International Central Nervous System Germ Cell Tumour symposium: laying the foundations for future consensus. Ecancermedicalscience. 2013;7:333. Epub 2013/07/19.

68. Kim CY, Choi JW, Lee JY, Kim SK, Wang KC, Park SH, et al. Intracranial growing teratoma syndrome: clinical characteristics and treatment strategy. J Neurooncol. 2011;101(1):109–15. Epub 2010/06/10.

69. Fujimaki T. Central nervous system germ cell tumors: classification, clinical features, and treatment with a historical overview. J Child Neurol. 2009;24(11):1439–45. Epub 2009/10/21.

Atypical Teratoid Rhabdoid Tumors

Lucie Lafay-Cousin, Douglas R. Strother,
Jennifer A. Chan, Jonathon Torchia,
and Annie Huang

Introduction

Atypical teratoid rhabdoid tumor (ATRT) is a subgroup of aggressive CNS embryonal tumors included in the WHO classification system of brain tumors for the first time in 2000. The appreciation of this unique entity began with observations from the first National Wilms Tumor Study of a rhabdomyosarcomatoid variant of Wilms tumor that had a markedly poor prognosis. Ultrastructural analysis of these tumors led to the designation of malignant rhabdoid tumor of the kidney. Subsequently, reports of renal rhabdoid tumors with metastases to the brain were reported. The first apparent case of a primary CNS rhabdoid tumor was reported in 1987 and the entity of ATRT was suggested the same year by Rorke et al. [1]. With the development and increased use of a specific diagnostic immunostain, ATRTs are increasingly recognized as a distinct embryonal CNS tumor of infancy and early childhood. ATRTs remain highly malignant tumors with dismal prognosis; clinical management is particularly challenged by the very young age of the patients and consequent increased vulnerability to treatment-related neurotoxicity. However, increasing reports of ATRT survivors after intensified multimodal regimens offer promise of better prospects for ATRT patients with newer therapeutic approaches.

L. Lafay-Cousin, M.D., M.Sc. (✉)
Department of Pediatrics, Division of Oncology,
Alberta Children's Hospital, Calgary, AB, Canada
e-mail: lucie.lafay-cousin@albertahealthservices.ca

D.R. Strother, M.D.
Departments of Oncology and Pediatrics, Section of
Oncology and Blood and Marrow Transplant,
Cumming School of Medicine and Alberta Children's
Hospital, Calgary, AB, Canada

J.A. Chan, M.D.
Department of Pathology & Laboratory Medicine,
University of Calgary, Calgary, AB, Canada

J. Torchia, M.Sc.
Department of Lab Medicine and Pathobiology,
Labatt's Brain Tumour Centre, SickKids, University
of Toronto, Toronto, ON, Canada

A. Huang, M.D., Ph.D.
Department of Cell Biology, The Hospital for Sick
Children, Toronto, ON, Canada

Epidemiology and Demographics

When the first American workshop that was focused on ATRT was held in 2001, approximately 130 cases of ATRT were identified in published literature [2]. Five years later, the number of reported cases had nearly doubled [3]. This jump reflects the increased awareness of the entity among neuropathologists and the availability of INI1 immunohistochemistry staining to assess embryonal neoplasms that might previously have been diagnosed as medulloblastoma or

K. Scheinemann and E. Bouffet (eds.), *Pediatric Neuro-oncology*,
DOI 10.1007/978-1-4939-1541-5_15, © Springer Science+Business Media New York 2015

supratentorial primitive neuroectodermal tumor (sPNET) [4].

The incidence of ATRT has not been precisely defined. Registries and clinical trials provide some suggestion but are inherently biased by their voluntary natures. Population-based series provide the best data, and from Austria and the United States, incidence rates are 1.38 and 0.89, respectively, per million person-years in children <15 years of age [5, 6]. The frequency of ATRT reported among CNS tumors also varies between series according to the age group described. While ATRT represents 1–2 % of all pediatric CNS tumors, they account for up to 20 % in children less than 36 months of age [2, 7]. Two-thirds of the children diagnosed with ATRT are less than 3 years of age at time of diagnosis [7–9]. The median age at diagnosis issued from population-based series is 16–18 months [6, 8, 10] while the median age reported from therapeutic series is slightly higher, approximately 24 months [7, 9, 11, 12]. This difference could be due to lower enrollment of the very young children with ATRT onto clinical trials, or a greater likelihood than older children to undergo palliative treatment at time of diagnosis [8]. ATRTs are extremely rare in adults with just over 30 cases reported to date.

There appears to be a male predominance, with 55–68 % of affected children being male [6, 9, 13]. Although there may be a slight predominance of tumor distribution in the supratentorial compartment, primary location in the posterior fossa is more common in children less than 24 months of age [6–9, 11, 13]. Primary location in the spine occurs in only 1–7 % of cases [7, 8, 14]. Leptomeningeal dissemination is present at initial diagnosis in 20–40 % of patients [9, 11, 13, 14]. When metastatic disease is located outside the CNS, concern for rhabdoid tumor predisposition syndrome should be raised, especially in very young infants [15]. The presence of metastatic disease at diagnosis has not consistently been associated with prognosis [11–13].

Given the highly aggressive natural history of these tumors, the usual duration of presenting symptoms is rather short, with a median time of 3 weeks [8]. Signs at presentation are not specific to ATRT but instead depend on tumor location and age of the patient. Young patients with posterior fossa tumors present with signs of hydrocephalus such as enlarged head circumference, vomiting, headache, and lethargy, while patients with supratentorial masses generally present with additional signs of motor or sensory deficits, seizures, or both [16].

Imaging Findings

There are no pathognomonic radiographic features for ATRT (Fig. 15.1). Their appearance is very similar in many aspects of those of other high-grade tumors such as medulloblastoma or sPNET. They often present as a large heterogeneous mass, containing necrosis, hemorrhage, and areas of high cellularity that are hypointense on T2-weighted images. Extensive surrounding edema and mass effect are often present. These tumors also demonstrate intense heterogeneous enhancement on post-contrast sequences. In their comparative review of 55 medulloblastoma and 19 ATRT cases, Koral et al. suggested that, although, both tumors display similar imaging characteristics on conventional MRI, cerebellopontine angle (CPA) involvement and intratumoral hemorrhage were more common in ATRT [17]. Some authors describe a thick, wavy, and irregular, heterogeneously enhancing wall surrounding a central cystic region as being highly specific, though not pathognomonic, for ATRT among pediatric supratentorial brain tumors [18] (Fig. 15.1). In light of the lack of specific imaging features, ATRT needs to remain in the differential diagnosis of highly cellular tumors, certainly in young children and irrespective of the tumor location.

Pathology

As described in Chap. 6, the consistent histologic feature of ATRT is the largely PNET-like expanses of poorly differentiated small round blue cells. Although classically described as having heterogeneous morphologies, including areas containing characteristic "rhabdoid" cells with eccentric nuclei, prominent nucleoli, and increased

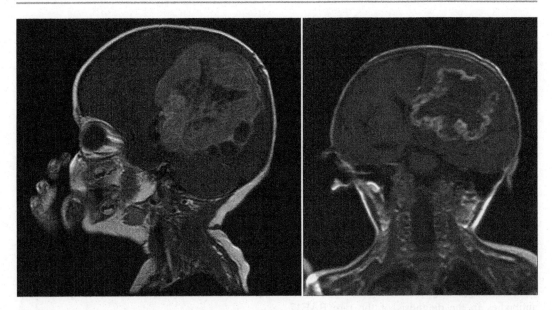

Fig. 15.1 Sagittal T1 + gadolinium and coronal T1 + gadolinium sequences of a left large parietal ATRT

amounts of eosinophilic cytoplasm, it is important to recognize that ATRT frequently does not contain obvious rhabdoid cells, despite the tumor's name. Recognition of this, as well as the fact that ATRT can occur throughout the neuroaxis, underscores the need to exclude the diagnosis of ATRT in any poorly differentiated CNS neoplasm in infants and children. In that regard, INI1 immunohistochemistry is particularly useful and readily available as a clinical test in many pathology laboratories. In nearly all cases, ATRT cells show loss of INI1 staining while normal cell constituents such as blood vessels and non-neoplastic-infiltrated brain serve as internal positive controls [19]. INI1-negative immunostaining is highly specific for ATRT and, therefore, an efficient diagnostic tool. However, Hasselblat et al. have recently reported a negative INI1 staining in cribriform neuroepithelial tumor (CRINET) [20].

Molecular Biology

The recognition of ATRT as a distinct pathological entity was initially supported by the recurrent association with chromosome 22 abnormalities involving monosomy or deletion/translocation involving the chromosome band 22q11.2 detected by conventional karyotype or fluorescent hybridization in situ (FISH) studies for submicroscopic deletion [21]. Subsequent positional cloning studies of this region lead to the identification of the tumor suppressor gene INI1/hSNF5/BAF47/SMARCB1; one of >10 members of the highly conserved ATP-dependent SWI/SNF chromatin-remodeling complex is required for transcriptional activation of many genes with fundamental roles in cell growth, differentiation, DNA repair, and other cellular processes [22]. Mutations of a gene involved in chromatin remodeling raises the possibility of epigenetic dysregulation as a major mechanism for oncogenesis [23]. However, the function of SMARCB1 and the mechanisms by which its loss leads to the development of rhabdoid tumors remain poorly understood. SMARCB1 is a demonstrated modulator of the cell cycle through downregulation of p16 and increased expression of cyclin D1 leading to a dysregulated CDHK4/Rb/E2F signaling axis [24]. Reintroduction of SMARCB1 into SMARCB1-deficient cell lines leads to cytoskeletal changes and ultimately apoptosis or cellular senescence and accumulation in the G0/G1 phase. The mechanism is believed to involve the loss of EZH2 inhibition by the SMARCB1-deficient SWI/SNF complex leading to derepression of Polycomb targets and aberrant activation of stem cell programs [25]. c-Myc is also dysregulated in ATRT through direct binding of SMARCB1. Loss of SMARCB1 is thought to disrupt c-myc-mediated repression of cyclin D1, further compounding loss of cell cycle control. Such studies have spawned interest in EHZ2 inhibitors as a potential therapeutic avenue. Other researchers have suggested that the loss of SMARCB1 results in chromosomal instability and may also be involved in the DNA damage response [26].

Biallelic alteration of SMARCB1 can be found in up to 94 % of ATRTs; however, a minority of cases has reported homozygous mutations involving another SWI/SNF chromatin-remodeling complex member—the ATPase subunit SMARCA4 (BRG1)—suggesting the usefulness of SMARCA4 antibodies in the diagnosis of the rare BAF47-positive ATRT [27].

Other than alterations in SMARCB1, the ATRT genome is highly stable and largely devoid of other recurrent mutations in other loci. Kieran et al. described the absence of canonical pathway mutations in rhabdoid tumor using a platform of 983 mutations encompassing 115 genes [28]. High-resolution genotyping array studies failed to identify copy number changes outside of chromosome 22. Similarly, a recent exome sequencing study conducted in 2012 by Lee et al. reported an overall somatic mutation rate of only 0.19 mutations/Mb, well below the rates observed for other known pediatric cancers [23]. Global gene expression studies have revealed distinct sub-clusters of ATRT. Birks et al. identified a sub-cluster of ATRT with a high expression of the BMP pathway genes (i.e., BMP4, SOST, BAMBI, MSX2), which correlated with a worse prognosis [29]. An independent study of ten rhabdoid tumors also demonstrated an enrichment of BMP signaling pathway genes suggesting an aberrant differentiation program and disruption of BMP signaling. This suggests the discovery of subgroup-specific treatment strategies will be important for future clinical investigation.

Germ-line mutations of SMARCB1 have been reported in up to 20–35 % in ATRT, but the true incidence of constitutional SMARCB1 mutations is not known [30, 31]. Patients with germ-line mutations are predisposed to rhabdoid tumor of the brain, kidney, and soft tissues and may present with multiple synchronous tumors. These children tend to be less than 1 year of age at the time of diagnosis and carry a worse prognosis [31]. In the vast majority of the cases, these SMARCB1 germ-line mutations are sporadic, but familial cases of ATRT have been reported [27]. Germ-line mutation of SMARCA4 has also been implicated in familial form of ATRT [32]. The pedigree analysis of this affected family supports an autosomal dominant inheritance with incomplete penetrance. The identification of asymptomatic carrier parents in this reported family highlights the need for systematic testing of all newly diagnosed ATRT patients for germ-line mutations [15].

Therapeutic Management

ATRTs are typically associated with a grim prognosis with estimated median survival times ranging from 8 to 16 months [2, 8, 9, 13, 14]. Because of the rarity of these tumors and a history of having been treated nonspecifically with other malignant tumors, there is no current standard of care for these tumors.

While in the early years of recognition of the entity, a significant number of patients only received palliative treatment and rapidly succumbed to their disease, in the most recent era, more aggressive and multimodality approaches have emerged and may be associated with a trend toward improved outcome [11]. These multimodality strategies variously include surgery, conventional chemotherapy, high-dose chemotherapy with hematopoietic stem cell support, intrathecal chemotherapy, and radiotherapy. The specific role of each individual modality, however, has not yet been clearly defined.

Surgery

There is strong evidence to show that complete tumor resection is associated with a more favorable outcome [6, 9, 33]. In the series reported by Chi et al., patients who underwent gross total

resection (GTR) of their tumors had a 2-year OS
of 91 ± 9 %, while those who underwent less than
a GTR had a median OS of 18 months [11].
Similarly, in the Canadian series, patients for
whom GTR was achieved had a 2-year OS of
60 ± 12.6 % compared to 21.7 ± 8.5 % for those
whose tumors were less than completely resected.
The invasive and vascular nature of these tumors
can limit the possibility of initial GTR, and the
rates of GTR reported in various series range
from 30 to 68 % [7, 8, 11, 13]. With the goal of
potentially maximizing the benefit of surgery,
treatment on the recently closed Children's
Oncology Group (COG) clinical trial for
ATRT, the first national cooperative group trial
exclusively for patients with ATRT, included a
recommendation for a second operation after two
courses of chemotherapy for those cases where
GTR of disease was not possible at diagnosis.

Conventional Chemotherapy

ATRT responds to chemotherapy, but the isolated
use of conventional-dose chemotherapy alone, as
used in the "baby-brain" strategies of the 1990s,
failed to cure most patients. In the second-generation
Pediatric Oncology Group (POG) "baby-brain"
protocol 9233/9234, complete response to chemotherapy was achieved in 21 % of the evaluable
patients, but the median survival time was only
6.7 months and none of the 36 patients survived
(Douglas Strother personal communication). Using
similar chemotherapy, the Children's Cancer Group
(CCG) 9921 protocol achieved a 29 % 5-year survival for its ATRT patients [34]. Based on several
case reports of successful treatment using conventional chemotherapy according to the Intergroup
Rhabdomyosarcoma Study protocol III (IRS-III)
for parameningeal rhabdomyosarcoma [35], the
group from Dana-Farber developed a specific protocol for ATRT using a modified IRS-III regimen
which utilized doxorubicin and dactinomycin that
are not typically used in other pediatric brain tumor
protocols. It also included intrathecal chemotherapy
and radiation; therefore, the distinct role of these
particular drugs is not known. Nonetheless, use of
this approach has been associated with a 58 %
objective response rate prior to radiation [11].

High-Dose Chemotherapy

In the most recent decade, high-dose chemotherapy
and hematopoietic stem cell rescue (HSCR) have
been reported in relatively small cohorts of patients
[33, 36, 37]. The most common regimen used single cycle of high-dose carboplatin, thiotepa, and
etoposide or 3 cycles of high-dose carboplatin and
thiotepa. Ginn et al. compiled 33 cases published of
patients treated with high-dose chemotherapy strategy. Fourteen of them also received radiation therapy at some point in their treatment. Overall, 20
patients were reported alive at a median follow-up
time of 50 months (5–105) [38]. In the Canadian
registry, 9 of 18 patients treated with high-dose chemotherapy were alive at a median follow-up time of
41 months. High-dose chemotherapy was associated with a significant survival benefit with a 2-year
OS of 47.9 ± 12.1 % versus 27.3 ± 9.5 % for the conventional chemotherapy group ($p=0.036$) [8].

Although definitive conclusions cannot be
made from these series because patient numbers
are very low, studies are not randomized, and the
use of therapy before and after high-dose consolidation is inconsistent, the results suggest that
consolidation with high-dose chemotherapy regimens to these patients is feasible and may provide
encouraging survival figures.

Intrathecal Chemotherapy

Because of the young age of children with ATRT,
the use of intrathecal chemotherapy for CNS prophylaxis, instead of craniospinal irradiation, has
been explored. Methotrexate, with or without
cytosine arabinoside, hydrocortisone, or both,
has preferentially been used. In the US ATRT
registry, 16 patients (38 %) received intrathecal
chemotherapy as part of the primary therapy. The
repeated use of IT methotrexate via Ommaya reservoir is a key component of the German HIT
SKK protocol for infant brain tumors, including
ATRT [39]. Similarly the Dana-Farber Cancer
Institute ATRT protocol also included iterative
injections of IT chemotherapy. The use of IT
is one component of these multimodality approaches; the small numbers of patients limit our

ability to assess its specific role for disease control. In one meta-analysis of published ATRT cases, Athale et al. reported a benefit in 2-year overall survival for patients treated with IT chemotherapy in combination with RT, compared to patients treated with RT alone or neither RT nor IT chemotherapy [14].

Radiation Therapy

As is the case with all other malignant brain tumors in very young children, the use of RT in ATRT raises serious concerns related to its significant long-term toxicity, primarily in terms of neurocognitive impairment. In the absence of a randomized study specifically addressing the role of radiotherapy, incorporation of radiation into most current strategies has been based on observations from retrospective series that suggest a survival benefit in children treated with some form of radiation. In the registry reported by Hilden, 13 patients (31 %) received radiation. Eight of the 13 survivors received primary radiation with a median survival of 48 months. The median age of irradiated patients was older than that of the entire registry cohort (47 months versus 24 months, respectively) [14]. In the recently updated experience from the St. Jude Children's Research Hospital, 19 children under 3 years of age received focal ($n = 13$) or craniospinal ($n = 6$) radiation, and six were alive without disease at the time of the report. All six survivors received focal radiation only after local progression of disease on chemotherapy. The 4-year PFS and OS rates for the entire cohort were 33.2 % ± 10 % and 53.5 % ± 10 %, respectively. Although treatment regimens were not uniform, nearly all patients younger than 3 years were treated with neoadjuvant, pre-irradiation chemotherapy. With these caveats, the investigators found that delay of radiation was associated with an increased risk of local and distant disease progression [12]. In a cohort of patients with a median age of 4.5 years, Chen et al. also reported increased time between diagnosis and radiation therapy to adversely affect outcome [40].

In contrast, and with many similar limitations of retrospective series, including multiple regimens of chemotherapy and various combinations of treatment modalities used, French investigators found no significant survival benefit for the patients who received adjuvant radiotherapy (16/58). While in their cohort, children younger than 2 years fared significantly worse than older children, the sub-analysis between adjuvant radiation and no radiation failed to show statistical significance ($p = 0.06$). They hypothesized that the underlying molecular biology of ATRT may be different in infants compared to older children. Germ-line mutation of INI1 seen with higher frequency in younger patients is associated with an earlier onset and more aggressive phenotype and may partially explain the poorer prognosis of the younger age group [13, 41]. Analyses from the Canadian registry showed that cure without radiation was possible. Among 16 patients treated with high-dose chemotherapy and no radiation, 9 (56 %) were long-term survivors at a median follow-up of 64 months [42]. If RT is used to treat ATRT, German data suggest that there is no survival difference between patients treated with radiation at diagnosis and those treated at the time of relapse (3-year OS 43 ± 14 % versus 31 ± 13 %, respectively, ($p = 0.314$)) [39].

Thus, the benefit of RT for patients with ATRT is still a matter of debate [3, 38]. Optimal doses and volumes of radiation have not been standardized. Nevertheless, radiation has been included in recent therapeutic strategies for ATRT. Given the very young age of the vast majority of these patients and the predominance of relapse at the primary site, priority has been given to focal radiation. Patient with localized disease are treated with focal RT while craniospinal irradiation is recommended for disseminated disease with doses varying with age [11, 43].

In the recently closed COG ACNS0333 protocol for patients with ATRT, the sequencing of RT and the prescribed doses and volumes were be based on (1) the age of the patient at the completion of induction chemotherapy, (2) primary tumor location (infratentorial vs. supratentorial), and (3) the extent of disease (localized vs. neuroaxis dissemination) [44].

Although there is also growing number of reports of long-term survivors cured without adjuvant radiation, we have not yet been able to identify these particular patients at diagnosis with conventional clinical criteria. Upcoming molecular characterization of CNS ATRT may provide insight and new prognostic factor to tailor therapy.

Multimodality Strategies

Although ATRTs are relatively rare tumors, prospective dedicated protocols for these tumors using multimodality strategies have recently been reported or are soon to be completed, namely, the Head Start experience, the Dana-Farber protocol, and the recently closed COG ACNS0333.

The Head Start I and II (HS) strategies consisted in 5 cycles of induction conventional chemotherapy (cis-platinum, etoposide, cyclophosphamide, vincristine, and high-dose methotrexate) followed by 1 cycle of myeloablative chemotherapy (etoposide, carboplatin, and thiotepa) with stem cell rescue. Maximal surgical resection was recommended either up front or on second-look surgery. Radiation therapy was planned in presence of residual disease before consolidation therapy. While none of the six patients treated on the HS I survived, three of the seven treated on the successor protocol HS II were alive at respectively 42, 54, and 67 months from diagnosis [33].

Twenty patients were prospectively treated on the DFCI ATRT protocol with a combination of maximal safe surgical resection, conventional chemotherapy based on the IRS-III regimen, repeated intrathecal chemotherapy, and age-based adapted radiation therapy. The systemic chemotherapy agents included vincristine, dactinomycin, cyclophosphamide, cis-platinum, doxorubicin, and DTIC or temozolomide for a total duration of treatment of 51 weeks. The 2-year PFS and OS were respectively 53 ± 13 % and 70 ± 10 %. Although the median overall survival had not been reached at time of publication, this protocol carries the highest survival rate at 2 years reported in a prospective manner [11].

The COG ACNS0333 protocol which recently reached accrual included an induction chemotherapy using vincristine, cis-platinum, cyclophosphamide, and high-dose methotrexate. Maximum safe surgical resection was recommended either up front or with a second-look surgery approach. Consolidation phase consisted in 3 cycles of high-dose carboplatin and thiotepa with stem cell rescue. The sequencing of radiation therapy, the prescribed doses, and volumes were age based as described in the radiation section [44]. The data still need to mature and the results on the 2-year EFS and OS endpoints of this strategy should be available in the next couple of years.

Pattern of Relapse and Survival

The prognosis of ATRT patients remains poor overall. The median time to progression in most series is only approximately 5 months from diagnosis [7, 8, 12]. Although not consistently reported in every series, it seems that the local relapse occurs most frequently, ranging from 42 to 72 % in smaller series [7, 8, 12]. Combined local and distant recurrences make up a sizable proportion of the remaining patients. For this reason, early local control with RT is advocated by some authors [12]. Recurrent disease, particularly following multimodality treatment, is essentially incurable. Pai Panandiker et al. described eight local relapses and six combined relapses among the 19 children who received chemotherapy prior to radiation, with a median time to relapse of 3.3 months from diagnosis [12].

Future Directions

Recent, more aggressive treatment strategies seem to be associated with a trend toward higher cure rate [8, 11, 36]. However, use of RT in this vulnerable age group is reason for concern. New alternative therapeutic pathways are needed and might be based on understanding of the molecular mechanisms underlying the development of this tumor. While the genetic alteration of SMARCB1 is well described, the rest of ATRT genome is uniquely silent compared to other brain tumors. These findings suggest that other novel mechanisms that have yet to be defined may be driving the oncogenesis of ATRT. Exploration of post-transcriptional mechanisms and the new generation of sequencing techniques may provide clues by identifying new therapeutic targets or new predictive markers that rationalize tailoring of therapy. Already, preclinical studies have shown that loss of the INI1 gene leads to increased expression of several other target genes such as cyclin D1, involved in cell cycle regulation; Aurora A kinase, implicated in mitosis and meiosis processes; and also insulin-like growth factor. The repression of the related signaling inhibitors or IGF inhibitor or EGFR inhibitors may provide new therapeutic weapons for the next generation of clinical trials for ATRT.

Conclusion

ATRTs remain very aggressive tumors with poor survival. However, recent multimodality strategies seem to be associated with a trend to improve outcome. Aside from the significant benefit of a complete surgical resection, the respective role of other modalities such as intrathecal chemotherapy or high-dose chemotherapy still needs to be determined. Also radiation is embedded in most of the current therapeutic protocols; the existence of long-term survivors treated without radiation is increasingly reported. Further identification of molecular markers may help to delineate the subgroup of patients who can be spared from radiation. A better understanding of the molecular pathways involved in the development of ATRT should lead through international collaboration in more tailored therapy to protect this vulnerable group of young patients from treatment-induced neurotoxicity.

References

1. Rorke LB, Packer RJ, Biegel JA. Central nervous system atypical teratoid/rhabdoid tumors of infancy and childhood: definition of an entity. J Neurosurg. 1996;85(1):56–65.
2. Packer RJ, et al. Atypical teratoid/rhabdoid tumor of the central nervous system: report on workshop. J Pediatr Hematol Oncol. 2002;24(5):337–42.
3. Squire SE, Chan MD, Marcus KJ. Atypical teratoid/rhabdoid tumor: the controversy behind radiation therapy. J Neurooncol. 2007;81(1):97–111.
4. Fleming AJ, et al. Atypical teratoid rhabdoid tumors (ATRTs): the British Columbia's Children's Hospital's experience, 1986–2006. Brain Pathol. 2012;22(5): 625–35.
5. Annual incidence of rhabdoid tumors among children <15, 2000–2008. Volume SEER 17. Bethesda: Surveillance, Epidemiology, and End Results (SEER) Program, SEER Stat version 7.06;2011.
6. Woehrer A, et al. Incidence of atypical teratoid/rhabdoid tumors in children: a population-based study by the Austrian Brain Tumor Registry, 1996–2006. Cancer. 2010;116(24):5725–32.
7. Tekautz TM, et al. Atypical teratoid/rhabdoid tumors (ATRT): improved survival in children 3 years of age and older with radiation therapy and high-dose alkylator-based chemotherapy. J Clin Oncol. 2005; 23(7):1491–9.
8. Lafay-Cousin L, et al. Central nervous system atypical teratoid rhabdoid tumours: the Canadian Paediatric Brain Tumour Consortium experience. Eur J Cancer. 2012;48(3):353–9.
9. Hilden JM, et al. Central nervous system atypical teratoid/rhabdoid tumor: results of therapy in children enrolled in a registry. J Clin Oncol. 2004;22(14): 2877–84.
10. Heck JE, et al. Epidemiology of rhabdoid tumors of early childhood. Pediatr Blood Cancer. 2013; 60(1):77–81.
11. Chi SN, et al. Intensive multimodality treatment for children with newly diagnosed CNS atypical teratoid rhabdoid tumor. J Clin Oncol. 2009;27(3):385–9.
12. Pai Panandiker AS, et al. Sequencing of local therapy affects the pattern of treatment failure and survival in children with atypical teratoid rhabdoid tumors of the central nervous system. Int J Radiat Oncol Biol Phys. 2012;82(5):1756–63.
13. Dufour C, et al. Clinicopathologic prognostic factors in childhood atypical teratoid and rhabdoid tumor of the central nervous system: a multicenter study. Cancer. 2012;118(15):3812–21.
14. Athale UH, et al. Childhood atypical teratoid rhabdoid tumor of the central nervous system: a meta-analysis of observational studies. J Pediatr Hematol Oncol. 2009;31(9):651–63.

15. Bruggers CS, et al. Clinicopathologic comparison of familial versus sporadic atypical teratoid/rhabdoid tumors (AT/RT) of the central nervous system. Pediatr Blood Cancer. 2011;56(7):1026–31.

16. Reddy AT. Atypical teratoid/rhabdoid tumors of the central nervous system. J Neurooncol. 2005;75(3): 309–13.

17. Koral K, et al. Imaging characteristics of atypical teratoid-rhabdoid tumor in children compared with medulloblastoma. AJR Am J Roentgenol. 2008; 190(3):809–14.

18. Au Yong KJ, et al. How specific is the MRI appearance of supratentorial atypical teratoid rhabdoid tumors? Pediatr Radiol. 2013;43(3):347–54.

19. Judkins AR, et al. Immunohistochemical analysis of hSNF5/INI1 in pediatric CNS neoplasms. Am J Surg Pathol. 2004;28(5):644–50.

20. Hasselblatt M, et al. Cribriform neuroepithelial tumor (CRINET): a nonrhabdoid ventricular tumor with INI1 loss and relatively favorable prognosis. J Neuropathol Exp Neurol. 2009;68(12):1249–55.

21. Biegel JA, et al. Monosomy 22 in rhabdoid or atypical tumors of the brain. J Neurosurg. 1990;73(5):710–4.

22. Roberts CW, Orkin SH. The SWI/SNF complex–chromatin and cancer. Nat Rev Cancer. 2004;4(2): 133–42.

23. Lee RS, et al. A remarkably simple genome underlies highly malignant pediatric rhabdoid cancers. J Clin Invest. 2012;122(8):2983–8.

24. Fujisawa H, et al. Cyclin D1 is overexpressed in atypical teratoid/rhabdoid tumor with hSNF5/INI1 gene inactivation. J Neurooncol. 2005;73(2):117–24.

25. Wilson BG, et al. Epigenetic antagonism between polycomb and SWI/SNF complexes during oncogenic transformation. Cancer Cell. 2010;18(4):316–28.

26. Klochendler-Yeivin A, Picarsky E, Yaniv M. Increased DNA damage sensitivity and apoptosis in cells lacking the Snf5/Ini1 subunit of the SWI/SNF chromatin remodeling complex. Mol Cell Biol. 2006;26(7):2661–74.

27. Hasselblatt M, et al. Nonsense mutation and inactivation of SMARCA4 (BRG1) in an atypical teratoid/rhabdoid tumor showing retained SMARCB1 (INI1) expression. Am J Surg Pathol. 2011;35(6):933–5.

28. Kieran MW, et al. Absence of oncogenic canonical pathway mutations in aggressive pediatric rhabdoid tumors. Pediatr Blood Cancer. 2012;59(7):1155–7.

29. Birks DK, et al. High expression of BMP pathway genes distinguishes a subset of atypical teratoid/rhabdoid tumors associated with shorter survival. Neuro Oncol. 2011;13(12):1296–307.

30. Bourdeaut F, et al. Frequent hSNF5/INI1 germline mutations in patients with rhabdoid tumor. Clin Cancer Res. 2011;17(1):31–8.

31. Biegel JA. Molecular genetics of atypical teratoid/rhabdoid tumor. Neurosurg Focus. 2006;20(1):E11.

32. Schneppenheim R, et al. Germline nonsense mutation and somatic inactivation of SMARCA4/BRG1 in a family with rhabdoid tumor predisposition syndrome. Am J Hum Genet. 2010;86(2):279–84.

33. Gardner SL, et al. Intensive induction chemotherapy followed by high dose chemotherapy with autologous hematopoietic progenitor cell rescue in young children newly diagnosed with central nervous system atypical teratoid rhabdoid tumors. Pediatr Blood Cancer. 2008;51(2):235–40.

34. Geyer JR, et al. Multiagent chemotherapy and deferred radiotherapy in infants with malignant brain tumors: a report from the Children's Cancer Group. J Clin Oncol. 2005;23(30):7621–31.

35. Zimmerman MA, et al. Continuous remission of newly diagnosed and relapsed central nervous system atypical teratoid/rhabdoid tumor. J Neurooncol. 2005; 72(1):77–84.

36. Finkelstein-Shechter T, et al. Atypical teratoid or rhabdoid tumors: improved outcome with high-dose chemotherapy. J Pediatr Hematol Oncol. 2010;32(5): e182–6.

37. Nicolaides T, et al. High-dose chemotherapy and autologous stem cell rescue for atypical teratoid/rhabdoid tumor of the central nervous system. J Neurooncol. 2010;98(1):117–23.

38. Ginn KF, Gajjar A. Atypical teratoid rhabdoid tumor: current therapy and future directions. Front Oncol. 2012;2:114.

39. von Hoff K, et al. Frequency, risk-factors and survival of children with atypical teratoid rhabdoid tumors (AT/RT) of the CNS diagnosed between 1988 and 2004, and registered to the German HIT database. Pediatr Blood Cancer. 2011;57(6):978–85.

40. Chen YW, et al. Impact of radiotherapy for pediatric CNS atypical teratoid/rhabdoid tumor (single institute experience). Int J Radiat Oncol Biol Phys. 2006; 64(4):1038–43.

41. Kordes U, et al. Clinical and molecular features in patients with atypical teratoid rhabdoid tumor or malignant rhabdoid tumor. Genes Chromosomes Cancer. 2010;49(2):176–81.

42. Lafay-Cousin L, Hawkins C, Fryer C, Bouffet E. Some infants with CNS ATRT can be cured without radiation. Neuro Oncol. 2012;14 Suppl 1:2.

43. Frühwald MC, Graf N. European Rhabdoid Registry. *EU-RHAB*. V2010. 29/07/2010; Available from: http://www.kinderkrebsstiftung.de/fileadmin/kinderkrebsinfo.de/EURHAB100729MS_ger.pdf. Accessed on 29 August 2013.

44. Clinical Trials (PDQ®). Combination Chemotherapy, Radiation Therapy, and an Autologous Peripheral Blood Stem Cell Transplant in Treating Young Patients With Atypical Teratoid/Rhabdoid Tumor of the Central Nervous System. National Cancer Institute. June 10, 2013. Available from: http://www.cancer.gov/clinicaltrials/search/view?cdrid=592812&version=HealthProfessional. Accessed on 29 August 2013.

Craniopharyngioma

16

David Phillips, Patrick J. McDonald, and Ute Bartels

Introduction

Craniopharyngiomas, although a tumor of benign histology, can take a morbid clinical course. They are thought to originate from squamous epithelial cells left over after partial involution of the hypophyseal-pharyngeal duct during formation of the anterior pituitary gland. By nature they are slow-growing, insidious intra- and suprasellar tumors that cause symptoms by local extension and injury to the adjacent pituitary, hypothalamic, and third ventricular regions or by raised intracranial pressure from mass effect or hydrocephalus.

While they can occur at any age, craniopharyngiomas typically present in a bimodal distribution, with one peak in childhood and another in adulthood. The histology, presentation, and clinical course of pediatric craniopharyngiomas differ in many respects from the adult version. Most importantly, craniopharyngiomas in childhood pose challenges in regard to treatment choices at young age that are associated with significant morbidities. The optimal treatment of these tumors remains controversial some 200 years after the first case was described.

Craniopharyngiomas were first identified and characterized in the latter half of the 1800s by a combination of pathologists, neurologists, and neurosurgeons. Clinically, patients presented with visual loss, diabetes insipidus, and brainstem compression, though Babinski also described a patient with "sexual infantilism and dystrophic adiposity." Halstead was the first to operate on a craniopharyngioma in 1909, followed by others who used either transnasal or transcranial approaches. In 1932, Cushing published the largest case series of the time, in which he popularized Charles Frazier's term craniopharyngioma for these tumors [1]. Surgical mortality was high, due to limited imaging and surgical techniques and lack of antibiotics and hormonal replacement therapies.

Advances in all these fields have improved the management of craniopharyngiomas. Diagnosis and treatment considerations have changed with improvements in MRI, CT, and intraoperative

D. Phillips, B.A.S.C. (Eng)., M.Sc.S.S., M.D., F.R.C.S.C.
Department of Neurosurgery, University of Manitoba, Winnipeg, MB, Canada

P.J. McDonald, M.D., M.H.Sc., F.R.C.S.C. (✉)
Department of Neurosurgery and Pediatrics, Winnipeg Children's Hospital, University of Manitoba, Winnipeg, MB, Canada
e-mail: pmcdonald@hsc.mb.ca

U. Bartels, M.D.
Department of Hematology/Oncology, The Hospital for Sick Children, Toronto, ON, Canada

neuronavigation. Medical and perioperative care is vastly superior to initial case series, with the primary improvement being in the neuroendocrinological management of these patients. Modern surgery is safer particularly with the aid of microsurgical techniques and neuro-endoscopy. Finally, radiotherapy, including stereotactic, conformal therapy and newer, directed chemotherapy agents, has enabled better control of these tumors over longer periods. Despite that, the management of craniopharyngiomas is still fraught with controversy and high morbidity rates, leaving room for improvement and innovation. Craniopharyngiomas remain, in Harvey Cushing's words, "the most formidable of intracranial tumors" [1].

Epidemiology

Craniopharyngiomas represent 2–4 % of all pediatric intracranial tumors [2]. Though the majority of craniopharyngiomas are found in adults, the distribution is bimodal, with a peak from 5 to 15 years and another at 45–60 years. Neonatal and intrauterine cases have been described but are rare.

Clinical Presentation

Children with craniopharyngiomas present in a variety of ways, related to the sellar and suprasellar location of these slow-growing tumors. They typically present with a combination of neuroendocrinological symptoms, visual impairment, hydrocephalus, hypothalamic disorder, or cranial nerve or brainstem dysfunction. One or more of these symptoms may be missed for an extended period, especially in younger patients. Rare craniopharyngiomas present as a nasopharyngeal, sphenoid, or exclusively third ventricular lesion, following the path of the hypophyseal-pharyngeal duct. Extremely rare craniopharyngiomas can occur in other parts of the brain, which can result in unusual clinical presentations.

Neuroendocrinological Symptoms

Common endocrine derangements present as diabetes insipidus, delayed or precocious puberty, growth deceleration, or hypothalamic obesity. Diabetes insipidus manifests in any age group as polyuria and polydipsia. Normal thirst mechanisms may be impaired by hypothalamic dysfunctions, leading to an exacerbation of electrolyte abnormalities in patients with diabetes insipidus. In adolescents, as presented in Babinski's first case report, a craniopharyngioma may only be discovered during a workup for delayed puberty. Alternatively, craniopharyngiomas can be associated with precocious puberty. Growth deceleration or stunted growth is a commonly missed symptom, often found only after workup for the patients' other presenting complaints. Further symptoms of hypopituitarism including central hypothyroidism, hypogonadism, and hypoadrenalism mandate a full endocrinologic assessment in a patient with presumed craniopharyngioma.

Hypothalamic obesity is associated with craniopharyngiomas that involve hypothalamic structures and may progress to morbid obesity due to further hypothalamic injury as a result of treatment. Tragically, this morbid obesity is essentially unresponsive to usual dietary or lifestyle modifications as the pathogenesis "involves the inability to transduce afferent hormonal signals of obesity" [3].

The obesity may be confounded by comorbid pituitary abnormalities. Substitution of growth hormone if necessary or manipulation of insulin secretion, e.g., with oral hypoglycemias may assist with weight control. While hyperphagia can be present, it is not the main culprit of the morbid obesity. Symptoms of autonomic, sleep, or memory derangements further indicate hypothalamic injury.

An alternate manifestation of hypothalamic damage is the "diencephalic syndrome," a failure to thrive despite appropriate nutritional intake. Children with this syndrome usually present emaciated, with hyperactivity, euphoria, and normal linear growth. The difference between these two presentations is thought to be hypothalamic invasion versus extrinsic compression, respectively [4, 5].

Visual Symptoms

Visual disturbance is a common feature of craniopharyngiomas, though a presenting complaint in a minority (30 %) of pediatric cases [6]. Children, especially when less than 5 years of age, are often unaware of visual loss, even if it has progressed significantly. The visual impairment may be discovered only after consultation for inattention, deteriorating school performance, or presumed clumsiness. Up to 20 % of children may be functionally blind by the time of presentation [7]. Visual field assessment, though difficult to perform in younger children, may reveal the classic bitemporal hemianopsia of chiasmatic compression, though asymmetric symptoms due to eccentric tumor growth are more common. Diplopia, decreased visual acuity or "blurriness," and fundoscopic abnormalities including pallor as a sign of optic atrophy are common. Serial ophthalmologic assessments in a child with craniopharyngioma are an essential part of diagnosis, surveillance, and management strategies.

Hydrocephalus

The classic triad of symptoms of increased intracranial pressure (ICP), consisting of headaches, nausea, and vomiting, will be present in children with obstructive hydrocephalus and is not specific for craniopharyngioma. Headache in intrasellar tumors may reflect dural stretch, not necessarily hydrocephalus. Hydrocephalus caused by a craniopharyngioma may present with acute symptoms or with a more protracted course of waxing and waning of symptoms. The most common cause of hydrocephalus in the setting of craniopharyngioma is tumor growth into the third ventricle causing obstruction at the foramen of Munro.

Other Presenting Symptoms

Cranial nerve palsies, brainstem signs, and ataxia are uncommon but may be present either due to focal compression or as a false-localizing sign in the setting of hydrocephalus. Rarely craniopharyngiomas cause seizures (likely due to temporal lobe involvement) or aseptic meningitis (due to cyst rupture). Mental status changes, which may appear in adults, are rare in children. Memory may be impaired due to involvement of the fornices and mammillary bodies. Sleep and thermoregulation can be altered in the setting of hypothalamic injury. Headaches may occur due to dural irritation, even in the absence of hydrocephalus.

Imaging Findings

Pediatric craniopharyngiomas are typically well-delineated tumors, mostly cystic in nature, with and without solid components (Fig. 16.1). The imaging modality of choice is MRI, though CT may be useful to identify calcifications and bony alterations. Calcifications are evident on CT scan in almost all of the pediatric adamantinomatous subtype. Craniopharyngiomas vary widely in size and sellar versus suprasellar location, though the former may demonstrate sellar enlargement and occasionally bony destruction. The tumor grows eccentrically, often with multiple lobules that can extend superiorly or posteriorly into the hypothalamus, third ventricle, or middle or posterior fossae. The optic chiasm and anterior carotid vessels can be stretched or displaced by this growth and are best seen on MRI. Peri-tumoral edema is uncommon.

Cystic contents are often proteinaceous and may appear as hyperintense on T1- and T2-weighted MRI compared to CSF. The solid tumor itself is hypo- to isointense on T1-weighted and heterogeneously hyperintense on T2-weighted MRI. There is typically heterogeneous enhancement of the solid component and often smooth enhancement of the cyst wall.

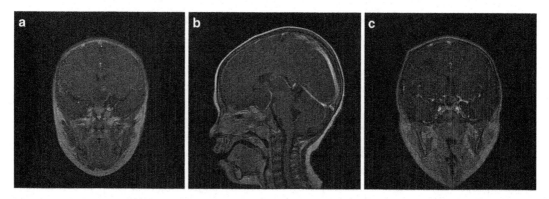

Fig. 16.1 Preoperative coronal (**a**) and sagittal (**b**) T1-weighted MR images following gadolinium infusion showing a predominantly cystic sellar and suprasellar craniopharyngioma in a 2 year old. Postoperative coronal (**c**) images showing a significant reduction in the size of the cyst after image-guided drainage and placement of an Ommaya reservoir

Neuroimaging must also characterize the degree and nature of hydrocephalus, if it is present, and is essential for planning operative approaches. Many centers use image navigation and intraoperative imaging as useful adjuvants for surgical management. Follow-up protocols have not been formally studied and are often based on personal or institutional preferences. Few case reports of antenatal diagnosis by ultrasound are available. Craniopharyngiomas may be discovered as incidental findings on neuroimaging for other indications.

While MRI and CT are quite characteristic for craniopharyngioma, there are some similar-appearing lesions, such as Rathke's cleft cyst, xanthogranuloma, dermoid or epidermoid cysts, germ cell tumors, and low-grade glioma, or some pituitary adenomas (potentially with calcified hemorrhagic infarction) that should be considered in the differential diagnosis.

Pathology/Biology

The anterior pituitary gland is formed during gestation by the infolding of nasopharyngeal cells. Remnants of these cells are thought to give rise to some pineal region tumors and cysts in addition to craniopharyngiomas. This pedigree explains their resemblance to adamantinoma (enamel-forming tumor) of the jaw and calcifying odontogenic cysts. This origin also explains how craniopharyngiomas can also appear in the nasopharynx or sphenoid bone, as these are along the path of the infolding cells. Few craniopharyngiomas arise solely in the third ventricle, putatively growing from rest cells (remnants of the infolding) in the tuber cinereum. An alternate theory of origin attributes craniopharyngiomas to metaplasia of pituitary adenoid cells.

There are two variants of craniopharyngioma, adamantinomatous and papillary, though transitional types cloud this distinction. Papillary craniopharyngiomas occur nearly exclusively in adults, can be easier to resect, recur less often, and calcify and form cysts less often. Both subtypes are histologically benign tumors and only exceptionally show malignant transformation or CNS seeding. The following description focuses on the pediatric, adamantinomatous type of craniopharyngioma.

Macroscopically, the majority of pediatric craniopharyngiomas are multilobular cystic tumor with or without a solid component. The cysts are filled with thick, gritty, "machine-oil" fluid brownish in appearance. It is this fluid that can cause an aseptic meningitis if spillage occurs. The walls of the cyst may have a smooth lining and can be calcified leading to an eggshell appearance. The solid portion of the tumor is

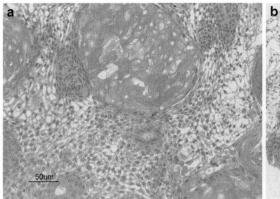 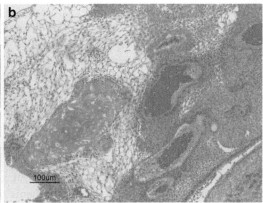

Fig. 16.2 (**a, b**) Cystic spaces are lined by neoplastic cells arranged in palisaded profiles. Cuboidal to columnar epithelium blends into looser central zones containing stellate cells. Calcification and clumps of "wet keratin" consisting of ghosts of keratinized cells are a prominent feature of the adamantinomatous variant of craniopharyngioma. Courtesy of Cynthia E. Hawkins

hard and gray and often has calcifications throughout making it crumbly. The tumor may be adherent to brain parenchyma, infundibulum, or optic pathway and may invaginate the third ventricle/foramen of Munro region.

Microscopically, craniopharyngiomas are microcystic, with cysts lined by squamous epithelial cells (Fig. 16.2). There may be a peripheral rim of palisading columnar cells. Sheets of cells keratinize and form anuclear ghost cells, creating "wet keratin." Areas of dystrophic calcification give the tumor its adamantinomatous name. Tumor cells may secrete fluid and cholesterol, forming clefts and necrotic debris, or the fluid may be retained in the cells creating a looser matrix in regions.

Tumor may interdigitate into the parenchyma without infiltration or causing frank invasion. The arachnoid may be absent in areas of significant gliosis or interdigitation.

Multinucleated giant cells may be present surrounding necrotic debris and cholesterol clefts; however, these are more typical for xanthogranuloma. The surrounding brain may show gliotic changes with Rosenthal fibers as a reactive process owing to the slow growth of these tumors. This should not be mistaken for pilocytic astrocytoma. Epidermoid and Rathke's cleft cyst may be raised in the differential diagnosis but should be distinguishable by the experienced neuropathologist. As the majority of adamantinomatous cra- niopharyngioma harbors a mutation of the β-catenin gene, nuclear accumulation of β-catenin can aid in the distinction.

Current Treatment

Optimal management of craniopharyngiomas remains one of the most hotly debated topics in pediatric neurosurgery, neuro-oncology, and endocrinology. While total resection may confer the best long-term prospect for cure, patients can be left with devastating hypothalamic and pituitary dysfunction [8]. Neurosurgeons have attempted to reduce patient morbidity using microsurgical techniques, transnasal, transventricular, or a variety of skull-base approaches with the assistance of newer technology such as endoscopy, intraoperative MRI and ultrasound, and image-guided navigation, all with varying degrees of success. Alternative approaches, aimed at protecting the visual system and treating hydrocephalus, have therefore been pioneered with resultant improvements in quality of life, but higher progression rates. These approaches include subtotal resection, cyst drainage including placement of Ommaya reservoirs, intracystic chemotherapy, and radiotherapy. Prospective data with sufficient patient numbers to support a specific management approach is limited.

Surgical

Neurosurgeons who manage craniopharyngiomas have a number of choices available to them. Firstly, the extent of resection must be decided upon. The UK Children's Cancer and Leukaemia Group consensus guidelines recommend total resection for tumors smaller than 2–4 cm without hypothalamic involvement or hydrocephalus in order to minimize postoperative worsening of pituitary, hypothalamic, and visual function [9]. Larger tumors, and those with hypothalamic involvement or hydrocephalus, are preferentially treated by subtotal resection followed by radiotherapy (according to age). Both of these approaches must be customized to the individual patient.

Upon deciding to proceed with surgery, multiple approaches are available. Transsphenoidal and endoscopic/endonasal surgeries approach the tumor through the sphenoid sinus and sella and may be extended through the diaphragm, planum sphenoidale, or the dorsum sella. It provides limited exposure to lateral and intraventricular tumor lobules, but may result in shorter hospital stays [10] (Fig. 16.3). Transcallosal or transventricular approaches are used to debulk tumors with extensive protrusion into the third ventricle; many centers use endoscopes to assist with these approaches. The limitation of a superior approach is access to infra-chiasmatic structures. Skullbase approaches provide multiple avenues for supra- and intrasellar tumors, with options to use pterional, subfrontal, frontolateral, or extended approaches for resection. Lateral approaches may not provide enough exposure of both optic nerves and intraventricular tumor lobules, and subfrontal (particularly bifrontal) approaches risk injury to both olfactory nerves and both inferior frontal lobes and have limited access to retrosellar regions and CSF cisterns. Ultimately, tumors with intrasellar, suprasellar, and/or intraventricular growth patterns may require combined approaches, capitalizing on the strengths of each in a staged or simultaneous manner.

Since craniopharyngiomas grow superiorly, they should have arachnoid dissection planes with overlying structures. Unfortunately, this is not always the case. Many will induce a gliotic rim that can provide a pseudo-dissection plane. Care must be taken to preserve the infundibulum, optic apparatus, and hypothalamus. As well, perforating arteries and superior hypophyseal arteries (supplying the optic chiasm) may be stretched and displaced superolaterally and should be preserved. Dissection may be simpler prior to cyst drainage. Gentle retraction of the capsule as opposed to the nervous tissue is essential. Exposure may be improved by drilling off the planum sphenoidale and/or optic strut. Entry into the frontal or sphenoid sinuses requires careful closure or exenteration.

Often a large cyst may be aspirated prior to or instead of surgical resection. Cyst aspiration may be done under direct visualization, endoscopically, transsphenoidally, or via stereotactic needle or drainage tube placement. Draining a cyst early may expose the dissection plane better or may be a sufficient treatment for hydrocephalus. Care must be taken to avoid spillage of the cyst contents to avoid aseptic meningitis. For cysts that will require repeated aspirations, one may insert a subcutaneous catheter and reservoir, such as an Ommaya or Rickham reservoir, and/or use intracavitary sclerosing therapy (see below). Prior to intracystic chemotherapy, most institutional protocols require instillation of contrast medium to ensure the agent does not leak out of the cyst.

Hydrocephalus adds an extra dimension to surgical management of craniopharyngiomas, often requiring a first operation to divert CSF or drain an enlarged cyst. Acute hydrocephalus is typically treated with an extraventricular drain, while subacute presentations may be treated with endoscopic or stereotactic cyst aspiration. Septal perforation is occasionally beneficial for significant involvement of the foramen of Munro. CSF shunting may be required for a subset of patients, though most surgeons will initially attempt to reestablish CSF drainage pathways prior to committing a patient to a shunt.

Surgical complications are unfortunately common in these complex tumors. The most common complication, as mentioned previously, is pituitary injury causing transient or

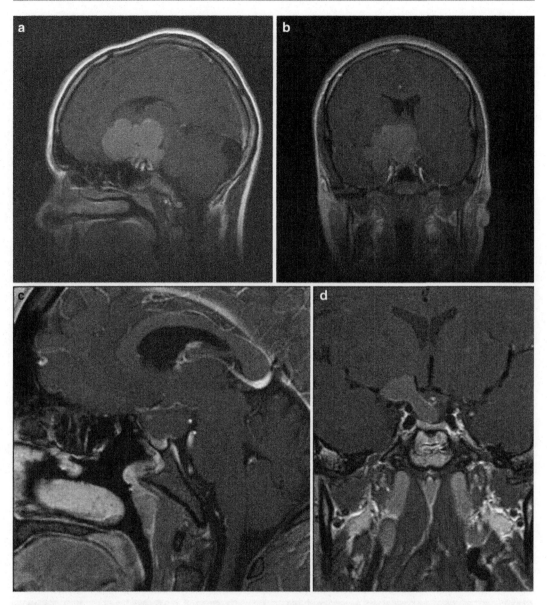

Fig. 16.3 Preoperative sagittal (**a**) and coronal (**b**) T1-weighted MR images following administration of gadolinium showing a multilobulated cystic craniopharyngioma in a 13 year old. Postoperative sagittal (**c**) and coronal (**d**) images showing reduction in the size of the cyst after endoscopic endonasal drainage

permanent hypopituitarism and diabetes insipidus. Hypothalamic injury is more common in patients with preoperative symptoms. Visual deterioration may occur due to manipulation of the optic chiasm or its vascular supply. Aseptic meningitis results from cyst content leakage and presents immediately, while septic meningitis takes a few days to develop. Communicating hydrocephalus can be a further complication of meningitis or occur despite reestablishment of the normal CSF pathways. Postoperative CSF leaks may be a sign of hydrocephalus or due to penetration of the sphenoid sinus, frontal sinus, or ventricular system; they may respond to temporary drainage via EVD or lumbar drain. Lastly, injury to the nerves or anterior circulation vascular structures may cause other focal neurological deficits, with anosmia and ageusia being common after subfrontal approaches.

Medical

Medical management comprises the bulk of care for craniopharyngioma patients due to hypothalamic, pituitary, and neurocognitive concerns pre- and postoperatively. Purely asymptomatic craniopharyngiomas with minimal to no suprasellar cystic extension may be followed without surgery, though cysts may enlarge at any time and cause symptoms. Systemic chemotherapy has limited efficacy in treating craniopharyngiomas, though some promise was seen in one trial of systemic interferon-α-2b [11].

Recent trials of intracystic bleomycin or interferon alpha have been shown to sclerose some cysts and induce shrinkage, with the best benefit risk profile favoring interferon [12] (Fig. 16.4). While bleomycin is neurotoxic and leakage may cause meningitis, cranial neuropathies, or even fatalities, interferon is used as an intrathecal treatment in leptomeningeal carcinomatosis, and therefore leakage outside the cyst does not pose the risk of CNS damage. This has particular application to young patients who are not yet candidates for radiotherapy or those who have failed prior cyst aspirations. Intracystic treatment does not affect the solid component of the tumor and only is beneficial to the cyst being treated.

Radiotherapy

In general, craniopharyngiomas are responsive to radiotherapy (RT) but limits relate to their proximity to adjacent critical, radiosensitive structures. Intracystic radiation via *beta*-emitting particles has been tried in the past with success at preventing cyst growth, but with unsatisfactory risks of injury to vision. It has therefore fallen out of favor. Radiation often prevents tumor progression, but risks injury to pituitary, optic, and hypothalamic structures and global brain development in the young. Ultimately, radiotherapy decreases the need for further surgery in incompletely resected (STR) craniopharyngiomas.

Conventional RT in combination with STR has shown similar control rates to gross total resection (GTR) (75–90 % progression-free survival) [13], with fewer rates of endocrinopathy and neurological deficit than GTR [8]. Typical management algorithms provide RT as an adjuvant to partially resected tumors in patients older than 5 years of age with current prospective research determining the benefit of immediate postoperative versus radiotherapy at the time of progression [5]. Repeated surgery, cyst drainage, or intracystic treatment may avoid or at least postpone radiotherapy. Approximately 10–20 % of patients who have received radiation will have cyst enlargement or regrowth requiring surgery [14].

Craniopharyngiomas remain highly radiosensitive, responding to focal doses of less than 10 Gy. The standard of care in children is

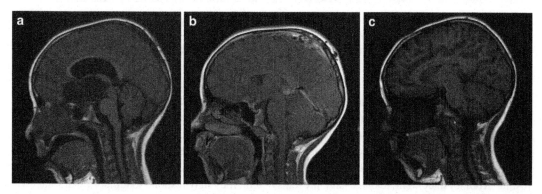

Fig. 16.4 Four-year-old girl with craniopharyngioma at diagnosis (**a**), 19 months after intracystic treatment with interferon alpha (**b**) and 2 years later (**c**). She remains in response and fully pituitary intact 5.5 years later

currently fractionated RT (54 Gy in 30 daily fractions) which can be delivered via stereotactic techniques (FSRT) or more commonly with daily image guidance to maximize positioning accuracy.

Many large series of stereotactic radiosurgery (SRS) via multi-collimator cobalt (Gamma Knife) or robot-mounted linear accelerators (LINAC) to treat craniopharyngiomas include both adult and pediatric patients. SRS provides high-dose radiation to the tumor volume with rapid falloff to the optic apparatus and hypothalamus [15, 16]. Because the long-term effects of SRS in young children have not been well studied, caution should be exercised before utilizing this treatment modality. Proton beam therapy has a similar potential to preserve structures adjacent to the tumor with promising preliminary results [17]. Tumor control rates exceed 90 % in some studies of radiosurgery.

Radiotherapy confers risk of pituitary and hypothalamic dysfunction, optic injury or neuritis, neurodevelopmental sequelae, and delayed risk of vascular injury or secondarily induced tumors [14]. Innovations in conformal RT and new types of RT may reduce long-term morbidities but likely won't eliminate these risks.

Outcome

Outcomes in craniopharyngioma are the key to comparing treatment modalities. The goal of treatment should be to provide the best quality-of-life outcome possible; cure is therefore only one aspect of this approach. Morbidity and impairment or retreatment are very important other factors. The major impacts on mortality are related to hydrocephalus, surgery-related infections, and hormonal derangements especially diabetes insipidus and cortisol insufficiency. Important factors affecting quality of life in craniopharyngiomas are vision, endocrinological and hypothalamic function, memory, school or work performance, and subsequent ability of an independent life. The need of multiple hospital visits, including management of blocked shunts, acute endocrinopathies, infections, and late radiation effects, negatively affects outcomes and interferes with quality-of-life factors as listed above. The controversy regarding goals of treatment should therefore be viewed in this light.

The prognosis for visual, endocrinologic, and hypothalamic outcome seems to depend primarily on preoperative status [10] and age at presentation as well as social insertion [18]. Surgical series aiming for GTR are associated with higher risks of injury [19], and long-term side effects of radiotherapy in young children are well documented. Due to the rarity of craniopharyngioma and its diverse presentation, the lack of prospective trials and publications that are often limited to institutional retrospective reviews, treatment strategies, and outcomes remains difficult to compare [20].

Recurrence

The frequency of craniopharyngioma recurrence is similar in patients who have received GTR or STR followed by RT [13], with tumor control rates in most series exceeding 90 % over 5 years [11]. Most recurrences become evident within the first 3 years.

The majority of patients requiring reoperation do so because of new cysts or cyst regrowth. Reoperation, cyst drainage, or placement of a subcutaneous catheter and reservoir for intracystic therapy may be reconsidered at this time and will depend on the initial interventions chosen. Radiotherapy may be used in selected cases. New symptoms or imaging findings may be due to prior radiation treatment as opposed to tumor recurrence. Craniopharyngiomas do not undergo dedifferentiation. Serial follow-up including imaging and visual and endocrine assessments are recommendable throughout childhood, and most institutions will continue with at least yearly MRIs for 10 years following diagnosis.

Neuroendocrine

Endocrine injury is possible even if the pituitary and its stalk are preserved at the time of operation or excluded from the radiation field [8]. The estimated rate of postoperative endocrinopathy is 37 %, with patients undergoing a GTR having a significantly higher risk [18]. Partial injury is better tolerated than total panhypopituitarism, as is older age (postpubertal) at the time of pituitary dysfunction. The anterior pituitary functions may be affected more than the posterior pituitary functions, as ADH may also be secreted by the hypothalamus or upper stalk. However, in cases of additional injury to the pituitary gland and hypothalamus, management of diabetes insipidus becomes even more challenging due to a dysfunctional hypothalamic thirst center.

Hypothalamic Dysfunction

Much of the chronic morbidity in childhood craniopharyngioma is related to hypothalamic dysfunction, in particular obesity. The hypothalamus is integral to homeostatic control of metabolism, weight and hunger, thirst, sleep, and arousal. Obesity after craniopharyngioma treatment is the most common complication, ranging from 30 to 77 % [3], especially if pretreatment hypothalamic involvement is present. Hypothalamic symptoms escalate proportionate to the extent and location of the hypothalamic injury pre- and posttreatment; there are no or minor symptoms when graded as 0^0 (no involvement) or I^0 (hypothalamic involvement anterior to the mammillary bodies) but significant hypothalamic symptoms when graded as II^0 (anterior and posterior hypothalamic involvement) [5]. Patients with hypothalamic dysfunction can be obese or cachectic and sedate or impulsive or may have disturbances of sleep or memory. Obesity may result in metabolic syndrome and sleep apnea and contributes to impaired quality of life.

Patients with hypothalamic injury have decreased energy and energy expenditure and continue to gain weight even with caloric restriction. The mechanism behind the weight gain is incompletely understood, but relates to leptin resistance and decreased sympathetic tone, among others [3]. Prevention of hypothalamic injury is the best treatment, helping to drive less

aggressive initial surgeries [6]. Octreotide may have some benefit, while other pharmaceutical intervention thus far had limited benefit.

Other hypothalamic sequelae can lead to behavioral and emotional pathology, difficulty interacting in society, and lack of independence. These patients can be severely handicapped and require significant support through childhood, adolescence, and into adulthood.

Future Directions

While optimal treatment strategies still need to be defined, there is evidence that less aggressive surgical approaches contribute to better quality of life in children affected by extensive craniopharyngioma. Intracystic treatment offers a less invasive strategy that may at least delay the need for radiation to an older, less vulnerable age. Highly conformal radiotherapy such as proton beam therapy or stereotactic radiosurgery may limit treatment-related morbidity. Comparisons and reliable conclusions in regard to optimal treatment strategies will be facilitated by achieving consensus on prospective data collection and multi-institutional cooperation and collaboration.

References

1. Barkhoudarian G, Laws ER. Craniopharyngioma: history. Pituitary. 2013;16(1):1–8.
2. Müller HL. Consequences of craniopharyngioma surgery in children. J Clin Endocrinol Metab. 2011;96(7): 1981–91.
3. Lustig RH. Hypothalamic obesity after craniopharyngioma: mechanisms, diagnosis, and treatment. Front Endocrinol (Lausanne). 2011;2:60.
4. Fleischman A, Brue C, Poussaint TY, et al. Diencephalic syndrome: a cause of failure to thrive and a model of partial growth hormone resistance. Pediatrics. 2005;115(6):e742–8.
5. Müller HL, Gebhardt U, Teske C, et al. Post-operative hypothalamic lesions and obesity in childhood craniopharyngioma: results of the multinational prospective trial KRANIOPHARYNGEOM 2000 after 3-year follow-up. Eur J Endocrinol. 2011;165(1):17–24.
6. Lopez-Serna R, Gomez-Amador JL, Barges-Coll J, et al. Treatment of craniopharyngioma in adults: systematic analysis of a 25-year experience. Arch Med Res. 2012;43(5):347–55.

7. van Effenterre R, Boch A. Craniopharyngioma. In: Tonn J, Westphal M, Rutka JT, editors. Oncology of CNS tumors. 2nd ed. Heidelberg: Springer; 2010. p. 559–70.

8. Clark AJ, Cage TA, Aranda D, Parsa AT, Auguste KI, Gupta N. Treatment-related morbidity and the management of pediatric craniopharyngioma. J Neurosurg Pediatr. 2012;10(4):293–301.

9. Mallucci C, Pizer B, Blair J, et al. Management of craniopharyngioma: the Liverpool experience following the introduction of the CCLG guidelines: introducing a new risk assessment grading system. Childs Nerv Syst. 2012;28(8):1181–92.

10. Chakrabarti I, Amar AP, Couldwell W, Weiss MH. Long-term neurological, visual, and endocrine outcomes following transnasal resection of craniopharyngioma. J Neurosurg. 2005;102(4):650–7.

11. Yeung JT, Pollack IF, Panigrahy A, Jakacki RI. Pegylated interferon-α-2b for children with recurrent craniopharyngioma. J Neurosurg Pediatr. 2012;10(6): 498–503.

12. Bartels U, Laperriere N, Bouffet E, Drake J. Intracystic therapies for cystic craniopharyngioma in childhood. Front Endocrinol (Lausanne). 2012;3:39.

13. Yang I, Sughrue ME, Rutkowski MJ, et al. Craniopharyngioma: a comparison of tumor control with various treatment strategies. Neurosurg Focus. 2010;28(4):E5.

14. Kiehna EN, Merchant TE. Radiation therapy for pediatric craniopharyngioma. Neurosurg Focus. 2010; 28(4):E10.

15. Kobayashi T. Long-term results of gamma knife radiosurgery for 100 consecutive cases of craniopharyngioma and a treatment strategy. Prog Neurol Surg. 2009;22:63–76.

16. Loeffler J, Shrieve D, Wen P, et al. Radiosurgery for intracranial malignancies. Semin Radiat Oncol. 1995;5(3):225–34.

17. Merchant TE. Clinical controversies: proton therapy for pediatric tumors. Semin Radiat Oncol. 2013;23(2):97–108.

18. Gautier A, Godbout A, Grosheny C, et al. Markers of recurrence and long-term morbidity in craniopharyngioma: a systematic analysis of 171 patients. J Clin Endocrinol Metab. 2012;97(4):1258–67.

19. Sughrue ME, Yang I, Kane AJ, et al. Endocrinologic, neurologic, and visual morbidity after treatment for craniopharyngioma. J Neurooncol. 2011;101(3):463–76.

20. Cohen M, Bartels U, Branson H, Kulkarni A, Hamilton J. Trends in treatment and outcomes of pediatric craniopharyngioma, 1975-2011. Neuro Oncol. 2013;15(6):767–74.

Rare Tumours of the Central Nervous System in Children

17

Adam J. Fleming

Introduction

According to the Central Brain Tumor Registry of the United States (CBTRUS), the incidence of all central nervous system (CNS) tumours in the 0–19-year-old paediatric range is approximately 4.8 in 100,000 population [1]. Therefore, tumours of the brain and spine are rare occurrences in children overall, regardless of the type. However, beyond the more commonly encountered paediatric CNS tumours lies the existence of a large number of *very rare* tumours, or *extremely rare* in some cases. In this chapter, we will highlight a few examples of the different types that occur at a frequency of less than 5 % of all paediatric CNS tumours. There is not enough room to cover every rare tumour type in this chapter, so a few have been selected as examples of tumours that present an interesting diagnostic dilemma, classification challenge, or clinical problem.

More importantly, we will outline a basic approach to rare tumours in children, with diagnostic and management considerations applicable to all tumour types.

A.J. Fleming, M.A.Sc., M.D., F.R.C.P.(C). (✉)
Division of Hematology/Oncology, The Montreal
Children's Hospital (McGill University Health
Center), Montréal, QC, Canada
e-mail: adam.fleming@muhc.mcgill.ca

Overview: Epidemiology

When dealing with small percentages within a small group of patients, one must apply caution in interpreting statistics for incidence or prevalence. Accurate statistics on incidence and prevalence require that a disease has been described in the past, is well recognized and reported by clinicians, and is rarely mistaken for other diseases. Tumours may become re-classified. Other tumours may not 'exist' as a separate entity until a diagnostic test becomes readily available to pathologists. Any time a tumour is described as a 'new' tumour type, these will effectively be removed from the statistics of whatever tumour it was previously classified as. In summary, if a tumour is very rare then one must re-evaluate the statistics over time as technologies evolve and definitions emerge.

Overview: Imaging and Pathology

As with all paediatric brain tumours, referral to a tertiary care specialized centre should be arranged as soon as possible, depending on the urgency and stability of the patient. It is extremely important to have *paediatric* neuro-oncology expertise in the neuroimaging, diagnostic surgery, and subsequent management decisions. A multidisciplinary team approach is necessary, as is emphasized throughout this book. Pathology specimens should be organized, reviewed, and reported by a neuropathologist with specialized training and

K. Scheinemann and E. Bouffet (eds.), *Pediatric Neuro-oncology*,
DOI 10.1007/978-1-4939-1541-5_17, © Springer Science+Business Media New York 2015

expertise in paediatric CNS tumours. It becomes particularly important for most neuropathologists to be able to seek consensus opinions when dealing with very rare tumours. Some rare tumour types may not yet have a World Health Organization grading or classification. Even when the pathology is challenging to define, certain general features such as metastases, mitotic index, neovascular proliferation, or invasion into surrounding tissues may help influence treatment strategies. The staging work-up will be guided in part by the general category of the tumour, indicating the need for other investigations (e.g. spinal imaging, a bone marrow biopsy, or a lumbar puncture to sample cerebrospinal fluid (CSF)).

Overview: Treatment

There are over 300 different CNS tumour subtypes in the 2007 WHO classification textbook. Often the description alone gives a clue as to the origins or family of tumours to which it belongs. There are those that exist within a larger family of tumours, as a rare subset of a more common type (e.g. ependymoblastoma, medulloepithelioma, and gliosarcoma). There are mixed groups of tumours, most commonly in the neuronal-glial category (ganglioglioma, dysembryoplastic neuroepithelial tumour, central neurocytomas). Other very rare tumours may stand alone from the major groupings (choroid plexus tumours). Oligodendrogliomas, astroblastoma, and papillary tumour of the pineal region are other examples that have unique features making them difficult to categorize under one of the larger groups. Finally, some 'benign' tumours lack malignant potential but can cause hormonal problems (pituitary adenomas). Case reports and small series in the literature may provide the only guidance for treatment, and expert opinion should be sought when appropriate. Does this tumour belong to a family of tumours that typically responds to radiation? Will a complete surgical resection offer a significant survival advantage? Is this tumour related to other categories that are sensitive to chemotherapy? The age of the patient and location in the CNS always influence the morbidity of

total resection. Large-field high-dose radiation can be devastating to the very young brain, regardless of the tumour type. For tumours that have disseminated throughout the CNS axis, aggressive surgery or focal radiation may not play a role in the treatment approach.

Overview: Outcomes

The prognostic outcome for patients with very rare tumours may be poorly described in the literature, if at all. Case series or case reports become vitally important as a reference basis for the paediatric neuro-oncology community worldwide. Whenever appropriate, clinicians should consider publishing the presentation and outcomes for very rare tumours, obtaining consent as required by local ethical review boards.

Specific Examples of Rare CNS Tumours in Childhood

Choroid Plexus Tumours

Our first example of a rare paediatric CNS tumour is the family of choroid plexus tumours (CPT). CPT refers to a tumour family that is generally thought of in two forms: a more 'benign' choroid plexus papilloma (CPP) and the malignant 'choroid plexus carcinoma' (CPC). The 2007 WHO categorizes another group called 'atypical choroid plexus papillomas' (aCPP), an intermediate grade in terms of malignant behaviour and response to therapy.

Epidemiology

CPTs occur in young children primarily. While we have included them as a 'very rare' tumour overall, they actually make up more than 10 % of all CNS tumours in the first year of life and are not a rare tumour to be diagnosed in an infant with a brain tumour. This age predisposition makes the treatment options difficult when considering radiation therapy, compounded by the fact that a

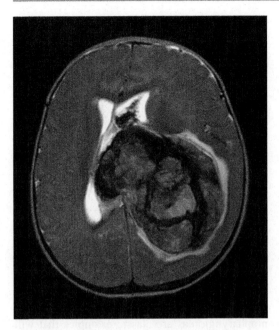

Fig. 17.1 Choroid plexus carcinoma in an infant (MRI T2-weighted image)

significant number of the higher-grade choroid plexus tumours are metastatic at diagnosis.

Imaging Findings

Choroid plexus tumours often have a characteristic appearance on neuroimaging with a distinctly irregular tumour margin and an inconsistent enhancing pattern. Their location is most commonly the lateral ventricles, followed by the fourth ventricle. Metastatic spread is not uncommon at diagnosis, especially with choroid plexus carcinomas. Hydrocephalus is typically present and often quite impressive (Fig. 17.1).

Pathology/Biology

Choroid plexus papillomas are classified as a WHO grade I (low-grade) tumour, while choroid plexus carcinoma is a WHO grade III (high-grade) tumour. The pathology for these tumours exists on a spectrum between papilloma and carcinoma. Cytokeratins and vimentin are expressed in both, while S-100 staining is more common in CPP than CPC. As expected, CPPs have a very

low mitotic index of activity, while CPCs show obvious signs of malignancy that include high cell division, nuclear pleomorphism, and necrotic areas [2]. The higher-grade CPCs are the CNS tumours with the strongest association with the genetic cancer predisposition syndromes related to p53 mutations. Therefore, all patients with a CPC should undergo a thorough family history and screening for the presence of hallmark cancer types, such as adrenocortical carcinomas or sarcomas in young family members. When suspicion is made of a familial cancer syndrome, referral for genetic counselling and appropriate screening tests should be made. Experienced genetic counsellors are crucial as the emotional and medical consequences of having a familial cancer predisposition are extensive. If a familial pattern is found, such as the *Li–Fraumeni* syndrome, published guidelines have demonstrated that careful screening and early detection can impart a survival benefit [3].

Current Treatment

For choroid plexus papillomas, surgical resection is the mainstay of treatment and attempts should be made to safely achieve gross total resection. Careful observation would follow, and there is no indication for radiation or chemotherapy in the upfront treatment of this subgroup.

Surgical resection remains important for choroid plexus carcinomas but is insufficient to cure this disease, and total resection often be limited by the haemorrhagic nature of these tumours. Radiation has been used in different settings for the treatment of CPCs, with consideration of craniospinal treatment given the metastatic potential of this subgroup. This may be considered for 'older' children (e.g. older than 3 years), but toxicities will be very significant for the younger population. In a population-based study by the Canadian Pediatric Brain Tumour Consortium, none of the infant CPC patients had been treated with radiation over a 15-year period (median age at diagnosis was 10 months old, with the oldest being 30 months old) [4]. While a specific chemotherapy regimen has yet to be defined for CPTs, there is evidence to suggest that intensive chemotherapy plays an important role for the malignant choroid plexus carcinomas [5]. The use of 'ICE' chemotherapy (ifosfamide, carboplatin, etoposide) in the neo-adjuvant setting has allowed a second-look surgical approach to be more feasible [5]. There is an ongoing investigation into the use of direct CSF chemotherapy (intraventricular or intrathecal) for this group of patients, perhaps thought to be more effective due to the location of the choroid plexus in the ventricular space. This can technically be done via lumbar puncture or more commonly with the use of an implanted device, such as an Ommaya reservoir.

Outcome

Patients with choroid plexus papilloma have a very good survival rate overall, even in the rare cases of metastatic disease. The long-term outcome for children has generally been greater than 90 %; a study of 21 CPP patients over a 15-year period in Canada showed 100 % survival [4].

On the other hand, CPC is known to carry a relatively poor prognosis, even with aggressive therapy. Gross total resection carries a dominant influence on prognosis; 5-year survival rates are close to 60 % with complete removal, compared to 20 % with partial resection alone [6]. In the patients with an incomplete resection, chemotherapy increases to the survival in the range of 40–60 % [5] [6].

Future Directions in Choroid Plexus Tumours

The rarity and poor prognosis of choroid plexus carcinoma has created a strong interest in international collaboration over the past two decades. This is an example of using well-designed clinical trials and registry data to maximize our understanding of a very rare disease, instead of relying only upon case reports. The type, timing, and intensity of chemotherapy will continue to be explored, and the question of which patients truly need radiation therapy is still under investigation.

At the same time, we need to continue to follow the choroid plexus papilloma patients to ensure that their very high survival rate holds up over time. As well, many other factors contribute to long-term neurocognitive deficits in children with choroid plexus tumours: the size of these aggressive tumours, long-standing hydrocephalus at diagnosis, and extensive or sometimes multiple surgeries. These patients should be followed closely long term and need to have access to neuropsychological testing and resources for academic rehabilitation.

Pituitary Adenomas

Several different tumour types can be localized in the suprasellar region; germ cell tumours and craniopharyngiomas are classic examples that will be discussed elsewhere in this book. As a group, tumours of the pituitary area are the most common CNS tumour type for older children in the 15–19 years age group [1]. *Pituitary adenomas* are one type that occur throughout adulthood and in rare circumstances occur in the postpubertal adolescence [7]. While they may have a benign histology, these tumours can be functionally harmful. Symptoms depend on the size and on hormonal secretion, with prolactinomas being the most common in children, followed by adrenocorticotropin-hormone-secreting and growth-hormone-secreting tumours [8]. Headaches, raised intracranial pressure, and visual field defects can result from any mass in this area, and elevated hormone levels will cause secondary problems (such as elevated prolactin levels leading to amenorrhoea and galactorrhoea). On neuroimaging, loss of the pituitary bright spot can provide an early sign that the pituitary stalk is being compressed. MRI may reveal a mass lesion, although adenomas can exist in both microadenoma and macroadenoma forms. Current treatment can involve surgical resection, with a transsphenoidal approach often considered. However, medical management is often needed for the endocrinopathies and may be a sufficient treatment for these tumours depending on whether other symptoms (e.g. hydrocephalus) are present. The appropriate use of dopamine agonists (bromocriptine, cabergoline) is sufficient for treating prolactinomas [9]. Once medical management is established and endocrinopathies have been addressed, overall prognosis is extremely good. Since this tumour occurs at a much greater frequency in adults than in children, this is an appropriate situation to consult adult medical oncology and surgical colleagues for advice on management strategies.

Astroblastoma

This very rare neuroepithelial glial tumour is included as an interesting CNS tumour that has been difficult to classify from a tumour grade perspective (Fig. 17.2). While the grading of rare tumours can often guide the clinician as to the best course of treatment, this is one of the few tumours listed in the WHO classification book that has not been assigned a specific grade. Although a tumour of its description was first described by Bailey and Cushing, it is felt to be 'premature to establish a WHO grade at this time' [2], which speaks to the rarity of its occurrence. These tumours have been reported at almost any age but typically appear in children and young adults. The imaging findings are quite striking, typically appearing as a large cystic area with a well-demarcated wall that enhances with MRI contrast. The pathology shows clear tumour margins and areas around blood vessels where tumour cells radiate outwards, anchored by cytoplasmic processes [2]. A variety of features have been described, ranging from anaplastic to a more well-differentiated form, and this information will be important for the clinician. In conjunction with the location and degree of resection, this could direct the choice for further adjuvant therapies including chemotherapy or radiotherapy. In the few literature case series and reports, a wide variety of treatment approaches have been used, including surgery alone, surgery followed by radiation, or the addition of many different chemotherapy treatments [10, 11]. Due to its rarity, a true prognosis is difficult to estimate but the limited data suggests an excellent prognosis overall.

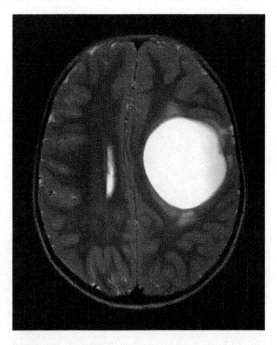

Fig. 17.2 Astroblastoma (axial MRI T2-weighted imaging)

Papillary Tumour of the Pineal Region

Most high-grade tumours presenting in the pineal region of children will turn out to be a form of primitive neuroectodermal tumour (PNET), referred to as a *pineoblastoma* in this location (Fig. 17.3). A much less common type is called *papillary tumour of the pineal region* (PTPR), which is considered to be a very rare tumour (less than 100 reported cases in the literature). This tumour serves as a reminder of how location can help define different types; there are a limited number of tumour types that will occur in this specific area, and the surgical approach may be very different between the histologies. The rarity of this tumour makes it challenging to estimate an incidence for this tumour, and case reports have described this tumour occurring in people of all ages. As with other tumours in this area, hydrocephalus is a common presenting symptom due to obstruction, and MRI is the ideal scan to define tumours in the pineal region. The MRI demonstrates a contrast-enhancing tumour with

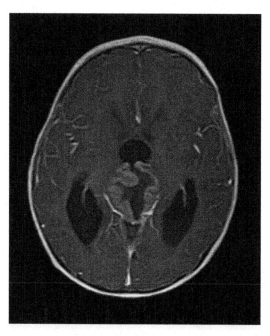

Fig. 17.3 High-grade papillary tumour of the pineal region (axial MRI with contrast, T1-weighted imaging)

high T2 signal. Immunohistochemistry is striking for reaction to keratin stains, along with vimentin, S-100, and focal GFAP expression. The WHO grading rests between grade II and grade III; therefore, the grade does not necessarily demonstrate the exact course of treatment. Treatments reported in the literature vary from surgical resection alone, to radiation (depending on the age), to attempts at chemotherapy if there is dissemination at diagnosis (in younger children). Relapse is relatively common, leading to a progression-free survival around 25 % with an average survival rate around 75 % [12].

Vestibular Schwannoma (Acoustic Neuroma)

Neurofibromatosis type I and type II are genetic syndromes that carry a predisposition for the formation of many different CNS tumours, both benign and malignant. The presence of bilateral vestibular schwannomas is one of the diagnostic criteria for neurofibromatosis type II (NF-2). This is one of the many examples of rare paediatric CNS tumours that can be linked to patients with an underlying genetic syndrome. Sometimes called 'acoustic neuromas', these are benign tumours arising from the 8th cranial nerve that can cause progressive hearing loss and deafness. NF-2 is an autosomal dominant genetic disorder occurring at an incidence of 1 per 25–40,000 people in the population [13]; about half of cases arise as a spontaneous mutation on chromosome 22 with no family history [14]. MRI imaging is usually performed after an acute hearing loss without other explanation, although other cranial nerves can become involved as well causing isolated deficits. Contrast-enhancing T1 imaging demonstrates these tumours well and the diagnosis can often be made on imaging, without a tissue biopsy. Vestibular schwannomas are benign tumours, so the treatment principle is typically to consider surgical resection (with an experienced skull-base neurosurgeon) or to use focal radiation. Depending on the size of the tumour, stereotactic radio-surgery may plan an important role. There has been research suggesting that medical therapy may play a role in stabilizing or even reversing the hearing loss with acoustic neuroma, for example, by targeting vascular endothelial growth factor (VEGF) receptors [15].

Mixed Glial-Neuronal Tumours

Certain tumours are difficult to categorize in the main subgroups of 'glial' vs. 'neuronal' CNS tumours and end up in their own category of 'mixed glial-neuronal tumours'. While most of the tumours in this category are typically considered to be 'low grade' with benign features, there are exceptions to every rule and rare anaplastic features and metastatic spread have been reported at some point for most tumours. Given the mix of cell types, a reasonable approach would be to consider elements of both the glial and neuronal families of tumours when considering treatment options for newly diagnosed or recurrent disease.

Dysembryoplastic Neuroepithelial Tumours

Dysembryoplastic neuroepithelial tumours (DNET) are low-grade (WHO grade 1) tumours that are most often diagnosed in young patients with seizure disorders that are refractory to anticonvulsants. They are very rare, representing less than 1 % of all paediatric CNS tumours, but are reported to be found in 10–20 % of children with localizable refractory seizures. These tumours are predominantly found in the supratentorial cortex, with the temporal lobe being the most common location (around 50 %) [16]. DNET (also referred to as 'DNTs') seems to be associated with cortical dysplasia and may be developmental in nature. On MRI imaging, an absence of high-grade features is the rule; they should not demonstrate mass effect, should not cause oedema, and should only have minimal contrast enhancement. The pathology also lacks malignant features, and the most typical feature is the appearance of the 'floating neuron' against an eosinophilic background. Consistent, recurrent genetic mutations have not been identified. Treatment is localization in preparation for epilepsy surgery and then complete or near-total resection. Seizure control is often much better after surgery, and local recurrence is reported but would be the rare exception for these lesions. Malignant transformation and atypical features have been reported [17]. As with any rare tumour, this should make one extremely cautious about the diagnosis and seek second opinions on the pathology whenever appropriate.

Ganglioglioma

Gangliogliomas are also in the category of 'mixed glial-neuronal tumour' and similar to DNETs are often diagnosed after a child presents with new seizures that are difficult to control (Fig. 17.4). Also occurring at a frequency of less than 1 % of paediatric CNS tumours, gangliogliomas are also found in approximately 20 % of patients who undergo epilepsy surgery.

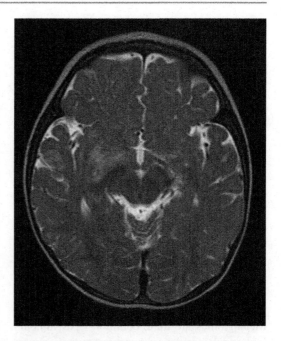

Fig. 17.4 Subtle features of a medial temporal lobe ganglioglioma (axial MRI T2-weighted image)

They can occur anywhere in the brain or spine and on MRI may have solid, cystic, or nodular components. Mass effect and enhancement on MRI are generally minimal to none. Genetic studies on GG samples reveal a high proportion of BRAF^{v600e} mutations, ranging from 18 [18] to 58 % [19], and there is suggestion that this may be associated with a worse prognosis [20]. Treatment is surgical resection, with an attempt for total resection whenever possible. For the most part, the prognosis for these low-grade tumours is excellent and local recurrence is rare. However, anaplastic features have been reported and unresectable tumours (e.g. brainstem) can pose a particular problem. Historically, unresectable progressive gangliogliomas have been treated in a similar fashion to low-grade gliomas, using a chemotherapy regimen for children and possibly radiation for older adolescents. Human clinical trials are under way using BRAF v600e inhibitors, which may show promise in a subset of unresectable gangliogliomas that test positive for this mutation.

Neurocytoma

Most commonly presenting as 'central' neurocyto-mas, these are rare WHO grade II tumours with a tendency to present in young adults or adolescents. They are classified as a neuroepithelial or 'mixed' neuronal-glial tumour. Neurocytomas are typically found in the supratentorial intraventricular areas, and patients will therefore often present with signs of worsening hydrocephalus. Surgical resection is the goal of treatment, and complete resection is essentially curative [21]. When total removal is not possible, focal radiation can be used to control the inevitable regrowth of these tumours.

Meningioma

Meningiomas are quite common CNS tumours in the adult population, but are extremely rare in children (Fig. 17.5). They are generally low-grade or 'benign' lesions, either found as an incidental MRI finding or through investigations for

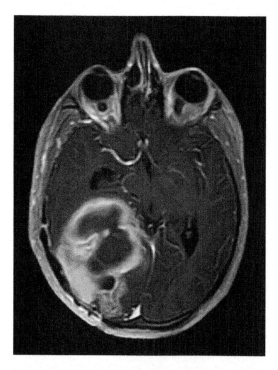

Fig. 17.5 Atypical meningioma in a paediatric patient, presenting with a history of mild headaches and visual changes (axial MRI contrast image)

new onset headaches. They are important for the paediatric neuro-oncology community to recognize since meningiomas can arise as a result of the damage from treatment doses of ionizing radiation. The increased risk of meningiomas continues for years and even decades after radiation therapy is given, and parents and paediatric patients need to understand the risk of developing a meningioma at some point to direct investigations if symptoms arise. Meningiomas require surgery whenever possible, and recurrence after complete resection is rare. There are 'atypical' meningiomas (WHO grade III) that would require closer follow-up after surgery and consideration of radiation therapy in cases of unresectable disease. Obviously, the best treatment is always prevention, and this is just one of many radiotherapy side effects that should emphasize the need to minimize radiation use in paediatric patients.

CNS Sarcoma

In adults, a large proportion of 'CNS' tumours will actually turn out to be metastases from extracranial solid tumours. On the contrary, metastases to the CNS in children are extremely rare. Occasionally, tumours that are normally found outside of the CNS can be found intracranially without an extracranial primary lesion. For example, Ewing's sarcoma (peripheral neuroepithelial tumour) can occur as a primary in the CNS without an extracranial site. Genetic analysis for the typical translocations (chromosome 22, e.g. t(11;22)) will be useful to distinguish this tumour from a CNS primitive neuroectodermal tumour (PNET), which shares some similar histologic features. A CNS sarcoma will often have a predilection for the calvarium, skull base, or meningeal surface and may have an extradural component [22]. Treatment would typically involve chemotherapy and a multimodal approach with radiation and surgery, similar to the treatment for extracranial lesions. While anthracycline chemotherapy is not used often to treat tumours of the CNS, it is an important part of sarcoma treatment and therefore may play a role in other CNS tumours [23].

Future Directions

For many of the tumours listed in this chapter, there will never be large therapeutic trials capturing one common group of patients. We must remember that paediatric tumours are rare to begin with, and there will always be subgroups that are described predominantly in case series or reports. Some tumour types have only been recently described; therefore, in older studies, these patients would have been included in whatever category they fit best, so their outcomes would have either 'brought down' or elevated survival curves. One example of this is with atypical teratoid rhabdoid tumour (ATRT); prior to its recognition as an entity in the early 2000s, it was understandably often diagnosed as medulloblastoma or PNET. Efforts have been made to re-analyze older samples and re-classify older tumour specimens with modern tests that are now widely available [24]. Finally, it is important to remember that as we advance in our understanding of CNS tumour molecular genetics, we will naturally move towards further subcategorization of all tumours. As an example, the name 'medulloblastoma' now refers to a tumour that is being considered to be at least four different subtypes, all of which may lead to a unique treatment strategy with unique outcomes [25]. A new understanding of driver mutations in glioblastoma multiforme is allowing us to subclassify this tumour more accurately and therefore understand the survival differences between these groups [26]. All the while, oncology is driving towards more 'personalized medicine', where each tumour is considered unique and attempts will be made to design treatments specifically for one patient. We are moving into an era where our sophisticated diagnostic tools will essentially be putting more tumours into the 'very rare' category, and no longer will we be able to necessarily rely on large clinical trials where every patient is treated in a similar fashion. Starting with the rarity of all paediatric CNS tumours, we face new challenges in how to study the clinical history and draw therapeutic conclusions for the very rare subtypes.

References

1. Dolecek TA, Propp JM, Stroup NE, Kruchko C. CBTRUS statistical report: primary brain and central nervous system tumors diagnosed in the United States in 2005–2009. Neuro Oncol. 2012;14 Suppl 5:v1–49.
2. Louis DN, Ohgaki H, Wiestler OD, et al. The 2007 WHO classification of tumours of the central nervous system. Acta Neuropathol. 2007;114:97–109.
3. Villani A, Tabori U, Schiffman J, et al. Biochemical and imaging surveillance in germline TP53 mutation carriers with Li–Fraumeni syndrome: a prospective observational study. Lancet Oncol. 2011;12: 559–67.
4. Lafay-Cousin L, Keene D, Carret AS, et al. Choroid plexus tumors in children less than 36 months: the Canadian Pediatric Brain Tumor Consortium (CPBTC) experience. Childs Nerv Syst. 2011;27: 259–64.
5. Lafay-Cousin L, Mabbott DJ, Halliday W, et al. Use of ifosfamide, carboplatin, and etoposide chemotherapy in choroid plexus carcinoma. J Neurosurg Pediatr. 2010;5:615–21.
6. Wrede B, Liu P, Wolff JE. Chemotherapy improves the survival of patients with choroid plexus carcinoma: a meta-analysis of individual cases with choroid plexus tumors. J Neurooncol. 2007;85:345–51.
7. Kane LA, Leinung MC, Scheithauer BW, et al. Pituitary adenomas in childhood and adolescence. J Clin Endocrinol Metab. 1994;79:1135–40.
8. Harrington MH, Casella SJ. Pituitary tumors in childhood. Curr Opin Endocrinol Diabetes Obes. 2012; 19:63–7.
9. Schlechte JA. Clinical practice. Prolactinoma. N Engl J Med. 2003;349:2035–41.
10. Zagzag D, Blanco C, Friedlander DR, Miller DC, Newcomb EW. Expression of p27KIP1 in human gliomas: relationship between tumor grade, proliferation index, and patient survival. Hum Pathol. 2003; 34:48–53.
11. Kantar M, Ertan Y, Turhan T, et al. Anaplastic astroblastoma of childhood: aggressive behavior. Childs Nerv Syst. 2009;25:1125–9.
12. Fevre-Montange M, Hasselblatt M, Figarella-Branger D, et al. Prognosis and histopathologic features in papillary tumors of the pineal region: a retrospective multicenter study of 31 cases. J Neuropathol Exp Neurol. 2006;65:1004–11.
13. Lu-Emerson C, Plotkin SR. The neurofibromatoses. Part 2: NF2 and schwannomatosis. Rev Neurol Dis. 2009;6:E81–6.
14. Propp JM, McCarthy BJ, Davis FG, Preston-Martin S. Descriptive epidemiology of vestibular schwannomas. Neuro Oncol. 2006;8:1–11.
15. Plotkin SR, Stemmer-Rachamimov AO, Barker 2nd FG, et al. Hearing improvement after bevacizumab in

patients with neurofibromatosis type 2. N Engl J Med. 2009;361:358–67.

16. Ozlen F, Gunduz A, Asan Z, et al. Dysembryoplastic neuroepithelial tumors and gangliogliomas: clinical results of 52 patients. Acta Neurochir. 2010;152: 1661–71.

17. Daghistani R, Miller E, Kulkarni AV, Widjaja E. Atypical characteristics and behavior of dysembryoplastic neuroepithelial tumors. Neuroradiology. 2013;55:217–24.

18. Schindler G, Capper D, Meyer J, et al. Analysis of BRAF V600E mutation in 1,320 nervous system tumors reveals high mutation frequencies in pleomorphic xanthoastrocytoma, ganglioglioma and extracerebellar pilocytic astrocytoma. Acta Neuropathol. 2011;121:397–405.

19. Koelsche C, Wohrer A, Jeibmann A, et al. Mutant BRAF V600E protein in ganglioglioma is predominantly expressed by neuronal tumor cells. Acta Neuropathol. 2013;125:891–900.

20. Dahiya S, Haydon DH, Alvarado D, Gurnett CA, Gutmann DH, Leonard JR. BRAF(V600E) mutation is a negative prognosticator in pediatric ganglioglioma. Acta Neuropathol. 2013;125:901–10.

21. Maiuri F, Spaziante R, De Caro ML, Cappabianca P, Giamundo A, Iaconetta G. Central neurocytoma: clinico-pathological study of 5 cases and review of the literature. Clin Neurol Neurosurg. 1995;97: 219–28.

22. Ibrahim GM, Fallah A, Shahideh M, Tabori U, Rutka JT. Primary Ewing's sarcoma affecting the central nervous system: a review and proposed prognostic considerations. J Clin Neurosci. 2012;19:203–9.

23. Chi SN, Zimmerman MA, Yao X, et al. Intensive multimodality treatment for children with newly diagnosed CNS atypical teratoid rhabdoid tumor. J Clin Oncol. 2009;27:385–9.

24. Fleming AJ, Hukin J, Rassekh R, et al. Atypical teratoid rhabdoid tumors (ATRTs): the British Columbia's Children's Hospital's experience, 1986–2006. Brain Pathol. 2012;22:625–35.

25. Jones DT, Jager N, Kool M, et al. Dissecting the genomic complexity underlying medulloblastoma. Nature. 2012;488:100–5.

26. Schwartzentruber J, Korshunov A, Liu XY, et al. Driver mutations in histone H3.3 and chromatin remodelling genes in paediatric glioblastoma. Nature. 2012;482:226–31.

Radiotherapy

18

Anne-Marie Charpentier, Carolyn Freeman,
David Roberge, and Pierre Rousseau

Introduction

Radiation therapy has long been regarded as a cornerstone of the treatment of children with CNS tumors. In the 1980s, increasing recognition of the possible long-term side effects of radiation, in particular the increased risk of secondary malignancies and the neurocognitive effects of radiation on the maturing brain, led to the development of treatment strategies in which the goal was to avoid or at least delay the use of radiation therapy, especially for children under the age of 3. While this was shown to be a successful approach in selected groups of patients, many of these studies actually underscored the important role that radiotherapy still plays. Major advances in radiation technology over the same time period now enable more focused and precise irradiation, with a promise for reduced long-term toxicity.

A.-M. Charpentier, M.D., F.R.C.P.C. (✉)
D. Roberge, M.D., F.R.C.P.C. • P. Rousseau, M.D.
Department of Radiation Oncology, CHUM
Notre-Dame Hospital, Montréal, QC, Canada
e-mail: anne-marie.charpentier.chum@ssss.gouv.qc.ca

C. Freeman, M.B.B.S., F.R.C.P.C., F.A.S.T.R.O.
Department of Radiation Oncology, McGill
University Health Centre, Montréal, QC, Canada

Basic Radiation Physics

X-rays are the type of radiation most commonly used in clinical practice. Their interaction with matter can only fully be understood by recognizing that they have both a wave (electromagnetic) and a quantum nature. X-ray beams used in radiation oncology are typically in the megavoltage (4–18 MV) range and are produced by a medical linear accelerator (linac). Each photon energy is characterized by a specific dose absorption profile, known as the percent depth dose (PDD) profile, along the central axis of the beam.

Therapeutic radiation can also be delivered through the use of particles: electrons, protons, neutrons, and heavy-charged particles. *Electrons* are small negatively charged particles that are produced by a standard linac. The major clinical advantage of electron beam therapy is a rapid dose drop-off at a depth that depends on the energy of the beam. Its role is, however, limited in CNS malignancies, except for its use in some centers for craniospinal irradiation. *Protons* are positively charged particles with a relatively high mass in comparison to electrons. Their use requires a dedicated complex and expensive unit. Proton therapy will be discussed in more details (see "Proton Therapy" section). Neutrons and heavy-charged particles are experimental modalities available only in a very small number of centers worldwide and for now of limited use in oncology.

K. Scheinemann and E. Bouffet (eds.), *Pediatric Neuro-oncology*,
DOI 10.1007/978-1-4939-1541-5_18, © Springer Science+Business Media New York 2015

Basic Radiobiology

DNA Damage

The biologic effect of radiation therapy is due to damage to DNA. All types of radiation interact with matter via either a direct or indirect action. In direct action, the radiation interacts directly with the critical cell target, while the indirect action is mediated through the creation within the cell of free radicals that initiate a chain of events leading to biologic damage. The latter predominates for irradiation by photons. Ionizing radiation can induce multiple types of damage including base damage, single- and double-strand breaks, and DNA–DNA and DNA-protein cross-links, of which the most lethal type is the double-strand breaks. While the rationale for combining chemotherapy and radiotherapy is most commonly to gain "spatial cooperation," with chemotherapy acting on distant micrometastases and radiotherapy killing tumor cells locally, a synergistic effect for cell death also occurs with several cytotoxic drugs, providing the rationale for the concurrent use of both modalities in the treatment of some CNS tumors.

The "Four Rs" of Radiobiology

In clinical practice, the biologic effect of the radiation is intrinsically related to the concept of dose fractionation, in which the goal is to deliver an effective tumoricidal dose while sparing normal tissues. Radiobiologically, this can be summarized with four terms, which are referred to as the "four Rs" of radiobiology: repair, redistribution, repopulation, and reoxygenation. Favoring normal tissue sparing, *repair* of sublethal damage to normal tissues occurs between each dose or "fraction" at a rate and with a capacity that depends on the specific tissue type; this is the basis of the hyperfractionation studies that explored dose escalation in pontine gliomas. During the interfraction interval, two factors influence tumor cell killing:

redistribution of cancer cells within the cell cycle to more radiosensitive phases and *reoxygenation* of any less radiosensitive hypoxic areas of the tumor. The fourth "R," *repopulation* of tumor cells, may result in a decrease in tumor control if the overall treatment time is prolonged, especially for a rapidly proliferating tumor. Avoidance of repopulation is the rationale underpinning studies of accelerated fractionation in medulloblastoma/PNET.

Planning

Children needing radiotherapy should be treated in centers with sufficient numbers of patients to ensure the required level of expertise, not only medical, but also technical and nursing. Preparation for the first visit to the radiation oncology department, often in a different hospital, is ideally done in an environment that is familiar to the child by nurses and play and child life specialists, with the help of printed and/or electronic material that can be referred to later by the child and/or parents [1]. Ideally, there will also be a friendly, familiar face—a nurse or radiation therapist—to greet the child and the parents in the radiation oncology department, show them the rooms where planning and treatment will take place, and introduce them to the staff that will be involved in their care. This preparation can be pivotal in encouraging a young child to lie still for the making of the immobilization device, for simulation, and for treatment itself.

Immobilization and Sedation

The greater precision of modern radiotherapy, often now using millimetric margins, mandates accurate setup for each of the typically 25–33 daily fractions and also immobility of the patient during the daily treatment that may take up to 45 min. Unexpected movements could have an impact on the chances of delivering a successful oncological treatment without complications. Consequently, a thermoplastic mask is almost always used. This is a mesh mask that is molded to the child's face after being immersed in a warm water bath or heated in an oven. The mask becomes rigid at room temperature and is then ready for use for imaging and treatment.

For children younger than age 4 or 5 years, daily anesthesia will almost always be necessary for all of these steps. This will require a skilled pediatric anesthesiology team with in-room equipment for anesthesia and monitoring. Other factors are recognized to contribute to the need for sedation or anesthesia, such as anxiety related to previous procedures, fear of radiation therapy equipment and immobilization devices, and separation from the parents, as well as the attitude of the parents toward radiation. Guidelines for the safety of the child under sedation are well described [2]. Sedation or anesthesia needs to be administered by a dedicated anesthesia team not only comfortable with the sedation protocol but also with the management of possible adverse reactions that include hypoxemia, hypoventilation, stridor, laryngospasm, and airway obstruction. It is reported that 1 of 65 procedures can result in a minor but potentially serious complication [3], but no delayed effects have been reported from daily sedation.

Planning CT Scan

The need for a planning CT scan for pediatric CNS tumors is well established. Children undergo the planning CT scan at the CT simulator in the radiation oncology department in the same position as the one that will be used for each daily treatment. The limits of the CT scan will generally encompass the whole brain, from the convexity to the cervical spine, to include the target volumes as well as the organs-at-risk. For craniospinal irradiation, the lower limit of the planning CT scan will go down to the pelvis, since the inferior border of the lower spinal field usually extends at least to the bottom of the S2 vertebral body.

Image Co-registration

In order for the radiation oncologist to delineate precisely the tumor, the planning CT scan will almost always be co-registered with diagnostic images, such as the pre- and/or postoperative MRI. In some radiation facilities, some of these images will be produced using a dedicated treatment planning MRI. The appropriate MRI sequences will depend on the clinical situation. Often a combination of sequences will be necessary; for example, axial T1 post-gadolinium and T2/FLAIR sequences together enable visualization of residual enhancing and non-enhancing tumor. Co-registration with metabolic/functional images, such as FDG-PET or MR spectroscopy and even tractography, is increasingly being studied. Applicability to CNS tumors is currently limited but of interest for targeting of metabolically active tumor, as well as for selective avoidance of critical pathways.

Contouring Target Volumes and Organs-at-Risk

Definition of target volumes and organs-at-risk is a critical part of the planning process. The first step is usually to delineate the *gross tumor volume* (GTV), which corresponds to macroscopic tumor. The *clinical target volume* (CTV) is then created to encompass the GTV and any areas at risk for potential microscopic tumor spread. While for certain tumors (e.g., ependymoma and craniopharyngioma) this area of suspected tumor infiltration may be tightly confined around the GTV, tumors with higher infiltrative potential such as high-grade astrocytoma require larger margins. Both GTV and CTV are anatomically defined volumes and independent of the treatment technique or modality used (e.g., photon or proton therapy). Uncertainties regarding the patient positioning and alignment of beams at each radiation treatment, and the possible changes in the size, shape, and position of the CTV within the patient, respectively the *setup margin* and the *internal margin*, are then taken into account to create the *planning target volume* (PTV). With modern radiotherapy using rigid immobilization and daily pretreatment image verification, a 2–5 mm margin from the CTV to the PTV is usually sufficient. The PTV is the geometrical volume to which the absorbed dose is prescribed.

Although all nontarget normal tissues can be considered as *organs-at-risk* (OAR), the concept in practice depends on the location of the CTV and the dose of radiation that will be given. The optic structures (optic nerves and chiasma), brainstem, and spinal cord are typically considered the main OARs when treating CNS tumors. Similar to the notion of PTV, a margin accounting for uncertainties and variations in the position of OAR can be created and is referred to as the *planning organ-at-risk volume* (PRV). This is most relevant to serial structures, such as the spinal cord. Recognizing the risks of late effects of radiation therapy and with the possibility now of more precise radiation delivery and even selective avoidance, increasing importance is now being given to other normal tissues such as the pituitary, hypothalamus, hippocampi, temporal lobes, supratentorial brain, and cochleae. Contouring these normal structures and evaluating and recording the dose delivered to them is helpful in planning appropriate follow-up (e.g., tests of neuroendocrine function depending on the dose to the pituitary and hypothalamus).

Techniques

3D-CRT

Three-dimensional conformal radiotherapy (3D-CRT) refers to the incorporation of 3D anatomic information acquired at CT simulation into planning and dose calculation in order to conform the dose as tightly as possible to the planning target volume with minimization of dose to OARs.

IMRT

In *intensity-modulated radiation therapy* (IMRT), the dose is conformed to the target by the use of beams with nonuniform dose fluences. Optimization of the plan is generally performed through "inverse planning," where the goals for target coverage and dose constraints on OARs are stated and used in planning, with the process continuing until minimization of the cost function.

Radiosurgery

Radiosurgery (RS) has a long history dating back to the 1940s at which time the term referred to a single large dose of radiation given with ablative intent. It took four decades for RS to become widely available with the use of modified linacs, and until the 1980s, the differences between radiosurgery and conventional radiation therapy were striking. In the years since, the improved dosimetry achieved using standard linacs and dedicated radiosurgery accelerators has blurred the distinction between conventional and stereotactic radiation and freed clinicians from the previous choice between a precise single fraction treatment and nonselective fractionated treatments. In addition, the image-guidance systems now available have completely eliminated the need for surgical frame placement and erased the last remaining difference between single fraction and fractionated delivery techniques. Currently, the working definition of RS is the precise application of radiation to a small intracranial target performed in a single or a limited number of sessions, up to a maximum of five (American Association of Neurological Surgeons/Congress of Neurological Surgeons) [4].

The devices currently used to deliver RS include dedicated and non-dedicated radiosurgery units. The prototypical dedicated radiosurgery device is the Leksell Gamma Knife®. The unit has gone through multiple revisions, but the basic principle has remained constant: multiple cobalt-60 sources (typically 192 or 201) are focused to a single point in space. Small circular collimators for each cobalt source are used to produce 4–18 mm spheres of radiation (called "shots"). While nonspherical shots can be produced on newer Perfexion™ units, the concept is still to pack shots into the target volume to produce a conformal dose distribution with a steep falloff. Although newer units hold the promise of noninvasive immobilization and image guidance, an invasive frame is currently necessary for immobilization and localization, almost always requiring general anesthesia in children and making the technique unsuitable for very young children with immature skulls.

The CyberKnife® mates a 6 MV x-band linac to a robotic arm. A purely image-guided device, the CyberKnife®, relies on stereoscopic planar imaging to target multiple noncoplanar, non-isocentric beams at targets inside or outside the head. The CyberKnife® is an inherently inverse-planned modality that uses beams collimated either with fixed conical collimators, a variable quasi-circular collimator, or, on newer units, a small multileaf collimator.

Since the mid-1980s, conventional isocentric linacs have been used for the delivery of radiosurgery requiring modifications to the units. Early modifications aimed at improving the mechanical accuracy of the couch and gantry used mechanical subsystems that supported the patient's head and sometimes the conical collimators. Current systems rely on the improved mechanics of modern linacs. With the increased use of stereotactic radiation, various modifications of gantry-based linacs have been incorporated into dedicated devices. Depending on the manufacturer and version of the product, the differences between these devices and modified linacs can be substantial or mainly cosmetic. What currently characterizes a stereotactic linac is the availability of features such as high output photon beams with reduced beam flattening, integrated image guidance, multileaf collimators with small leaf size, add-on conical collimators, a precise mechanical isocenter, and radiosurgery planning software.

Although cranial RS is most commonly used in oncological applications, the occasional child will be treated for a vascular or functional condition (e.g., to obliterate an arteriovenous malformation or reduce seizures from a hypothalamic hamartoma). In oncology, RS has been applied to a number of benign and malignant intracranial tumors (Table 18.1). In certain cases, RS is meant to exploit the biology of a large single fraction (Fig. 18.1), and in others the use of a single frac-

Table 18.1 Oncological applications of radiosurgery (RS) for pediatric patients with CNS tumors will typically fit one of the following three paradigms

1. RS alone to exploit the biology of large single doses of radiation in low-grade tumors
2. RS as an adjunct to more conventionally fractionated radiation to escalate tumor dose
3. RS to treat recurrent tumors after prior radiation

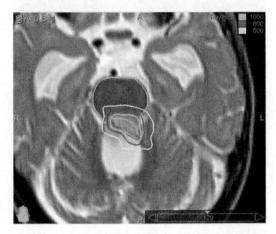

Fig. 18.1 Radiosurgery boost after conventional intensity-modulated radiotherapy for an ependymoma. Note the dose avoidance of the brainstem. The 1,000, 800, and 500 cGy isodose lines are shown

tion is a convenient way to provide high-dose radiation in a timely manner for patients in a palliative setting (e.g., recurrence or metastases).

Evidence to support the use of RS in the pediatric population is limited [5, 6], and no comparative trials can be expected in the small heterogeneous patient population of children with small, well-defined tumors amenable to radiosurgery. Although published results are generally favorable, RS carries a small risk of symptomatic radiation necrosis. The anti-VEGF antibody bevacizumab may be a new option for selected cases of necrosis refractory to steroids [7].

Special Techniques

Craniospinal Irradiation

One of the most complex and time- and resource-consuming techniques performed in radiotherapy departments, craniospinal irradiation (CSI), is

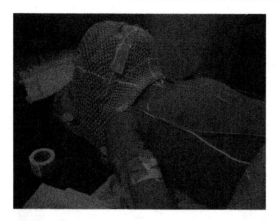

Fig. 18.2 A 3-year-old patient being treated under anesthesia for craniospinal irradiation. Note the thermoplastic immobilization device fixed to the treatment couch

made easier through the use of CT simulation combined with modern treatment planning and delivery.

Patient Positioning and Immobilization
CSI has traditionally been delivered to patients in the prone position, but most modern techniques are designed with treatment in the supine position. The supine position is more comfortable and, if anesthesia is required, safer because of better airway control (Fig. 18.2). Immobilization is essential but technique specific. While use of a thermoplastic mask is routine, full-body immobilization devices are variably used now, with emphasis shifting from immobilization to daily volumetric image guidance (e.g., using Tomotherapy®).

Target Volume Definition
The CTV for CSI consists of the whole brain and spinal cord and the overlying meninges. Careful target volume definition is critical, both to avoid recurrence in underdosed areas and to reduce the risk of late effects. For the brain, thin-slice CT simulation is essential to ensure adequate coverage of the CTV in the subfrontal region. Co-registration of a postoperative T2-weighted MRI to the planning CT is helpful in ensuring coverage of CSF along lower cranial nerve roots and in delineating the lateral aspect of CTV for the spine field that includes the

extension of the meninges along the nerve roots to the lateral aspects of the spinal ganglia. A T1-weighted sequence usually better identifies the caudal limit of the target volume which could be higher or lower than the traditional lower border for the spine field of the bottom of the S2 foramina.

Treatment Planning and Delivery
With traditional 2D CSI planning technique based on bony anatomy, large volumes of normal nontarget tissues are exposed to radiation. The move to CT simulation and 3D planning has reduced the field size in most patients. The use of IMRT results in further reductions of dose to structures directly anterior to the spine at the expense of increased low-dose exposure [8]. Further improvements to both can be achieved using daily image guidance that permits the use of smaller PTV margins.

There are many issues that need to be addressed in designing a CSI technique, most especially field matching in the cervical region and dose homogeneity throughout the target volume. Using modern tools for treatment planning and delivery, it is possible to greatly simplify the technique and substantially reduce planning and delivery times (Fig. 18.3a) [9]. In general, when posterior beams are used, 6 MV photons provide satisfactory target coverage. A variation of dose along the spinal axis of greater than 10 % will require the use of dose compensation that can be achieved using multileaf collimation. Helical tomotherapy techniques further simplify planning and treatment by avoiding the need for junctions and improving conformality to the target (Fig. 18.3b) [10].

Proton Therapy
Protons interact with matter differently from the high-energy X-rays routinely used in radiotherapy. A proton beam deposits a large proportion of its energy over a range of a few millimeters in the so-called Bragg peak with no exit dose. Although the entrance dose is increased when the Bragg peak is spread out to cover the target volume, the integral dose is still substantially reduced in comparison with photon beams (typically by a

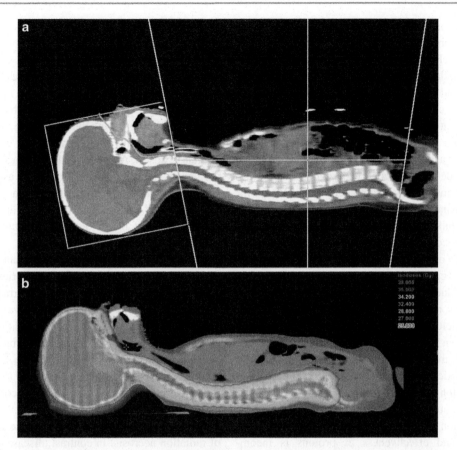

Fig. 18.3 (**a**): In a 3D CSI technique, lateral opposed fields are used to treat the brain and a direct posterior field is used to cover the spinal axis. The field junction over the cervical cord usually is moved weekly ("feathered") to avoid over- or underdosage. The supine position is more comfortable for the patient and safer if sedation or anesthesia is required. In the technique shown, fixed field parameters are used which greatly facilitates treatment planning and delivery (Parker IJROBP 2006). (**b**): An example of an IMRT technique using TomoTherapy®. The absence of junctions is a major advantage of this technique. Note the excellent conformality to the target volume and significant high-dose sparing of structures anterior to the target (Parker IJROBP 2010)

factor of 1.5–3). In pediatric radiotherapy, it is this reduction in integral dose as well as sparing of OARs from low and intermediate radiation doses that motivates the use of protons. The dose to OARs can be reduced quite dramatically, the most striking example being that of craniospinal radiation where exit dose to the thyroid, breasts, heart, and liver can be completely eliminated. In a Swedish planning study of craniospinal radiation, the lifetime risk of secondary cancer was estimated at 30 % for intensity-modulated photons as compared with only 4 % for intensity-modulated protons [11]. In a planning study of optic glioma, craniopharyngioma, and medulloblastoma, a dose-cognitive effect model predicted higher IQ scores and/or academic reading scores following proton treatment [12]. In other situations, long-term benefits may be expected from dose sparing of OARs such as the pituitary gland and hypothalamus, the optic apparatus, and cochleae.

Although protons have been used to treat cancer since 1954, the availability of the modality has been very limited and few children have been treated. As an example, a 2004 report from the Loma Linda University Medical Center reported on the first three patients treated with proton craniospinal radiation (from 2001 to 2003) [13]. With such small and relatively recent series, few clinical data are available to support the benefits predicted by dose models. A comparison of patients of all ages treated in Boston from 1974 with matched photon patients from the SEER database has been published in abstract form [14]. At a median follow-up of more than 6 years, the crude rate of second malignancies was 6.4 % for proton patients compared with 12.8 % for photon patients. Of the 503 proton patients in this study, only 15 were children and none had developed secondary malignancies. As new facilities become operational and better data are collected, we are beginning to see prospective reports showing reduced acute toxicity in pediatric CNS patients, notably health-related quality of life and ototoxicity [15, 16]. However, these reports suffer from the lack of an unbiased comparable photon-treated group, and accurate estimates of late toxicity and cancer induction will require much longer follow-up.

Although very attractive, the implementation of proton therapy does have caveats. The relative biological effectiveness of protons is incompletely characterized and varies, for example, by cell line. The proton dose distributions will likely be less forgiving to contouring errors, positioning variations and intra-treatment variations in patient contours/density. The unique dosimetry also poses new clinical questions such as the effect of sharp gradients on bone growth. Despite the lack of clinical evidence, the ASTRO Emerging Technology Committee's 2012 review of proton beam therapy noted that "the rationale for using PBT in posterior fossa tumors, optic pathway tumors, and brainstem lesions is compelling" and that "future clinical studies reporting on the outcome of patients treated with protons will decide how widespread protons become for pediatric CNS tumors" [17]. In practice, it is expected that the percentage of pediatric CNS tumors treated with proton therapy will increase yearly as new facilities come on line, confidence with the technology grows, and more clinical data become available.

Re-irradiation

Re-irradiation may be an option for some children with CNS tumors although the literature is scarce. This is partly explained by the fact that doses received by OARs during the first course of radiotherapy are typically high, approaching accepted tolerance doses. As well, pediatric oncologists may not be familiar with re-irradiation as a possible treatment option, with chemotherapy being the therapeutic strategy most often used at time of relapse. Most of the evidence thus comes from single institution experiences.

The largest series is that of Merchant et al. who in 2008 reported a retrospective series of 38 pediatric patients who underwent re-irradiation for recurrent ependymoma, using a variety of techniques including radiosurgery, focal fractionated radiation, and craniospinal irradiation, depending on the time period and the location and extent of disease at recurrence [18]. The median time to failure after the first course of radiotherapy was 19 months. Six patients treated with RS did poorly, four dying of disease and one of radiation necrosis. In contrast, disease control was high for patients with local relapse reirradiated using focal fractionated RT and for patients re-irradiated using CSI. Most notably, 4-year event-free survival was 53 %±20 % among 12 patients with metastatic failure treated with CSI. Despite total combined doses as high as 120 Gy, toxicity was limited to two patients with symptomatic radiation necrosis and one with a secondary malignancy.

More recently, the group from The Hospital for Sick Children/Princess Margaret Hospital similarly reviewed their experience with re-irradiation for pediatric ependymoma [19]. Eighteen patients received full-dose (≥54 Gy and/or craniospinal) re-irradiation at time of relapse. Overall survival (OS) was significantly better for re-irradiated children (3-year OS 81 % vs. 7 %). As in the Merchant study, re-irradiation was also associated with a longer time to second progression in comparison to time to first progression, raising the possibility that re-irradiation might change the natural history of recurrent pediatric ependymoma.

Despite limited, largely anecdotal evidence, re-irradiation may also be considered in other situations, for example, curative intent re-treatment for patients with radiosensitive tumors such as germinoma where initial radiation may have delivered only low or moderate doses. It can also be considered for palliation in other patients such as those with progressive diffuse intrinsic pontine gliomas who may obtain a useful symptomatic reprieve. Factors that need to be considered prior to re-treatment include the general condition of the patient, the interval from the first treatment, and the location and extent of the recurrent disease.

Acute Side Effects of Radiation Therapy

Postoperative complications, pretreatment general status, and treatment approach (e.g., induction chemotherapy and/or concurrent chemotherapy), as well as requirements for daily sedation, fasting, poor nutritional status, and medication used for symptom control can all contribute to the general status of the patient during radiation therapy.

Acute side effects due to radiation itself are observed in most children (Table 18.2), albeit with significant variability. In general, the larger the volume treated (i.e., partial brain, whole brain, or craniospinal), the greater the likelihood of acute side effects. While the majority of acute symptoms are self-limiting, the use of anti-nausea medication (e.g., 5-HT3 antagonists) or steroids (e.g., dexamethasone) might be required for the child presenting more severe nausea, vomiting, or headache as a consequence of radiation-induced cerebral edema. Premedication with an oral or intravenous 5-HT3 antagonist 30–60 min before each RT fraction is commonly administered prophylactically for radiation therapy with a high emetogenic potential, such as CSI. Steroids might also be required for patients presenting with a significant amount of residual tumor, or for children treated for brainstem glioma, situations where neurologic symptoms may worsen

Table 18.2 Acute side effects that might be experienced by the child during radiation therapy

Skin	Irritation varying from erythema to hyperpigmentation, dry or moist desquamation
Hair loss	Limited to the entry or exit of radiation beams
CNS	Headache, nausea, vomiting
Ear	External otitis or serous otitis media
Parotid gland	Acute parotiditis
Eye	Noninfectious conjunctivitis
Hematological	Leucopenia, thrombocytopenia, anemia
Gastrointestinal	Nausea, vomiting, poor appetite, esophagitis, diarrhea
Constitutional	Weight loss, fatigue, anxiety, sleep disturbance, difficulty with concentration

early in the RT course. While dexamethasone is an effective drug used during radiation therapy for CNS malignancies, tapering should be performed as soon as possible because of the morbidity associated with its long-term or high-dose use, including weight gain, myopathy, insomnia, hyperglycemia, susceptibility to infection, etc. When long-term use of steroids is expected, a gastric antacid is usually prescribed in order to avoid gastrointestinal associated toxicity.

Hematological toxicity with requirement for blood transfusions is usually not encountered with radiation to the brain only if no concurrent chemotherapy is given, but can be seen during the course of craniospinal irradiation where a significant portion of the bone marrow is irradiated in the vertebral bodies, and so blood counts should be monitored at least weekly during CSI. Treatment interruptions should be avoided if at all possible in order to not jeopardize treatment.

The somnolence syndrome is an early-delayed effect of radiation therapy. Best described and studied in children requiring whole-brain irradiation for the prevention of meningeal relapse in acute lymphoblastic leukemia, it consists of a variable degree of drowsiness, associated with low-grade fever and occasionally symptoms of increased intracranial pressure such as nausea and headache. It commonly appears about 1 month after completion of radiation therapy and lasts about 10 days. This is thought to result from transient demyelination of nerve fibers, as the turnover of myelin of 6 weeks would correspond to the time of onset and resolution of symptoms. Somnolence syndrome after partial brain irradiation has been reported [20]. Whether this is secondary to a high dose of radiation to a specific region of the brain such as the reticular activating system in the midbrain or to the whole-brain dose resulting from the multiple beams used to treat a focal lesion is unclear.

Late effects of radiation therapy and combined modality treatment are discussed in the "Long-Term Sequelae" and "Neurocognitive Outcome" chapters.

Future Directions

Important progress has taken place in radiotherapy over the past two decades. Better target volume definition and improved precision of treatment with sparing of nontarget tissues have been important in the treatment of children with CNS tumors. Radiotherapy practice has evolved through prospective studies of partnerships such as the Children's Oncology Group. These trials have often involved questions concerning radiation dose or volume and several have been practice-changing. The more widespread availability of new technologies and new modalities such as protons as well as modulators of radiation effect are exciting avenues for the future, offering even greater potential for differential effects on tumor and normal structures and as a result the positive effects of radiotherapy on tumor control with fewer long-term adverse effects than in the past.

References

1. Willis D, Barry P. Audiovisual interventions to reduce the use of general anaesthesia with paediatric patients during radiation therapy. J Med Imaging Radiat Oncol. 2010;54(3):249–55.

2. McFadyen JG, Pelly N, Orr RJ. Sedation and anesthesia for the pediatric patient undergoing radiation therapy. Curr Opin Anaesthesiol. 2011;24(4):433–8.

3. Cravero JP, Beach ML, Blike GT, Gallagher SM, Hertzog JH, Pediatric Sedation Research C. The incidence and nature of adverse events during pediatric sedation/anesthesia with propofol for procedures outside the operating room: a report from the Pediatric Sedation Research Consortium. Anesth Analg. 2009; 108(3):795–804.

4. Barnett GH, Linskey ME, Adler JR, Cozzens JW, Friedman WA, Heilbrun MP, et al. Stereotactic radiosurgery–an organized neurosurgery-sanctioned definition. J Neurosurg. 2007;106(1):1–5.

5. Hodgson DC, Goumnerova LC, Loeffler JS, Dutton S, Black PM, Alexander 3rd E, et al. Radiosurgery in the management of pediatric brain tumors. Int J Radiat Oncol Biol Phys. 2001;50(4):929–35.

6. Stauder MC, Ni Laack N, Ahmed KA, Link MJ, Schomberg PJ, Pollock BE. Stereotactic radiosurgery for patients with recurrent intracranial ependymomas. J Neurooncol. 2012;108(3):507–12.

7. Levin VA, Bidaut L, Hou P, Kumar AJ, Wefel JS, Bekele BN, et al. Randomized double-blind placebo-controlled trial of bevacizumab therapy for radiation necrosis of the central nervous system. Int J Radiat Oncol Biol Phys. 2011;79(5):1487–95.

8. Parker W, Filion E, Roberge D, Freeman CR. Intensity-modulated radiotherapy for craniospinal irradiation: target volume considerations, dose constraints, and competing risks. Int J Radiat Oncol Biol Phys. 2007; 69(1):251–7.

9. Parker WA, Freeman CR. A simple technique for craniospinal radiotherapy in the supine position. Radiother Oncol. 2006;78(2):217–22.

10. Parker W, Brodeur M, Roberge D, Freeman C. Standard and nonstandard craniospinal radiotherapy using helical TomoTherapy. Int J Radiat Oncol Biol Phys. 2010;77(3):926–31.

11. Mu X, Bjork-Eriksson T, Nill S, Oelfke U, Johansson KA, Gagliardi G, et al. Does electron and proton therapy reduce the risk of radiation induced cancer after spinal irradiation for childhood medulloblastoma? A comparative treatment planning study. Acta Oncol. 2005;44(6):554–62.

12. Merchant TE, Hua CH, Shukla H, Ying X, Nill S, Oelfke U. Proton versus photon radiotherapy for common pediatric brain tumors: comparison of models of dose characteristics and their relationship to cognitive function. Pediatr Blood Cancer. 2008;51(1): 110–7.

13. Yuh GE, Loredo LN, Yonemoto LT, Bush DA, Shahnazi K, Preston W, et al. Reducing toxicity from craniospinal irradiation: using proton beams to treat medulloblastoma in young children. Cancer J. 2004; 10(6):386–90.

14. Chung CS, et al. Comparative analysis of second malignancy risk in patients treated with proton therapy

versus conventional photon therapy. Int J Radiat Oncol Biol Phys. 2008;72(1 Suppl):S8. Abstract 17.

15. Moeller BJ, Chintagumpala M, Philip JJ, Grosshans DR, McAleer MF, Woo SY, et al. Low early ototoxicity rates for pediatric medulloblastoma patients treated with proton radiotherapy. Radiat Oncol. 2011;6:58.

16. Kuhlthau KA, Pulsifer MB, Yeap BY, Rivera Morales D, Delahaye J, Hill KS, et al. Prospective study of health-related quality of life for children with brain tumors treated with proton radiotherapy. J Clin Oncol. 2012;30(17):2079–86.

17. Allen AM, Pawlicki T, Dong L, Fourkal E, Buyyounouski M, Cengel K, et al. An evidence based review of proton beam therapy: the report of ASTRO's

emerging technology committee. Radiother Oncol. 2012;103(1):8–11.

18. Merchant TE, Boop FA, Kun LE, Sanford RA. A retrospective study of surgery and reirradiation for recurrent ependymoma. Int J Radiat Oncol Biol Phys. 2008;71(1):87–97.

19. Bouffet E, Hawkins CE, Ballourah W, Taylor MD, Bartels UK, Schoenhoff N, et al. Survival benefit for pediatric patients with recurrent ependymoma treated with reirradiation. Int J Radiat Oncol Biol Phys. 2012;83(5):1541–8.

20. Kelsey CR, Marks LB. Somnolence syndrome after focal radiation therapy to the pineal region: case report and review of the literature. J Neurooncol. 2006;78(2):153–6.

Chemotherapy

19

Joan Lee and Donna L. Johnston

Introduction

Chemotherapy is effective in the treatment of many childhood malignancies, and brain tumors are no exception. A variety of chemotherapeutic agents have proven to be effective for most types of brain tumors, and the role of chemotherapy varies from delaying the timing of radiation therapy, stabilizing tumors, reducing radiation doses, or even avoiding radiation therapy altogether. Chemotherapy has been shown to improve survival for many pediatric brain tumors including medulloblastoma, germ cell tumor, astrocytoma, and others.

This section will review the many chemotherapeutic agents that are effective in treating pediatric brain tumors, as well as various methods of delivery of chemotherapy to penetrate the central nervous system (CNS).

J. Lee, B.Sc.Phm. (✉)
Department of Pediatrics, Division of Hematology/
Oncology, McMaster Children's Hospital,
Hamilton, ON, Canada
e-mail: leejo@hhsc.ca

D.L. Johnston, M.D., F.R.C.P.C., F.A.A.P.
Department of Pediatrics, Division of Hematology/
Oncology, Children's Hospital of Eastern Ontario,
University of Ottawa, Ottawa, ON, Canada

Chemotherapy Agents

Alkylating Agents

Alkylating agents are a group of compounds that primarily function by substituting alkyl groups for hydrogen ions. The resulting carbonium ions react with DNA, RNA, and proteins of susceptible molecules, thereby causing abnormalities and interfering with normal cell function.

Alkylating agents are cell-cycle nonspecific. They are classified according to their chemical structure and bonding mechanism. The most commonly used agents for pediatric CNS tumors include nitrosoureas, platin compounds, and nitrogen mustards. Procarbazine and temozolomide are drug derivatives that function as alkylating agents.

Nitrosoureas

Lomustine (CCNU) and carmustine (BCNU) and their metabolites interfere with DNA, RNA, and protein synthesis through alkylation and carbamylation. These agents are also able to form cross-links with DNA and subsequently cause DNA damage. Lomustine is taken orally with good oral bioavailability while carmustine is administered intravenously. Both agents readily cross the blood–brain barrier.

The main dose limiting toxicity of nitrosoureas is myelosuppression. Pulmonary fibrosis can also develop with higher doses and is dependent on cumulative dosing. Renal toxicity and renal failure are rare and are associated with prolonged use

K. Scheinemann and E. Bouffet (eds.), *Pediatric Neuro-oncology*,
DOI 10.1007/978-1-4939-1541-5_19, © Springer Science+Business Media New York 2015

and/or high cumulative doses. Transient elevation of liver function tests have been reported with carmustine and hepatotoxicity may be seen with higher doses but is generally reversible.

Lomustine has long been used as part of combination chemotherapy for medulloblastoma. It is also often incorporated into chemotherapy regimens targeted at lower grade gliomas (LGGs). Based on encouraging results from adult trials, lomustine was recently trialed in a phase II study for high grade gliomas (HGGs) through the Children's Oncology Group (COG). Compared to lomustine, carmustine is not as commonly utilized due to its inferior toxicity profile. However, carmustine has been used as part of myeloablative chemotherapy for stem cell rescue in recurrent and/or progressive brain tumors.

Platin Compounds (Heavy Metals)

Platinum agents, namely cisplatin and carboplatin, inhibit DNA replication by binding to DNA and forming intra- and inter-strand cross-links that result in DNA breakage. Myelosuppression is dose limiting and these agents commonly cause nausea and vomiting—both acute and delayed. Platinums can cause nephrotoxicity, ototoxicity, and neurotoxicity with peripheral neuropathy. However, as carboplatin is an analog of cisplatin with a different structural configuration, these toxicities are less pronounced with its use. Caution should still be taken when carboplatin is used in combination with other nephrotoxic drugs. Furthermore, hypersensitivity reactions to carboplatin have been documented.

Cisplatin has been identified as one of the most active single agents for medulloblastoma and it is particularly effective when used in combination chemotherapy. It has shown positive results when added to adjuvant chemotherapy for medulloblastomas. Using carboplatin as a radiosensitizing agent during radiation for high risk medulloblastomas/PNET has shown encouraging results [1]. In high doses, carboplatin is used as part of myeloablative chemotherapy with stem cell rescue for recurrent CNS tumors. Carboplatin is also becoming increasingly utilized as part of combination chemotherapy for LGGs.

Nitrogen Mustards

Cyclophosphamide and ifosfamide are inactive in their parent form and require hepatic activation via the P450 pathway. The active metabolites form cross-links with DNA of susceptible molecules to inhibit DNA replication. The primary toxicity of nitrogen mustards is myelosuppression and hemorrhagic cystitis. SIADH and infertility have been associated with nitrogen mustards. Ifosfamide is also associated with neurotoxicity including encephalopathy, hallucinations, somnolence, and seizures. In general, ifosfamide encephalopathy is reversible.

In recent years, using cyclophosphamide-based regimens for high risk medulloblastoma has resulted in significant improvements in outcome. High-dose cyclophosphamide has also been utilized in conjunction with stem cell rescue for newly diagnosed medulloblastoma [2] and recurrent CNS tumors. Ifosfamide has been incorporated into multiagent chemotherapy regimens targeted at HGGs and pontine gliomas [3]. Its role has been most prominent in treating recurrent and/or progressive brain tumors.

Procarbazine

Taken orally, procarbazine is a derivative of hydrazine and functions as a cell-cycle nonspecific, alkylating agent. Although its exact mechanism of action is unknown, it likely acts by inhibiting DNA, RNA, and protein synthesis as well as producing free radicals that cause direct DNA damage. Procarbazine is a weak MAO inhibitor and caution should be taken for patients who may be concurrently using drugs affected by MAOI.

Common toxicities include myelosuppression, flu-like symptoms, and neurological effects such as headache, anxiety, and insomnia. Nausea and vomiting is frequently experienced. Hypertensive crisis secondary to MAO inhibition is rare. Secondary malignancies, azoospermia, and sterility have also been associated with procarbazine.

Procarbazine has been previously incorporated into multiagent regimens for LGGs and medulloblastoma. Such combinations include the TPCV regimen consisting of thioguanine, procarbazine, lomustine, and vincristine as well as the eight-in-one-day regimen (vincristine, methylprednisolone, cisplatin, lomustine, hydroxyurea, procarbazine, cytarabine, and cyclophosphamide). It has also been studied as a single agent and as part of combination chemotherapy for HGGs. However, it has not shown significant survival benefits in pediatric HGGs [4].

Temozolomide

Temozolomide is an imidazotetrazine derivative of dacarbazine and functions as an alkylating agent. The parent form of the drug requires chemical conversion to its active form 5-(3-methyl-1-triazeno)imidazole-4-carboxamide (MTIC). It exhibits antineoplastic activity via methylation of DNA. The drug is typically taken orally with excellent bioavailability, approaching 100 %, and has good penetration of the blood–brain barrier. Overall, temozolomide is well tolerated. The most commonly seen toxicities are leucopenia, thrombocytopenia, and gastrointestinal side effects including nausea, vomiting, constipation, and diarrhea. The dose limiting toxicity is myelosuppression.

Temozolomide is typically dosed from 150 to 200 mg/m^2/day×5 days of a 28-day treatment cycle. Starting doses generally begin at 150 mg/m^2/day and may be increased to 200 mg/m^2/day in the absence of grade 3/4 toxicities. When used concurrently with radiation, lower doses of 90 mg/m^2/day have been utilized [5].

In recent years, temozolomide has been widely studied for the treatment of HGGs. In adults, the addition of temozolomide to radiation therapy for newly diagnosed glioblastomas has demonstrated benefits. However, the results have not been as favorable in pediatrics. In a single-arm, nonrandomized phase II study, Cohen and colleagues did not find a significant improvement in outcome when adding temozolomide to radiation therapy and as a single adjuvant therapy following radiation for newly diagnosed high grade glioma or diffuse intrinsic pontine glioma (DIPG) [5, 6]. Currently, the role of temozolomide in pediatric HGGs has yet to be determined.

Temozolomide is also being increasingly utilized for recurrent and/or progressive HGGs and LGGs. Among these cases, disease stability or partial response to temozolomide has been reported [7, 8]. Of note, patients with prior exposure to alkylators appeared to demonstrate suboptimal response that may indicate drug resistance to temozolomide [7]. An underexpression of the 0^6-methylguanine-DNA-methyltransferase (MGMT) repair gene, the main mechanism of temozolomide resistance, appears to be associated with an improved outcome [5, 9]. Future research is ongoing to investigate the role of temozolomide in combination regimens with other chemotherapy agents.

Topoisomerase Inhibitors

Etoposide

Etoposide is an epipodophyllotoxin that is cell-cycle specific and functions by stabilizing the topoisomerase II-DNA complex. Through this interaction, it prevents DNA unwinding and consequently induces arrest in the G2 phase. Etoposide also exhibits antineoplastic activity by inhibiting microtubular assembly through tubulin binding. It can be given both orally and intravenously. Due to its large molecular size, it is not effective at crossing the blood–brain barrier. Major toxicities associated with etoposide include myelosuppression, hypotension, nausea, and vomiting. Although hypersensitivity reactions have also been seen with its use, these reactions are not as common.

Etoposide is typically a standard component of regimens used for treating high-grade tumors, including medulloblastomas, ependymomas, supratentorial PNET, and HGGs [9]. It is also given in high doses for myeloablative chemotherapy with autologous stem cell rescue for recurrent CNS tumors. Given orally, etoposide is well absorbed and well tolerated and has demonstrated activity in disseminated, recurrent medulloblastoma [10] and recurrent ependymoma [11]. Etoposide was also given orally concurrent with and following radiation for diffuse intrinsic brain stem glioma, but results showed no improvement in survival [12].

Plant Alkaloids

Vinca alkaloids, namely vincristine and vinblastine, are derived from the periwinkle plant. Vinorelbine is a semisynthetic derivative of vinca alkaloids. These agents are cell-cycle specific and function by binding to tubulin in S and M phases, thereby preventing polymerization and causing metaphase arrest and cell death. Since plant alkaloids are metabolized by CYP P450 enzymes in the liver, caution should be taken when using drugs that are metabolized via the same pathway. This may include antiepileptic drugs frequently prescribed for neuro-oncology patients.

Vinca alkaloids commonly cause gastrointestinal side effects and peripheral neuropathy. Rarely, they have been associated with SIADH. Myelosuppression is more prominent with the use of vinblastine and vinorelbine. In addition, transient elevations of liver function tests may be seen with vinorelbine.

Vincristine has been used extensively in combination with other chemotherapy agents for LGGs, HGGs, and medulloblastomas. It remains a key component of standardized treatment of medulloblastoma and is used in conjunction with radiation therapy as well as a part of adjuvant chemotherapy following radiotherapy [9]. Recently, Bouffet and colleagues reported on the use of single-agent vinblastine for refractory or recurrent LGGs. In this study, vinblastine demonstrated clinical activity and there was an overall 5-year EFS of 42 % [13]. Current research is ongoing to better define the role of vinca alkaloids for LGGs.

Antimetabolites

Methotrexate is a folic acid analog that binds reversibly to dihydrofolate reductase, which converts folic acid to tetrahydrofolic acid. This effectively reduces the pool of reduced folates that is necessary for purine and thymidylate synthesis and, in turn, inhibits DNA and RNA synthesis. Methotrexate is specific to the S-phase of the cell cycle. Significant toxicities include myelosuppression and mucositis.

Neurotoxicity becomes more common in high-dose therapy, intrathecal or Ommaya administration. Skin reactions can occur but are uncommon.

Use of high-dose methotrexate prior to radiotherapy for HGGs and DIPG in a phase II trial has been reported [14]. It has also been given by intravenous and intraventricular administration as part of combination chemotherapy for localized medulloblastomas [9, 15] and has shown promising results when added to induction therapy for high risk or disseminated medulloblastomas [16]. The Children's Oncology Group is currently investigating into the role of methotrexate for the treatment of PNET and high risk medulloblastomas in a phase III trial.

Recombinant Humanized Monoclonal Antibody

Bevacizumab

Bevacizumab is a recombinant humanized monoclonal antibody that selectively binds to human vascular endothelial growth factor (VEGF). This prevents VEGF from binding to its receptors on endothelial cell surfaces, thereby reducing blood vessel formation in tumors and subsequent tumor growth.

Commonly reported adverse effects include myelosuppression, fatigue, diarrhea, stomatitis, asthenia, anorexia, and abdominal pain. Hypertension is also common but can be controlled with oral antihypertensives. Hypertensive crisis or hypertensive encephalopathy is rare. Significant but uncommon toxicities include gastrointestinal perforation, hemorrhage, deep vein thrombosis, and arterial thromboembolism. Infusion-related and hypersensitivity reactions can occur and manifest as anaphylactic-like symptoms. Bevacizumab has been associated with fistulae, congestive heart failure, and infections and can cause impaired wound healing. Proteinuria has been reported with ranging severities and may be dose dependent. Urinalysis is recommended at baseline and throughout treatment.

Bevacizumab has shown promising results when used in combination with irinotecan for children with multiply recurrent LGGs [17].

Children with recurrent LGGs who received bevacizumab-based therapy demonstrated either rapid clinical response or disease stability while on treatment [18]. Unfortunately, the Pediatric Brain Tumor Consortium found that bevacizumab showed minimal efficacy when utilized for recurrent ependymoma [19], malignant glioma, and diffuse brainstem glioma [20]. Currently, the Children's Oncology Group is investigating the role of bevacizumab for newly diagnosed HGGs, recurrent and refractory medulloblastomas, and PNET (Table 19.1).

Blood–Brain Barrier

The blood–brain barrier is a dynamic interface separating the brain from the circulatory system. The blood–brain barrier is formed by specialized endothelial cells and regulates the transport of essential molecules from the circulation to the brain, while also protecting the brain from harmful chemicals. This barrier also limits the ability of many systemically administered chemotherapy agents to penetrate into the central nervous system. In general, small molecules and those that are lipophilic are more likely to cross the blood–brain barrier than those that are large and lipophobic. There are mechanisms such as blood–brain barrier disruption, intra-arterial chemotherapy injection, intrathecal chemotherapy administration, or intratumoral chemotherapy administration that have been utilized to overcome the blood–brain barrier.

Blood–brain barrier disruption has been utilized in several pediatric brain tumor studies. Recently, osmotic disruption using mannitol infusion followed by intra-arterial carboplatin or methotrexate was used to treat adult and pediatric embryonal and germ cell tumors [21]. This preliminary study showed promising survival outcome. Another study disrupted the blood–brain barrier using intra-arterial mannitol injection followed by intracarotid chemotherapy and was effective in treating a large number of children with a variety of brain tumors including germ cell tumors and PNETs [22]. Other methods of blood–brain barrier disruption

have been attempted and some have been shown to provide effective therapy for a variety of adult tumors.

Intrathecal Chemotherapy

Intrathecal administration of chemotherapy is another method of bypassing the blood–brain barrier to deliver chemotherapy within the central nervous system. Many agents have been investigated for a variety of brain tumors. Intrathecal liposomal cytarabine has been used with success in children with ependymoma, primitive neuroectodermal tumor, medulloblastoma, and atypical teratoid rhabdoid tumor [23]. As well, intrathecal mafosfamide and etoposide have been used successfully in children with similar tumor types [24]. Finally, there is extensive information on the use of intrathecal chemotherapy in medulloblastoma and directions for future agents warranting study have been established [25].

Intra-Ommaya Therapy

Ommaya reservoirs have been directly placed into the lateral ventricle to prevent repeated lumbar punctures for intrathecal chemotherapy. These provide easy access to the intrathecal space and eliminate the need for conscious sedation for lumbar punctures to be performed. Ommaya reservoirs have also been placed into the cysts of craniopharyngiomas in order to deliver chemotherapy agents intratumorally [26, 27]. The two agents that have previously been successfully utilized using this method of drug delivery are bleomycin [27] and alpha interferon [26].

Bleomycin
Bleomycin has been used successfully in the treatment of cystic craniopharyngioma. It is given via an Ommaya reservoir surgically implanted into the cyst. A review of 24 patients utilized a dose of at least 3 mg of bleomycin every other day with a dose of 5 mg in giant craniopharyngiomas [27]. This was repeated for a total dose of 30–150 mg. This therapy was found

Table 19.1 Clinical pharmacology of commonly used chemotherapy agents

Drug	Mechanism of action	Common toxicities	Less common toxicities	Dose ranges	Penetration of blood–brain barrier
Intravenous					
Vincristine	Vinca alkaloid	Constipation, diarrhea, peripheral neuropathy	SIADH, paralytic ileus, seizures, severe jaw pain	1.5–2 mg/m^2/dose (maximum dose = 2 mg)	Not significant
Vinblastine	Vinca alkaloid	Myelosuppression, leucopenia, constipation, peripheral neuropathy, paresthesias	SIADH, neurotoxicity, severe jaw pain, bronchospasm, shortness of breath	6 mg/m^2/dose qweek	Poor
Vinorelbine	Vinca alkaloid	Neuropathy, anemia, neutropenia, constipation, diarrhea, nausea, vomiting, fatigue, fever, elevation of AST, injection site reaction	SIADH, rash, pain, dyspnea, bronchospasm, tachycardia, hypo-/hypertension	30 mg/m^2/dose	Yes (limited to animal studies)
Cisplatin	Platinum—alkylating agent	Ototoxicity, tinnitus, nephrotoxicity, nausea, emesis, myelosuppression, electrolyte disturbances, taste disturbance	Peripheral neuropathy, visual impairment, seizures	60–75 mg/m^2/dose each cycle	Not readily
Carboplatin	Platinum—alkylating agent	Nephrotoxicity, nausea, emesis, myelosuppression, LFT elevation, electrolyte disturbances	Peripheral neuropathy, ototoxicity, hypersensitivity reactions	560 mg/m^2/dose qmonth; 175 mg/m^2/dose qweek *Myeloablative:* 1,200–1,500 mg/m^2/cycle *Radiosensitizer:* 30–45 mg/m^2/dose	Yes
Carmustine	Nitrosourea—alkylating agent	Myelosuppression, nausea and vomiting, elevation of liver function tests	Pulmonary toxicity, renal toxicity, renal failure, reversible hepatotoxicity	150–200 mg/m^2/dose q6–8weeks *Myeloablative:* 300–600 mg/m^2/cycle	Yes—readily
Cyclophosphamide	Nitrogen mustard—alkylating agent	Hemorrhagic cystitis, myelosuppression, nausea, vomiting, mucositis, nasal and/or sinus congestion	Cardiac dysfunction (high doses), hepatotoxicity, SIADH, gonadal suppression, sterility	400–1,800 mg/m^2 *Myeloablative:* 2 g/m^2/dose	Limited
Ifosfamide	Nitrogen mustard—alkylating agent	Myelosuppression, nausea, vomiting, hemorrhagic cystitis, hematuria, encephalopathy	Coma, SIADH, infertility, renal dysfunction, hepatic dysfunction	1–2 g/m^2/day × 3–5 days q3–4weeks	Yes—subtherapeutic
Etoposide	Topoisomerase II inhibitor	Myelosuppression, nausea, vomiting, hypotension	Type 1 hypersensitivity reaction, hepatotoxicity	*Intravenous:* 100 mg/m^2/day *Oral:* 50 mg/m^2/day × 14–21 days *Myeloablative:* 750–1,500 mg/m^2/cycle	Poor/limited

Methotrexate	Antimetabolite	Myelosuppression, mucositis, neurotoxicity (high dose, intrathecal, Ommaya)	Skin reactions	*Intravenous*: 4–15 g/m^2/dose 400 mg/kg/dose/cycle (medulloblastoma) *Intrathecal*: 6–12 mg/dose; age dependent *Intraventricular*: 2 mg/dose	Yes—variable
Bevacizumab	Angiogenesis—recombinant humanized monoclonal antibody	Myelosuppression, hypertension, fatigue, diarrhea, anorexia, asthenia, proteinuria, stomatitis, abdominal pain	Fistula, hypertensive crisis, arterial thromboembolic events, hemorrhage, hypersensitivity or infusion-related reaction, impaired wound healing, congestive heart failure, infections	10 mg/kg/dose q2weeks	N/A
Oral					
Lomustine	Nitrosourea—alkylating agent	Myelosuppression, nausea and vomiting	Pulmonary toxicity, renal toxicity, renal failure	100–130 mg/m^2 q6weeks	Yes—readily
Temozolomide	Nonclassic alkylating agent	Myelosuppression (leucopenia, thrombocytopenia), nausea, vomiting, constipation, diarrhea, fatigue, headache	Rash, pruritus, peripheral edema, asthenia, neuropathy	150–200 mg/m^2/day on day 1–5 of 28-day cycle *Radiosensitizer*: 90 mg/m^2/dose	Yes—variable
Procarbazine	Nonclassic alkylating agent	Myelosuppression, nausea and vomiting, flu-like symptoms, neurological symptoms	Hypertension, secondary malignancies, gonadal suppression, sterility	60 $mg/m^2/day \times 14$ days	Yes

to effectively treat the tumor in 70 % of cases. Documented side effects secondary to this intra-Ommaya bleomycin include blindness [27] and vasculopathy [28]. Documented side effects are attributed to leakage of the bleomycin out of the cyst. Other side effects include headache and vomiting [27].

Alpha Interferon

Alpha interferon has also been used successfully to treat cystic craniopharyngioma. It also is given via an intracystic Ommaya reservoir. The dose used in a recent review was 3,000,000 units three times per week for a total of 36,000,000 units [26]. This review of 19 patients revealed that patients received 1–4 cycles of the interferon and the tumor reduction was 60–98 %. Documented side effects were headache, fever, depression, eyelid erythema, and chronic fatigue syndrome. Overall this therapy was very well tolerated, and continues to be used effectively.

Conclusion

There are many chemotherapy agents that have been effectively utilized in the therapy of pediatric brain tumors. Effective agents include many alkylating agents, vinca alkaloids, topoisomerase inhibitors, antimetabolites, and angiogenesis inhibitors. Chemotherapy for brain tumors can be given by various routes, including orally, intravenously, intrathecally, and via an Ommaya reservoir. Novel modes of delivery include via novel strategies for blood–brain barrier disruption. There are many clinical trials ongoing, examining novel agents for therapy for this patient population.

References

1. Jakacki RI, Burger PC, Zhou T, Holmes EJ, Kocak M, Onar A, et al. Outcome of children with metastatic medulloblastoma treated with carboplatin during craniospinal radiotherapy: a Children's Oncology Group phase I/II study. J Clin Oncol. 2012;30:2648–53.
2. Gajjar A, Chintagumpala M, Ashley D, Kellie D, Kun LE, Merchant TE, et al. Risk-adapted craniospinal radiotherapy followed by high-dose chemotherapy and stem-cell rescue in children with newly diagnosed medulloblastoma (St Jude Medulloblastoma-96): long-term results from a prospective, multicentre trial. Lancet Oncol. 2006;7:813–20.
3. Wolff JE, Driever PH, Erdlenbruch B, Kortmann RD, Rutkowski S, Pietsch T, et al. Intensive chemotherapy improves survival in pediatric high-grade glioma after gross total resection: results of the HIT-gBM-c protocol. Cancer. 2010;116:705–12.
4. Chintagumpala MM, Friedman HS, Stewart CF, Kepner J, McLendon RE, Modrich PL, et al. A phase II window trial of procarbazine and topotecan in children with high-grade glioma: a report from the children's oncology group. J Neurooncol. 2006;77:193–8.
5. Cohen KJ, Pollack IF, Zhou T, Buxton A, Holmes EJ, Burger PC, et al. Temozolomide in the treatment of high-grade gliomas in children: a report from the Children's Oncology Group. Neuro Oncol. 2011;13:317–23.
6. Cohen KJ, Heideman RL, Zhou T, Holmes EJ, Lavey RS, Bouffet E, Pollack IF. Temozolomide in the treatment of children with newly diagnosed diffuse intrinsic pontine gliomas: a report from the Children's Oncology Group. Neuro Oncol. 2011;13:410–6.
7. Gururangan S, Fisher MJ, Allen JC, Herndon II JE, Quinn JA, Reardon DA, et al. Temozolomide in children with progressive low-grade glioma. Neuro Oncol. 2007;9:161–8.
8. Lashford LS, Theisse P, Jouvet A, Jaspan T, Couanet D, Griffiths PD, et al. Temozolomide in malignant gliomas of childhood: a United Kingdom Children's Cancer Study Group and French Society for Pediatric Oncology Intergroup study. J Clin Oncol. 2002;20:4684–91.
9. Gottardo NG, Gajjar A. Chemotherapy for malignant brain tumours of childhood. J Child Neurol. 2008;23:1149–59.
10. Ashley DM, Meier L, Kerby T, Zalduondo FM, Friedman HS, Gajjar A, et al. Response of recurrent medulloblastoma to low-dose oral etoposide. J Clin Oncol. 1996;14:1922–7.
11. Sandri A, Massimino M, Mastrodicasa L, Sardi N, Bertin D, Basso ME, et al. Treatment with oral etoposide for childhood recurrent ependymomas. J Pediatr Hematol Oncol. 2005;27:486–90.
12. Korones DN, Fisher PG, Kretschmar C, Zhou T, Chen Z, Kepner J, Freeman C. Treatment of children with diffuse intrinsic brain stem glioma with radiotherapy, vincristine and oral VP-16: a Children's Oncology Group phase II study. Pediatr Blood Cancer. 2008;50:227–30.
13. Bouffet E, Jakacki R, Goldman S, Hargrave D, Hawkins C, Shroff M, et al. Phase II study of weekly vinblastine in recurrent or refractory pediatric low-grade glioma. J Clin Oncol. 2012;30:1358–63.
14. Wolff JE, Kortmann RD, Wolff B, Pietsch T, Peters O, Schmid HJ, Rutkowski S, Warmuth-Metz M, Kramm C. High dose methotrexate for pediatric HGG: results of the HIT-GBM-D pilot study. J Neurooncol. 2011;102:433–42. doi:10.1007/s11060-010-0334-2. Epub 2010 Aug 8.

15. von Bueren AO, von Hoff K, Pietsch T, Gerber NU, Warmuth-Metz M, Deinlein F, et al. Treatment of young children with localized medulloblastoma by chemotherapy alone: results of the prospective, multi-center trial HIT 2000 confirming the prognostic impact of histology. Neuro Oncol. 2011;13:669–79.

16. Chi SN, Gardner SL, Levy AS, Knopp EA, Miller DC, Wisoff JH, et al. Feasibility and response to induction chemotherapy intensified with high-dose methotrexate for young children with newly diagnosed high-risk disseminated medulloblastoma. J Clin Oncol. 2004; 22:4881–7.

17. Packer RJ, Jakacki R, Horn M, Rood B, Vezina G, MacDonald T, Fisher MJ, Cohen B. Objective response of multiply recurrent low-grade gliomas to bevacizumab and irinotecan. Pediatr Blood Cancer. 2009;52:791–5.

18. Hwang EI, Jakacki RI, Fisher MJ, Kilburn LB, Horn M, Vezina G, Rood BR, Packer RJ. Long-term efficacy and toxicity of bevacizumab-based therapy in children with recurrent low-grade gliomas. Pediatr Blood Cancer. 2013;60:776–82.

19. Gururangan S, Fangusaro J, Poussaint TY, Onar-Thomas A, Gilbertson RJ, Vajapeyam S, et al. Lack of efficacy of bevacizumab 1 irinotecan in cases of pediatric recurrent ependymoma—a Pediatric Brain Tumour Consortium study. Neuro Oncol. 2012;14:1404–12.

20. Gururangan S, Chi SN, Poussaint TY, Onar-Thomas A, Gilbertson RJ, Vajapeyam S, et al. Lack of efficacy of bevacizumab plus irinotecan in children with recurrent malignant glioma and diffuse brainstem glioma: a Pediatric Brain Tumour Consortium study. J Clin Oncol. 2010;28:3069–75.

21. Jahnke K, Kraemer DF, Knight KF, Fortin D, Bell S, Doolittle ND, Muldoon LL, Neuwelt EA. Intraarterial chemotherapy and osmotic blood-brain barrier disruption for patients with embryonal and germ cell tumours of the central nervous system. Cancer. 2008;112:581–8.

22. Dahlborg SA, Petrillo A, et al. The potential for complete and durable response in nonglial primary brain tumours in children and young adults with enhanced chemotherapy delivery. Cancer J Sci Am. 1998;4: 110–24.

23. Lassaletta A, Lopez-Ibor B, Mateos E, Gonzalez-Vicent M, Perez-Martinez A, Sevilla J, Diaz MA, Madero L. Intrathecal liposomal cytarabine in children under 4 years with malignant brain tumours. J Neurooncol. 2009;95:65–9.

24. Slavc I, Schuller E, Falger J, Gunes M, Pillwein K, Czech T, Dietrich W, Rossler K, Dieckmann K, Prayer D, Hainfellner J. Feasibility of long-term intraventricular therapy with mafosfamide (n=26) and etoposide (n=11): experience in 26 children with disseminated malignant brain tumours. J Neurooncol. 2003;64:239–47.

25. Conroy S, Garnett M, Vloeberghs M, Grundy R, Craven I, Walker D. Medulloblastoma in childhood: revisiting intrathecal therapy in infants and children. Cancer Chemother Pharmacol. 2010;65:1173–89.

26. Dastoli PA, Nicacio JM, Silva NS, Capellano AM, Toledo SRC, Ierardi D, Cavalheiro S. Cystic craniopharyngioma: intratumoural chemotherapy with alpha interferon. Arq Neuropsiquiatr. 2011;69:50–5.

27. Mottolese C, Stan H, Hermier M, Berlier P, Convert J, Frappaz D, Lapras C. Intracystic chemotherapy with bleomycin in the treatment of craniopharyngiomas. Childs Nerv Syst. 2001;17:724–30.

28. Cho WS, Kim SK, Wang KC, Phi JH, Cho BK. Vasculopathy after intracystic bleomycin administration for a recurrent cystic craniopharyngioma. J Neurosurg Pediatr. 2012;9:394–9.

Targeted Therapies in Paediatric Brain Tumours

20

John-Paul Kilday, Nada Jabado, and Eric Bouffet

Introduction

Although significant improvements in survival have been achieved during recent decades, results of treatment in paediatric brain tumours are still unsatisfactory. For some tumours, such as diffuse intrinsic pontine gliomas (DIPG), the 5-year survival rate is less than 5 % and no progress in improving this outcome has been achieved in the past 20 years despite numerous clinical trials. Another concern is the long-term sequelae of treatments (surgery, radiation and chemotherapy) that clearly save life, but carry their own burden on quality of life. Advancement in molecular biology has provided new insight into abnormal cellular functions and many pathways have been identified that could potentially be targeted with novel agents. Targeted inhibition in oncology was first successfully applied in chronic myeloid leukaemia (CML), a condition driven by the BCR-ABL1 gene fusion [1]. While cytotoxic chemotherapy was associated with less than 15 % complete cytogenetic response, selective inhibition of the ABL1 tyrosine kinase by imatinib alone was found to result in over 75 % complete cytogenetic response.

The last decade has witnessed an explosion of new compounds for the treatment of cancer, using molecules aimed at targeting pathways specific for cancer cells. When the first compounds became available, the molecular pathogenesis of most childhood brain tumours was still poorly understood. For instance, in addition to BCR-ABL, imatinib also inhibits the c-KIT and PDGFR tyrosine kinases, and preclinical work had shown that inhibition of PDGF/PDGFR negatively affected glioma cell proliferation. Therefore the first clinical studies in paediatric neuro-oncology logically tested imatinib. The results of these early studies proved disappointing, despite evidence showing that PDGFR was expressed in several paediatric brain tumours. With increasing knowledge of the molecular pathogenesis of CNS tumour in childhood, a number of agents have now been tested, thereby contributing to our evolving understanding of targeted therapies in this context. This chapter reviews current developments in such targeted therapy for childhood brain tumours.

J.-P. Kilday, M.B.Ch.B., M.R.C.P.C.H., Ph.D.
Pediatric Brain Tumor Program, Department of Hematology/Oncology, Hospital for Sick Children, Toronto, ON, Canada

N. Jabado, M.D., Ph.D.
Department of Pediatrics, McGill University Health Center/McGill University, Montréal, QC, Canada

E. Bouffet, M.D. (✉)
Department of Hematology/Oncology,
The Hospital for Sick Children, University of Toronto, Toronto, ON, Canada
e-mail: eric.bouffet@sickkids.ca

K. Scheinemann and E. Bouffet (eds.), *Pediatric Neuro-oncology*,
DOI 10.1007/978-1-4939-1541-5_20, © Springer Science+Business Media New York 2015

Key Signalling Pathways in Paediatric CNS Tumours

Signalling pathways known to be upregulated in paediatric CNS tumours include PI3K (phosphoinositide 3-kinase), AKT, RAS/MEK, Notch, Sonic Hedgehog and Wnt, amongst others. The tumour cells use these pathways to perpetuate proliferation and survival and evade apoptosis. Although many of these pathways are also used by normal (non-malignant) cells, it is the reliance of the tumour cells on these pathways for survival that makes them potential targets for cancer treatment. The specific description of these pathways is beyond the scope of this review, and most information that relates to current knowledge of molecular pathogenesis and signalling pathways is available in disease-specific chapters.

Phase I and II Studies

The Children Oncology Group (COG), the Pediatric Brain Tumor Consortium (PBTC) and the Innovative Therapies for Children with Cancer (ITCC) Consortium have conducted and published several phase I and II studies of molecularly targeted agents that have enrolled paediatric brain tumour patients. Results of these studies are detailed in Table 20.1 (and reviewed in [2]). A phase I study of the farnesyl transferase inhibitor lonafarnib enrolled 53 patients with various brain tumour diagnoses and observed one partial response and nine cases of stable disease. One patient with recurrent high-grade glioma experienced a complete response in a phase I study of the selective Integrin αvβ3 and αvβ 5 antagonist cilengitide [3]. Two low-grade glioma patients showed partial response in a phase I study of lenalidomide, an anti-angiogenic agent [4]. Despite occasional observations of stable disease, no response was seen in the phase I or II studies of gefitinib, everolimus, temsirolimus, lapatinib, imatinib, cloretazine, tipifarnib, MK0752 and semaxanib that enrolled a total of 314 patients [2, 5–7]. Overall, minimal efficacy has been demonstrated for these single agents tested in the context of phase I or II

studies. The exception seems to be rapamycin, an mTOR inhibitor, and Sonic Hedgehog (SHH) inhibitors which have shown evidence of activity in tuberous sclerosis patients with subependymal giant cell astrocytomas and SHH-driven medulloblastoma, respectively (see below). Outside these specific contexts, there is currently no proven role for molecular targeted therapy as monotherapy in paediatric neuro-oncology.

Trials of Targeted Therapy in Specific Tumour Types

Medulloblastoma

The last decade has witnessed major progress in understanding the biology behind the clinical and histologic differences seen in medulloblastoma. Results of several transcriptional profiling studies from various cooperative groups have demonstrated that medulloblastoma consists of at least four different biological subgroups with divergent clinical and biological presentations and behaviour. The 4 groups, Wnt (Group 1), Sonic Hedgehog (SHH; Group 2), Group 3 and Group 4, differ in their demographics, histology, DNA copy-number aberrations and clinical outcome [8]. The identification of these molecular subgroups has triggered great interest in the identification of targeted therapies for each specific subgroup. So far, these studies have identified the SHH and Wnt pathways as potential molecular targets in medulloblastoma. The molecular pathogenesis of groups 3 and 4 medulloblastoma is still poorly understood and efforts are ongoing to develop accurate mouse models.

So far, most efforts to support translational developments have focused on the development and evaluation of SHH inhibitors. Tumours in the SHH group are associated with mutations in genes PTCH, SMO or SUFU. Aberrant activation of the SHH signalling pathway causes increased cell proliferation and is linked to the development of several types of cancer, in particular medulloblastoma, where activating or inactivating mutations in genes that regulate the SHH pathway have been identified in approximately

Table 20.1 Results of molecularly targeted therapies in paediatric brain tumours

Study type	Drug	BSG	Ependymoma	Medulloblastoma/sPNET	HGG	LGG	Other	Total	Outcome	References
Phase I	Gefitinib	3 (2 SD)	1					4	2 SD	[30]
Phase I	Lonafarnib	7	9	8	18		11	53	1 PR, 9 SD	[2]
Phase I	Cilengitide	5	8 (2 SD)	4 (1 SD)	9 (1 CR 1 SD)		7 (2 SD)	33	1 CR, 6 SD	[3]
Phase I	Semaxanib	3	4	1	9 (3 SD)		6 (2 SD)	23	5 SD	[2]
phase II	Tipifarnib	41	0	18	38			97	6 SD	[2]
Phase II	Imatinib		5 (1 SD)	8 (2 SD)	2	3 (1 SD)	1	19	4 SD	[31]
Phase II	Imatinib	4 (1 SD)		2 (1 SD)	1	1 (1 SD)	4	12	3 SD	[32]
Phase I	Imatinib	14			35			49	no response	[2]
Phase I	Cloretazine	5	9	10 (1 SD)	14 (1 SD)		3 (2 SD)	41	4 SD	[2]
Phase I	Erlotinib	6	6	2	12	1	2	19	8 SD	[13]
Phase II	Bevacizumab + irinotecan	16 (5 SD)	13 (2 SD)		18 (8 SD)			47	15 SD	[12, 33]
Phase II	Nimotuzumab	21 (1 PR, 10 SD)						21	1 PR 10 SD	[15]
Phase I	Everolimus	3 (1 SD)	4 (1 SD)	3	5 (1 SD)	4 (1 SD)	1	20	4 SD	[24]
Phase II	Temsirolimus	11 (5 SD)			6 (2 SD)			17	7 SD	[25]
Phase I	Lenalidomide	2	9	6	6	26 (2 PR)	2	51	2 PR, 23 SD	[4]
Phase I	MK0752	6	8 (1 SD)	4	3 (1 SD)		2	23	2 SD	[5]
Phase	Lapatinib		14 (4 SD)	17 (3 SD)	13			44	7 SD	[6, 7]

HGG high-grade glioma, *BSG* brainstem glioma, *sPNET* supratentorial primitive neuroectodermal tumour, *SD* stable disease, *PR* partial response, *Ref* reference

30 % of tumours. From early murine work, treatment of medulloblastoma in Ptc1($\pm$) p53($-/-$) mice with the SMO inhibitor HHAntag showed promising results. Following a high-throughput development cell-based screen for novel compounds capable of blocking SHH-activated gene transcription, several compounds were identified with potent activity. GDC-0449 (Vismodegib, Genentech) was the first-in-class small-molecule antagonist of the SHH receptor tested in medulloblastoma patients [9]. Another compound, LDE225 (Erismodegib, Novartis), was subsequently tested in clinical trials. Both drugs have shown activity in recurrent paediatric and adult medulloblastoma. A phase II trial of GDC-0449 is ongoing in children with recurrent or refractory medulloblastomas with evidence of activation of the Hedgehog signalling pathway. Likewise, a phase III trial of LDE225 has also recently opened for patients with SHH-pathway-activated medulloblastoma. The primary objective of the latter study is to compare the efficacy of LDE225 versus temozolomide in patients who have relapsed after prior standard-of-care therapy, including craniospinal radiotherapy with no prior temozolomide. This trial will also have two non-randomised, uncontrolled arms, one for paediatric patients aged less than 6 years who have not received radiotherapy as part of their initial treatment and one for adult and paediatric patients who have received prior craniospinal radiation with temozolomide as part of their primary therapy.

High-Grade Gliomas

Historically paediatric high-grade gliomas (HGGs) were thought to be similar to adults. However, there is increasing evidence that childhood HGGs have important differences when compared to their adult counterparts. PTEN mutation, EGFR amplification and EGFRvIII mutations are relatively rare in paediatric HGGs; they frequently show chromosome 1q gain and focal amplification of PDGFRA. In contrast, adult tumours frequently show focal amplification of EGFR and gain of chromosomes 7 and loss of 10q [10]. Unlike adult glioblastomas, paediatric HGGs also lack IDH1 mutations. While data on

this lack of EGFR amplification have gradually become evident, several trials have investigated EGFR inhibitors in paediatric HGGs. A phase I trial of erlotinib given concurrently with radiation enrolled 23 newly diagnosed high-grade glioma patients, including 20 cases below the age of 18 years. No objective radiologic responses to therapy were observed in patients with measurable disease and no correlation was found between markers of PI3K/AKT pathway activation and response to erlotinib [11]. Based on encouraging responses observed in a phase I trial of cilengitide [3], a phase II study was designed for paediatric patients with recurrent and progressive HGGs. The results of this study are pending. Bevacizumab, a VEGF monoclonal antibody inhibitor, has been used in combination with irinotecan in a PBTC HGG study. No sustained objective responses were observed in 16 evaluable patients, although eight patients demonstrated sustained stable disease for a period of 12 weeks or longer [12]. An international, phase II open-label, randomised study of bevacizumab in children with newly diagnosed supratentorial, infratentorial or peduncular high grade gliomas is now recruiting patients.

Diffuse Intrinsic Pontine Glioma (DIPG)

Despite multiple clinical trials of chemotherapy schedules (before and/or during and/or after radiation; low dose metronomic; intensive or high-dose chemotherapy with autologous stem cell rescue) and radiation techniques (hypo-, normo- or hyperfractionation), the outcome of this tumour is still devastating and no improvement in survival has been achieved over the last three decades. Post-mortem tissue collection was initiated in Canada, the USA and the Netherlands to address the lack of tumour material for research and to allow identification of new targets. These studies have shown a distinct genetic and methylation profile of DIPG as compared with other paediatric and adult high-grade gliomas. At the gene expression level, DIPG are mainly characterised by frequent amplification of the PDGF receptor, PDGFR. Other amplifications have been described involving the hepatocyte growth factor receptor MET, IGF receptor 1 (IGF1R), EGF receptors (EGFR, ERBB4 and EGFRv3), poly-ADP-ribose polymerase (PARP), VEGFA and associated downstream pathways including the PI3KAkt-phosphomammalian target of rapamycin (mTOR). In this context, several trials of small-molecule inhibitors have been conducted in recent years (reviewed in [2]).

Because of the role of PDGF in gliomagenesis and the frequent overexpression of PDGFR alpha in paediatric anaplastic astrocytoma, imatinib was the first agent incorporated into DIPG trials. A phase I/II study conducted by the Pediatric Brain Tumor Consortium enrolled 35 patients [2]. In this trial, the initial design was to administer imatinib in conjunction with radiation therapy. However, because of concerns regarding the incidence of intra-tumoural haemorrhage during irradiation, the protocol was amended to exclude patients with evidence of haemorrhage on MRI scan prior to irradiation, and imatinib treatment was started two weeks after completion of radiotherapy, provided that there was no evidence of intralesional blood on the post-irradiation MRI scan. This trial reported a 1-year event-free and overall survival rate of 24.3 % and 45.5 %, respectively, a result similar to that observed in previous DIPG studies of radiation with or without chemotherapy. This dampened enthusiasm for the development of further studies.

Although gene amplification of EGFR is uncommon in DIPG, overexpression of EGFR is nevertheless often detected. Two trials of EGFR inhibitors were conducted: one using gefitinib during and after radiation, and a trial of erlotinib that mandated histological confirmation of malignant brainstem gliomas [13, 14]. Both studies reported mild and reversible toxicity. Event-free and overall survival in these trials were consistent with the results of previous studies. However, intriguingly, anecdotal cases of long-term survivors were reported. For instance in the gefitinib study, three patients out of 43 cases remained progression free with 36 months of follow-up.

In addition to EGFR directed tyrosine kinase inhibitors, monoclonal antibodies that block EGFR have also been used in clinical trials. Bode et al. reported in 2006 the results of a phase II study of nimotuzumab, a monoclonal antibody that binds to and inhibits EGFR [36]. At the end of a 6-week induction period, one partial response and nine cases of stable disease were observed out of 21 DIPG patients. At the end of the consolidation phase (week 21), the trial reported three partial responses. Unfortunately, the promising results of this experience were not confirmed in a subsequent study of nimotuzumab combined with radiation in newly diagnosed DIPG patients [15].

With respect to other agents, the PBTC conducted a phase I followed by a phase II trial of tipifarnib, a farnesyl transferase inhibitor that had shown promising anti-neoplastic activity in a preclinical model with the ability to reverse radiation resistance in human glioma cells. In the initial phase I study, 17 DIPG patients were enrolled and no unexpected toxicity was observed; in particular there was no observation of intra-tumoural haemorrhage [2]. The subsequent phase II study enrolled 40 eligible DIPG patients and reported a median progression-free survival of 6.8 months and a median overall survival of 8.3 months [34]. Similarly, Broniscer reported the results of a phase I study of vandetanib administered during and after radiotherapy [35]. This small-molecule inhibitor of VEGFR2 and EGFR had shown activity against high-grade glioma cell lines and an orthotopic xenograft. Twenty-one DIPG patients were enrolled in this study that reported survival rates similar to other trials (Table 20.2).

The negative results of these initial trials of targeted therapy in DIPG did not alter the enthusiasm to test other compounds. The limited penetration of drugs through the intact blood–brain barrier was one of the explanations for the lack of success of early trials, while the use of isolated single agents was another limitation of these unsuccessful experiences. Recently the results of the first trial using a rational combination of small-molecule inhibitors targeting key pathways in DIPG were reported. In this trial, a combination of vandetanib and dasatinib was used concurrently with radiation. This study pointed out that the CSF exposure of vandetanib and dasatinib in the treated population was modest. However, the 1-year overall survival rate of 52 % compared favourably with those seen in previous

Table 20.2 Results of molecularly targeted therapies in paediatric brain tumours with diffuse intrinsic pontine gliomas

Drug	Trial	Number of patients	1 year EFS	1 year OS	Median EFS	Median OS	Patients alive >2 years	References
Imatinib	Phase I/II	35	24.3 ± 7.1 %	45.5 ± 8.7 %,			2	[2]
Tipifarnib	Phase I	17	9.4 ± 6.3 %	36.4 ± 16.7 %			NA	[2]
Tipifarnib	Phase II	40	12.9 % ± 4.9 %	34.3 ± 7.4 %	5.9	8.9	1	[34]
Gefitinib	Phase II	44	20.9 + 5.6 %	56.4 + 7.6 %	7.4		3 (at 3 years)	[14]
Erlotinib	Phase I	21			8	12	NA	[13]
Vandetanib	Phase I	21	21.4 % ± 11 %	37.5 % ± 10.5 %			3	[35]
Vandetanib and dasatinib	Phase I	25	52 ± 10 %				2	[16]

EFS event-free survival, *OS* overall survival, *Ref* reference

studies [16]. This experience and anecdotal reports of long-term survivors in other trials of targeted therapies suggest that biopsies and molecular testing of paediatric DIPG are critical to the rational utilisation of targeted agents.

Ependymomas

As there is no convincing role for chemotherapy in the treatment of ependymoma using conventional agents, the need for targeted treatment is even more crucial in this disease than in other paediatric brain tumours. Analysis of paediatric ependymoma specimens has reported a high expression of members of the receptor tyrosine kinase family, such as ERBB2, ERBB4 and EGFR in over 75 % of specimens studied [17]. Gilbertson et al. showed that activation of ERBB receptor signalling in cultured ependymoma cells resulted in AKT phosphorylation and cellular proliferation, demonstrating the importance of this pathway in ependymomas. In addition, cellular proliferation was blocked in a dose-dependent manner using an ERBB2 inhibitor [17].

As with ERBB2 and ERBB4, overexpression of EGFR is also common in intracranial ependymoma. In an evaluation of immunohistochemical markers from a large cohort of patients with ependymoma, Korshunov and colleagues reported that 43 % stained for EGFR. High-grade tumours were more likely to be EGFR positive (61 %) compared with 25 % of low-grade tumours [18].

Two trials of ERBB/EGFR inhibitors were recently conducted in patients with recurrent ependymoma. The first trial was a randomised study of erlotinib, the oral EGFR inhibitor with co-inhibitory activity against ERBB2, versus oral etoposide. The second trial was a single-arm phase II study of the combination of lapatinib and bevacizumab. Unfortunately, neither of the two trials met their primary efficacy end point.

Transcriptional profiling of large cohorts of ependymoma has recently pointed out the heterogeneity and complexity of this tumour, identifying several molecular subgroups [19, 20]. Efforts are ongoing to identify potential targets for these specific subgroups.

Subependymal Giant Cell Astrocytoma

Tuberous sclerosis complex (TSC) is an autosomal dominant genetic disorder characterised by the development of benign tumours in multiple organ systems, including the brain, skin, kidney, lung, heart and retina. Most patients with TSC present with mutations in either of two identified tuberous sclerosis genes—TSC1 (hamartin) or TSC2 (tuberin). These genes encode proteins that form the hamartin-tuberin tumour suppressor complex, which limits the activation of the mammalian target of rapamycin (mTOR) complex 1. This protein kinase regulates protein synthesis, cell growth and proliferation such that when the TSC genes are deficient, mTOR complex 1 is constitutively upregulated, leading to abnormal cellular growth, proliferation and protein synthesis.

Up to 15 % of TSC patients develop subependymal giant cell astrocytomas (SEGAs). SEGAs are low-grade astrocytomas that are usually located in the lateral ventricles near the foramen of Monro, causing obstructive hydrocephalus. They do not respond to low-grade glioma chemotherapy or radiation and require surgical resection when they show evidence of symptomatic growth.

Inhibition of the mTOR pathway initially focused on the use of sirolimus (rapamycin), a drug the USA's Food and Drug Administration Agency (FDA) approved in 1999 because of its immunosuppressant properties to prevent rejection in organ transplantation. The first report of successful use of mTOR inhibitor in TSC-associated SEGA described five individuals who all exhibited regression of their lesions [21]. This experience triggered significant interest, not only in the field of TSC, but also in other conditions in which the PI3K/AKT/mTOR pathway is upregulated.

An open label study of another mTOR inhibitor, everolimus, enrolled 28 SEGA patients, including 22 cases below 18 years of age, with evidence of tumour progression. Out of 27 evaluable patients, 21 demonstrated a reduction of tumour volume by at least 30 % on central review, including nine patients who had a reduction of 50 % or more. This trial also reported significant reduction in the degree of hydrocephalus and parenchymal dysplasia observed [22]. Subsequent to this trial, a larger double-blind, placebo-controlled randomised study was conducted, comparing oral everolimus and placebo. One hundred and seventeen patients were enrolled (78 in the everolimus stratum and 39 in the placebo). Twenty-seven patients in the everolimus arm demonstrated a reduction in the total volume of the target SEGA of 50 % or more versus none in the placebo arm [23].

All these studies also showed that regrowth of SEGA after discontinuation of treatment is frequent. However, resistance of SEGA to mTOR inhibitors has not been reported, and patients who show evidence of progression following discontinuation of treatment can be treated successfully with the same agent. Interestingly, the use of mTOR inhibitor in TSC patients has also demonstrated reductions in co-morbid skin lesions and kidney tumours. Several trials are ongoing to investigate the effect of mTOR inhibitors in epilepsy and neurocognitive impairments associated with tuberous sclerosis complex.

Currently, the activity and benefit of mTOR inhibitors have only been demonstrated in TSC-associated SEGA; evidence of activity in other paediatric CNS tumours is still lacking. In a phase I study of everolimus in 20 patients with various recurrent CNS tumours, no objective response was observed [24]. Similarly, no response was seen in a phase II study of temsirolimus that enrolled 17 paediatric high-grade glioma patients. However, seven patients (including five with recurrent/progressive DIPG) demonstrated stable disease for a period of 12 weeks [25]. Based on evidence that neurofibromatosis type 1 associated tumours demonstrate increased mTOR activity, trials of mTOR inhibitors are currently ongoing for NF1 patients with recurrent and refractory low-grade gliomas.

Low-Grade Gliomas

Low-grade gliomas (LGGs) constitute the largest group of brain tumours in the paediatric population. However, this group is heterogeneous and include various tumour types, although pilocytic astrocytomas account for the largest subgroup. Recent studies have suggested large biological differences amongst these tumours, including alterations in different signalling pathways. The most common alterations so far identified involve aberrations in BRAF that have been identified in both adult and paediatric LGGs. Pilocytic astrocytomas commonly demonstrate a duplication in chromosome 7q34 which includes BRAF, a downstream gene in the RAS-MAPK pathway. This gain is typically the result of a tandem duplication between BRAF and KIAA1549, producing a novel fusion oncogene. There is evidence that this fusion confers a less aggressive clinical phenotype and is therefore associated with better outcome [26]. Whether this fusion represents a potential target is still unclear. In a phase II study of sorafenib (a multi-kinase inhibitor targeting BRAF, VEGFR, PDGFR and c-kit) in children with recurrent/refractory low-grade gliomas, Karajanis et al. reported a high rate of early progression that may indicate a potential growth-stimulating effect, possibly via paradoxical ERK activation [27]. Although less common, mutations of BRAF are also observed in paediatric LGGs. In a study analysing the presence of BRAFV600E mutations in 1,320 CNS tumours, this mutation was identified in approximately 9 % of pilocytic astrocytomas. The frequency of this mutation was higher in some subtypes of LGGs, especially ganglioglioma (18 %) and pleomorphic xanthoastrocytomas (66 %). A recent report on a successful management of a patient with ganglioglioma harbouring this mutation illustrates the importance of early identification of patients likely to benefit from BRAF inhibitors [28].

Other inhibitors of the Ras/Raf/MAP kinase signalling cascade are in LGG clinical trials. A phase I study of AZD6244, a small-molecule inhibitor of the MAP kinase MEK1 and 2, is ongoing, in children with recurrent or refractory lesions. Finally, interesting results were reported with the use of bevacizumab in patients with recurrent LGGs [29]. Clinical trials are ongoing to confirm these promising data.

Future Directions

With the exception of TSC, single targeted agents have yet to demonstrate clinical benefit in paediatric brain tumour patients. It is clear from clinical experience and laboratory studies that targeting a single pathway is unlikely to be successful, because tumour cells engage other mechanisms to escape the effects of treatment. Thus, most targeted agents will only be successful when combined with other agents, either chemotherapeutic drugs or other small-molecule inhibitors. The other challenge in treating brain tumours is

the CNS penetration of the drugs. We still have limited information on the blood–brain barrier penetration of most small-molecule inhibitors and when this information is available, there is evidence that the CSF exposure of small molecules is modest. More work needs to be done to appreciate whether the limited activity observed so far with small-molecule inhibitors is due to the drugs themselves or to the poor CNS penetration that affects anti-tumour activity.

Overall, we are still in the infancy of a new and exciting era that is aiming at targeting specific pathways or mutations rather than using a "one drug/one protocol fits all" approach. It is clear that such a methodology adds to the complexity of patient management in paediatric neuro-oncology. However, we can hope that this approach will at last alter the dismal outcome of conditions such as DIPG or high-grade gliomas. Whether targeted therapies will also transform the management of highly curable conditions such as low-grade gliomas or even medulloblastoma is still unclear.

References

1. Druker BJ, Talpaz M, Resta DJ, Peng B, Buchdunger E, Ford JM, Lydon NB, Kantarjian H, Capdeville R, Ohno-Jones S, Sawyers CL. Efficacy and safety of a specific inhibitor of the BCR-ABL tyrosine kinase in chronic myeloid leukemia. N Engl J Med. 2001;344:1031–7.
2. Bouffet E, Tabori U, Huang A, Bartels U. Possibilities of new therapeutic strategies in brain tumors. Cancer Treat Rev. 2010;36:335–41.
3. MacDonald TJ, Stewart CF, Kocak M, Goldman S, Ellenbogen RG, Phillips P, Lafond D, Poussaint TY, Kieran MW, Boyett JM, Kun LE. Phase I clinical trial of cilengitide in children with refractory brain tumors: Pediatric Brain Tumor Consortium Study PBTC-012. J Clin Oncol. 2008;26:919–24.
4. Warren KE, Goldman S, Pollack IF, Fangusaro J, Schaiquevich P, Stewart CF, Wallace D, Blaney SM, Packer R, Macdonald T, Jakacki R, Boyett JM, Kun LE. Phase I trial of lenalidomide in pediatric patients with recurrent, refractory, or progressive primary CNS tumors: Pediatric Brain Tumor Consortium study PBTC-018. J Clin Oncol. 2011;29:324–9.
5. Fouladi M, Stewart CF, Olson J, Wagner LM, Onar-Thomas A, Kocak M, Packer RJ, Goldman S, Gururangan S, Gajjar A, Demuth T, Kun LE, Boyett JM, Gilbertson RJ. Phase I trial of MK-0752 in children

with refractory CNS malignancies: a pediatric brain tumor consortium study. J Clin Oncol. 2011; 29:3529–34.

6. Fouladi M, Stewart CF, Blaney SM, Onar-Thomas A, Schaiquevich P, Packer RJ, Gajjar A, Kun LE, Boyett JM, Gilbertson RJ. Phase I trial of lapatinib in children with refractory CNS malignancies: a Pediatric Brain Tumor Consortium study. J Clin Oncol. 2010; 28:4221–7.

7. Fouladi M, Stewart CF, Blaney SM, Onar-Thomas A, Schaiquevich P, Packer RJ, Goldman S, Geyer JR, Gajjar A, Kun LE, Boyett JM, Gilbertson RJ. A molecular biology and phase II trial of lapatinib in children with refractory CNS malignancies: a pediatric brain tumor consortium study. J Neurooncol. 2013;114: 173–9.

8. Taylor MD, Northcott PA, Korshunov A, Remke M, Cho YJ, Clifford SC, Eberhart CG, Parsons DW, Rutkowski S, Gajjar A, Ellison DW, Lichter P, Gilbertson RJ, Pomeroy SL, Kool M, Pfister SM. Molecular subgroups of medulloblastoma: the current consensus. Acta Neuropathol. 2012;123:465–72.

9. Rudin CM, Hann CL, Laterra J, Yauch RL, Callahan CA, Fu L, Holcomb T, Stinson J, Gould SE, Coleman B, LoRusso PM, Von Hoff DD, de Sauvage FJ, Low JA. Treatment of medulloblastoma with hedgehog pathway inhibitor GDC-0449. N Engl J Med. 2009;361:1173–8.

10. Jones C, Perryman L, Hargrave D. Paediatric and adult malignant glioma: close relatives or distant cousins? Nat Rev Clin Oncol. 2012;9:400–13.

11. Broniscer A, Baker SJ, Stewart CF, Merchant TE, Laningham FH, Schaiquevich P, Kocak M, Morris EB, Endersby R, Ellison DW, Gajjar A. Phase I and pharmacokinetic studies of erlotinib administered concurrently with radiotherapy for children, adolescents, and young adults with high-grade glioma. Clin Cancer Res. 2009;15:701–7.

12. Gururangan S, Chi SN, Young Poussaint T, Onar-Thomas A, Gilbertson RJ, Vajapeyam S, Friedman HS, Packer RJ, Rood BN, Boyett JM, Kun LE. Lack of efficacy of bevacizumab plus irinotecan in children with recurrent malignant glioma and diffuse brainstem glioma: a Pediatric Brain Tumor Consortium study. J Clin Oncol. 2010;28:3069–75.

13. Geoerger B, Hargrave D, Thomas F, Ndiaye A, Frappaz D, Andreiuolo F, Varlet P, Aerts I, Riccardi R, Jaspan T, Chatelut E, Le Deley MC, Paoletti X, Saint-Rose C, Leblond P, Morland B, Gentet JC, Meresse V, Vassal G. Innovative Therapies for Children with Cancer pediatric phase I study of erlotinib in brainstem glioma and relapsing/refractory brain tumors. Neuro Oncol. 2011;13:109–18.

14. Pollack IF, Stewart CF, Kocak M, Poussaint TY, Broniscer A, Banerjee A, Douglas JG, Kun LE, Boyett JM, Geyer JR. A phase II study of gefitinib and irradiation in children with newly diagnosed brainstem gliomas: a report from the Pediatric Brain Tumor Consortium. Neuro Oncol. 2011;13:290–7.

15. Bode U, Massimino M, Bach F, Zimmermann M, Khuhlaeva E, Westphal M, Fleischhack G. Nimotuzumab treatment of malignant gliomas. Expert Opin Biol Ther. 2012;12:1649–59.

16. Broniscer A, Baker SD, Wetmore C, Pai Panandiker AS, Huang J, Davidoff AM, Onar-Thomas A, Panetta JC, Chin TK, Merchant TE, Baker JN, Kaste SC, Gajjar A, Stewart CF. Phase I trial, pharmacokinetics, and pharmacodynamics of vandetanib and dasatinib in children with newly diagnosed diffuse intrinsic pontine glioma. Clin Cancer Res. 2013;19:3050–8.

17. Gilbertson RJ, Bentley L, Hernan R, Junttila TT, Frank AJ, Haapasalo H, Connelly M, Wetmore C, Curran T, Elenius K, Ellison DW. ERBB receptor signaling promotes ependymoma cell proliferation and represents a potential novel therapeutic target for this disease. Clin Cancer Res. 2002;8:3054–64.

18. Korshunov A, Golanov A, Timirgaz V. Immunohistochemical markers for prognosis of ependymal neoplasms. J Neurooncol. 2002;58:255–70.

19. Johnson RA, Wright KD, Poppleton H, Mohankumar KM, Finkelstein D, Pounds SB, Rand V, Leary SE, White E, Eden C, Hogg T, Northcott P, Mack S, Neale G, Wang YD, Coyle B, Atkinson J, DeWire M, Kranenburg TA, Gillespie Y, Allen JC, Merchant T, Boop FA, Sanford RA, Gajjar A, Ellison DW, Taylor MD, Grundy RG, Gilbertson RJ. Cross-species genomics matches driver mutations and cell compartments to model ependymoma. Nature. 2010;466:632–6.

20. Witt H, Mack SC, Ryzhova M, Bender S, Sill M, Isserlin R, Benner A, Hielscher T, Milde T, Remke M, Jones DT, Northcott PA, Garzia L, Bertrand KC, Wittmann A, Yao Y, Roberts SS, Massimi L, Van Meter T, Weiss WA, Gupta N, Grajkowska W, Lach B, Cho YJ, von Deimling A, Kulozik AE, Witt O, Bader GD, Hawkins CE, Tabori U, Guha A, Rutka JT, Lichter P, Korshunov A, Taylor MD, Pfister SM. Delineation of two clinically and molecularly distinct subgroups of posterior fossa ependymoma. Cancer Cell. 2011;20:143–57.

21. Franz DN, Leonard J, Tudor C, Chuck G, Care M, Sethuraman G, Dinopoulos A, Thomas G, Crone KR. Rapamycin causes regression of astrocytomas in tuberous sclerosis complex. Ann Neurol. 2006;59: 490–8.

22. Krueger DA, Care MM, Holland K, Agricola K, Tudor C, Mangeshkar P, Wilson KA, Byars A, Sahmoud T, Franz DN. Everolimus for subependymal giant-cell astrocytomas in tuberous sclerosis. N Engl J Med. 2010;363:1801–11.

23. Franz DN, Belousova E, Sparagana S, Bebin EM, Frost M, Kuperman R, Witt O, Kohrman MH, Flamini JR, Wu JY, Curatolo P, de Vries PJ, Whittemore VH, Thiele EA, Ford JP, Shah G, Cauwel H, Lebwohl D, Sahmoud T, Jozwiak S. Efficacy and safety of everolimus for subependymal giant cell astrocytomas associated with tuberous sclerosis complex (EXIST-1): a multicentre, randomised, placebo-controlled phase 3 trial. Lancet. 2013;381:125–32.

24. Fouladi M, Laningham F, Wu J, O'Shaughnessy MA, Molina K, Broniscer A, Spunt SL, Luckett I, Stewart CF, Houghton PJ, Gilbertson RJ, Furman WL. Phase I study of everolimus in pediatric patients with refractory solid tumors. J Clin Oncol. 2007;25:4806–12.

25. Geoerger B, Kieran MW, Grupp S, Perek D, Clancy J, Krygowski M, Ananthakrishnan R, Boni JP, Berkenblit A, Spunt SL. Phase II trial of temsirolimus in children with high-grade glioma, neuroblastoma and rhabdomyosarcoma. Eur J Cancer. 2012;48: 253–62.

26. Hawkins C, Walker E, Mohamed N, Zhang C, Jacob K, Shirinian M, Alon N, Kahn D, Fried I, Scheinemann K, Tsangaris E, Dirks P, Tressler R, Bouffet E, Jabado N, Tabori U. BRAF-KIAA1549 fusion predicts better clinical outcome in pediatric low-grade astrocytoma. Clin Cancer Res. 2011;17:4790–8.

27. Karajannis M, Fisher MJ, Milla SS, Cohen KJ, Legault G, Wisoff JH, et al. Phase II Study of Sorafenib in children with recurrent/progressive low-grade astrocytomas. Neuro Oncol. 2012;14:101–5.

28. Rush S, Foreman N, Liu A. Brainstem ganglioglioma successfully treated with vemurafenib. J Clin Oncol. 2013;31:e159–60.

29. Hwang EI, Jakacki RI, Fisher MJ, Kilburn LB, Horn M, Vezina G, Rood BR, Packer RJ. Long-term efficacy and toxicity of bevacizumab-based therapy in children with recurrent low-grade gliomas. Pediatr Blood Cancer. 2013;60:776–82.

30. Geyer JR, Stewart CF, Kocak M, Broniscer A, Phillips P, Douglas JG, Blaney SM, Packer RJ, Gururangan S, Banerjee A, Kieran MW, Kun LE, Gilbertson RJ, Boyett JM. A phase I and biology study of gefitinib and radiation in children with newly diagnosed brain stem gliomas or supratentorial malignant gliomas. Eur J Cancer. 2010;46:3287–93.

31. Baruchel S, Sharp JR, Bartels U, Hukin J, Odame I, Portwine C, Strother D, Fryer C, Halton J, Egorin MJ, Reis RM, Martinho O, Stempak D, Hawkins C, Gammon J, Bouffet E. A Canadian paediatric brain tumour consortium (CPBTC) phase II molecularly targeted study of imatinib in recurrent and refractory paediatric central nervous system tumours. Eur J Cancer. 2009;45:2352–9.

32. Geoerger B, Morland B, Ndiaye A, Doz F, Kalifa G, Geoffray A, Pichon F, Frappaz D, Chatelut E, Opolon P, Hain S, Boderet F, Bosq J, Emile JF, Le Deley MC, Capdeville R, Vassal G. Target-driven exploratory study of imatinib mesylate in children with solid malignancies by the Innovative Therapies for Children with Cancer (ITCC) European Consortium. Eur J Cancer. 2009;45:2342–51.

33. Gururangan S, Fangusaro J, Young Poussaint T, Onar-Thomas A, Gilbertson RJ, Vajapeyam S, Gajjar A, Goldman S, Friedman HS, Packer RJ, Boyett JM, Kun LE, McLendon R. Lack of efficacy of bevacizumab + irinotecan in cases of pediatric recurrent ependymoma–a Pediatric Brain Tumor Consortium study. Neuro Oncol. 2012;14:1404–12.

34. Haas-Kogan DA, Banerjee A, Poussaint TY, Kocak M, Prados MD, Geyer JR, Fouladi M, Broniscer A, Minturn JE, Pollack IF, Packer RJ, Boyett JM, Kun LE. Phase II trial of tipifarnib and radiation in children with newly diagnosed diffuse intrinsic pontine gliomas. Neuro Oncol. 2011;13:298–306.

35. Broniscer A, Baker JN, Tagen M, Onar-Thomas A, Gilbertson RJ, Davidoff AM, Pai Panandiker AS, Leung W, Chin TK, Stewart CF, Kocak M, Rowland C, Merchant TE, Kaste SC, Gajjar A. Phase I study of vandetanib during and after radiotherapy in children with diffuse intrinsic pontine glioma. J Clin Oncol. 2010;28:4762–8.

36. Bode U, Buchen S, Janssen G, Reinhard T, Warmuth-Metz M, Bach F, Fleischhack G. Results of a phase II trial of h-R3 monoclonal antibody (nimotuzumab) in the treatment of resistant or relapsed high-grade gliomas in children and adolescents. J Clin Oncol 2006;24:63S (abstract).

High-Dose Chemotherapy/Stem Cell Transplantation (HDSCT)

21

Victor Anthony Lewis and Shahrad Rod Rassekh

Introduction

Treatment of CNS tumors relies on the expertise of neurosurgeons to obtain as complete as possible a resection of the tumors to facilitate best outcomes. Radiation treatment (RT) despite its long-term effects on cognition and growth remains an additional modality. Increasing recognition of side effects from radiation has directed the development and enhancement of chemotherapy regimens for responsive tumors. The use of chemotherapy for a variety of brain tumors may permit delay of RT and decrease long-term side effects. Within specific entities, it may even allow omission of RT. As can be seen in previous chapters, the use of chemotherapy has had a significant impact on how brain tumors are treated today.

Sensitivity to chemotherapeutic agents and their demonstrated benefits has lead to consideration of higher doses of such agents with the use of stem cell support (HDCST) to maintain

V.A. Lewis, M.D.
Department of Pediatrics, Alberta Children's
Hospital, Calgary, AB, Canada

S.R. Rassekh, M.D., M.H.Sc. (✉)
Division of Pediatric Oncology, Department of
Pediatrics, British Columbia's Children's Hospital,
Vancouver, BC, Canada
e-mail: rrassekh@cw.bc.ca

dose intensity in order to improve outcomes. This chapter discusses the use of HDSCT for brain tumors.

Chemotherapy Regimens

In the mid 1980s, Finlay's [1] group advanced a series of regimens for the treatment of brain tumors. Finlay used thiotepa, a lipophilic agent that has excellent penetration into the CSF and achieves concentrations equivalent to that in plasma [2]. Myelosuppression, particularly with thrombocytopenia, is generally seen at lower doses, while mucositis, neurologic toxicities, and skin hyperpigmentation are seen at higher doses. Thiotepa in combination with other agents still forms the backbone of many successful regimens for brain tumors. Initial toxic mortality (TRM) with 900 mg/m^2 of thiotepa and 1,500 mg/m^2 of etoposide was unacceptable at 16 % [1]. Since that initial experience, better patient selection, an improved delivery, and dose adjustments of medications, e.g., use of Calvert correction to dose carboplatin [3], combination with other agents, e.g., busulfan, carmustine, etc., have decreased TRM [4, 5]. Treatment-related toxicity, however, remains an ongoing concern with older individuals. Response rates as high as 50 %, with a progression-free survival (PFS), have been seen in patients with high-grade astrocytoma. Similarly patients with recurrent medulloblastoma treated with thiotepa 300 mg/m^2/day, carboplatin

500 mg/m^2/day, and etoposide 250 mg/m^2/day, each for 3 days, showed a 35 % (8 of 23 patients) PFS at a median of 35 months after stem cell rescue (range, 10–63 months). Thiotepa has been combined with other drugs such as busulfan [6, 7] and cyclophosphamide [8, 9] to obtain reasonable survival in recurrent brain tumors.

The children's cancer group (CCG) study CCG99703 defined the maximum-tolerated dose (MTD) for thiotepa for the recently completed ACNS0333 study that treated infants with atypical teratoid rhabdoid tumors and the ACNS0334 study that is treating patients with medulloblastoma. The thiotepa MTD was defined at 10 mg/kg (300 mg/m^2/day for children >36 months). Carboplatin was given based on the Calvert correction [3]. Three tandem transplants, given approximately 21–28 days apart, provide the dose intensity speculated to provide long-term survival benefit.

The pediatric oncology group (POG) as well as scientists at Duke University investigated the use of melphalan in HDCST regimens and published their early experience. TRM was high (4 of 19 children) in the POG experience [10]. This decreased when the accompanying cyclophosphamide was fractionated into multiple doses each day maintaining the same overall dose [11]. Melphalan has also been combined with busulfan and separately with carboplatin and etoposide. TRM was found to be lower in those experiences.

Very specifically for treatment of medulloblastoma, the scientists at St. Jude have advanced a new treatment approach that is discussed in the following section. Suffice to say that HDCST has a possible niche in treatment of high-risk tumors in order to improve overall survival (OS) and event-free survival (EFS) [12].

Hematopoietic Stem Cell Transplant for Medulloblastoma

Natural History

The epidemiology of medulloblastoma and primitive neuroectodermal tumors (PNET) is discussed in Chap. 12. Improved surgical resections using advanced magnetic resonance imaging guidance, advancements in chemotherapy, more effective radiation therapy techniques, and better supportive care have substantially improved outcomes of children with medulloblastoma and PNET in the recent past [13]. In addition to age, amount of residual tumor after definitive resection, and presence of metastatic disease, there is new evidence that identifies histologic subtypes and molecular mechanisms that substantially impact outcome [14]. Given the significant improvement in adjuvant modalities, the extent of surgery needs to be weighed against possible neurological damage from this modality. Radiation to the posterior fossa with a boost to the tumor bed is an essential part of treatment but causes significant long-term deficits in younger children. The addition of chemotherapy to radiation has the advantage of improved survival rates as well as allowing decreases or delays in radiation treatment [15]. The use of chemotherapy has permitted omission of radiation in a specific low-risk subgroup of patients [16, 17].

Although 80 % of children with localized MB are likely to be cured with recent therapy combinations albeit with deficits, the cure rates for disseminated disease patients, those having supratentorial PNETs, and those with recurrent disease remain poor [18].

Use of High-Dose Chemotherapy

The experience with high-dose chemotherapy with stem cell rescue is derived mostly from patients with recurrent or high-risk medulloblastoma. Patients with recurrent MB/PNET treated with conventional treatments have a cure rate of less than 5 % [18]. High-dose chemotherapy with stem cell rescue in such patients might be a viable option as shown by the early work of Finlay et al. [1].

The initial experience in patients with recurrent MB/PNET utilized various combinations that included agents such as thiotepa, busulfan, cyclophosphamide, platinum drugs, and etoposide to obtain event-free survivals of 20–50 %. All regimens were myeloablative in nature and regimen-related toxicity was substantial. Patients, who had failure at only their primary site, were more likely to be survivors over the long term compared with those who had metastatic disease [10].

Gajjar et al. have nicely reviewed the recent experience with HDCT in patients with recurrent disease. They report results on 231 patients with recurrent disease with 202 having received radiation prior to relapse. Heterogeneity within the treated groups makes interpretation of results difficult. Comparing patients who received HDCST with those who did not, there is a slight benefit seen in EFS. Those receiving radiation in their previous treatment regimen fared poorly compared to those who had not been radiated. Of 159 patients who received HDCST, 35 disease-free survivors were reported (22 %). Of these 159 HDCST recipients, 133 relapsed after having received RT in their previous treatment. Among the latter, disease-free survival was 17.3 % [18].

Strother et al. [19] used HDCST with peripheral blood stem cell support following craniospinal radiation in 53 patients with newly diagnosed medulloblastoma or sPNET. Chemotherapy consisted of cyclophosphamide ($4,000$ mg/m^2), cisplatin (75 mg/m^2), and vincristine for each cycle. High-risk patients received topotecan on a phase II window. The 2-year PFS for standard and high-risk patients were 93.6 % and 73.7 %, respectively. Longer-term data from the same study includes a total of 134 patients (86 average risk, 48 high risk) and was reported by Gajjar et al. [12]; there were no treatment-related deaths in the cohort. Five-year OS was 85 % (95 % CI 75–94) in patients with average-risk status and 70 % (95 % CI 54–84) in the high-risk group. The EFS for the average and high-risk groups were 83 % (CI 73–93) and 70 % (CI 55–85) ($p=0.046$), respectively. Disease histology had an impact on outcomes with classic histology showing an EFS of 84 % (CI 74–95), and anaplastic tumors had an EFS of 57 % (CI 33–80) $p=0.04$. In the authors' own experience, the OS and EFS for average-risk patients receiving this treatment at his institution have remained at 100 % at 3 years.

Conclusions

The mainstay of treatment for MB/PNET is surgery with an attempt to obtain as complete as possible a resection followed by radiation and chemotherapy. Treatment of patients with high-risk disease and especially recurrent disease remains a challenge. The use of HDCST may add benefit in such cases. However, its use in frontline therapy of average-risk medulloblastoma, even with impressive results shown by Stother et al. and Gajjar et al., remains debatable and will be assessed in the follow-up study that will use the same regimen without stem cell rescue after chemotherapy cycles.

Hematopoietic Stem Cell Transplant for Ependymoma

Natural History

Ependymoma and its epidemiology are addressed in Chap. 8 of this textbook. The mainstays of therapy for ependymoma are surgery and radiation therapy, and the response of this tumor to chemotherapy is questionable. Overall survival rates have been disappointing with 5-year overall survival and progression-free survival of 50–64 % and 23–45 %, respectively [20]. The extent of surgical resection is a critical prognostic factor, yet practically, children with infratentorial ependymoma often have tumors that are difficult to resect due to their adherence to the brainstem and extension of tumor into the cerebellar pontine angle or down the cervical spine. The standard approach for the therapy of ependymoma is the use of RT to the tumor site. Recent advances in RT using conformal approaches are now considered standard treatment for children over the age of 12 months with 3-year progressive-free survival of approximately 70 % [21]. Short-term outcomes of cognitive function suggest that this treatment has acceptable results, but long-term results are still being evaluated.

Given the concerns of RT to very young children, numerous trials have investigated the role of chemotherapy for the treatment of ependymoma with mixed results [22]. A review by Bouffet et al. of all phase 2 studies in ependymoma showed disappointing results with only 11 % showing a response to single-agent chemotherapy with less than 5 % showing complete responses, with the best results seen with cisplatin [23]. However, the POG infant tumor trial had 48 children with ependymoma enrolled on it and nearly half of the 25 evaluable young children showed a partial or complete response to two courses of vincristine and cyclophosphamide, with a 5-year progression-free survival of 27 % [15, 18]. The use of HDCST in this tumor has thus been investigated.

Use of High-Dose Chemotherapy

A phase 2 study investigated autologous stem cell transplantation following conditioning with busulfan 150 mg/m^2/day for 4 days followed by thiotepa 300 mg/m^2/day for the next 3 days in 16 children with refractory or relapsed ependymoma. Half of the subjects had previously received RT and all had measureable disease. None of the subjects had a radiologic response of over 50 % and only three subjects were survivors with all three getting gross total resections and local radiation. There was significant toxicity of the skin and the gastrointestinal tract, and there was one treatment-related death [24].

The "Head Start" protocols were designed to use intensive chemotherapy and autologous stem cell transplantation to replace or delay radiation therapy. Children younger than 3 were eligible for the Head Start 1 and 2 protocols, and the protocols also allowed older children to enroll provided that they had incompletely resected disease (age 3–6 on Head Start 1 and age 3–10 on Head Start 2). Those with neuraxis dissemination were allowed to enter the arm of the study containing high-dose methotrexate on Head Start 2. Five cycles of induction therapy were given containing vincristine, cyclophosphamide, etoposide, and cisplatin. Those with disseminated disease enrolled on Head Start 2 also received high-dose methotrexate. Stem cells were collected

after the first or second cycles of induction chemotherapy. There were 29 children under the age of 10 years of age who were enrolled on this study. The estimated 5-year EFS and OS were 12 % (±6 %) and 38 % (±10 %), respectively [25]. There was a TRM of 10.3 % on this protocol, mostly in the early phases of the study. Interestingly, four of the five children with metastatic disease are long-term survivors with the only death being one who died of toxicity. The radiation-free survival of those on this study was only 8 %, and of the 12 survivors, only 3 did not receive radiation. The authors concluded that HDCST using this protocol showed disappointing results [25].

The Head Start 3 protocol investigated those under the age of 10 with newly diagnosed ependymoma and 19 subjects were enrolled. Similar to the above trials, five cycles of induction therapy were delivered followed by a sixth cycle comprising HDCST. Children between 6 and 10 or those with residual disease would receive RT. This study found different outcomes between those with supratentorial tumors and those with infratentorial tumors. The 3-year EFS and 3-year OS were a remarkable 86 % (±13 %) and 100 %, respectively, for the supratentorial group. This was in contrast with those with infratentorial disease who had a PFS and OS of 27 % (±13 %) and 73 % (±13 %), respectively. All three subjects with residual disease with supratentorial tumors achieved a CR with chemotherapy, compared to only one of the six with infratentorial residual disease. The study concluded that intensive induction and consolidation chemotherapy should be explored further in trials for supratentorial ependymoma [26].

The Australia and New Zealand collaborative group studied a heterogeneous group of children as part of their ANZCCSG BabyBrain99 study for infants with malignant brain tumors. Thirty-three children with malignant tumors under the age of 3 were enrolled in the study that followed primary resection with 4 cycles of induction chemotherapy. A second-look surgery could be offered at cycle 4 of treatment followed by consolidation therapy using carboplatin (AUC 12 mg/mL/min) over 4 days and melphalan 4.6 mg/kg on day 5 with autologous stem cell support. The children would then receive involved-field irradiation 6 weeks postrecovery. Twenty-two of the 33 children received all the courses including the stem cell transplant. There were six subjects with ependymoma included in the cohort, and they had the best outcomes of any of the tumor types with a 5-year EFS of 67 % [27].

A recent report from Korea investigated the feasibility and effectiveness of tandem HDCSTs in children under the age of 3 years. They enrolled five patients who were given 6 cycles of induction chemotherapy followed by tandem transplants [28]. RT was deferred in all children until after the age of 3 years, and all patients were alive at time of publication. The preparative regimen for the autologous transplant included carboplatin 500 mg/m^2/day for 3 days, followed by 3 days of thiotepa 300 mg/m^2/day and etoposide 250 mg/m^2/day for the first transplant, followed by a second transplant with cyclophosphamide 1,500 mg/m^2/day for 4 days and melphalan 60 mg/m^2/day for 3 days. They allowed a 12-week interval between the two transplants in order to prevent toxic deaths. One of the five who had a supratentorial tumor was alive without recurrence at 62 months and did not receive any radiation. Three of the five subjects had measureable disease going into the first transplant, and two of these three went into a complete remission following the tandem transplants. Overall four of the five remained alive and disease free, although only the one with supratentorial lesion avoided radiation. The investigators concluded that tandem transplants is feasible in young patients with anaplastic ependymoma, was well tolerated, and requires further investigation in a larger trial [28].

Conclusions

HDCST in children with supratentorial ependymoma shows promise and needs to be investigated further in larger studies. This is not the case with those who have infratentorial tumors or recurrent disease. Surgery is still the standard approach with chemotherapy being utilized to facilitate a second-look surgery.

Hematopoietic Stem Cell Transplant for High-Grade Glioma

Natural History

Despite improvements in surgery, radiation, and chemotherapy, the prognosis for children diagnosed with malignant high-grade glioma (HGG) remains very poor with the majority developing disease progression soon after diagnosis and dying from their brain tumor. Compared to those with glioblastoma multiforme (GBM), those with anaplastic astrocytoma have a slightly better prognosis with better overall survival and longer time to progression, yet the majority will also die of disease progression [29]. Given the poor outcomes with present standards, many studies have investigated the role for chemotherapy for HGG including the use of high-dose chemotherapy and autologous stem cell transplantation. Proponents of HDCST for malignant glioma suggest that high doses of chemotherapy are more likely to be efficacious for a few different reasons including: to overcome the protective role of the blood brain barrier, to increase the dose-dependent killing of glioma cells, and to reduce the volume of residual disease in an effort to reduce the volume of radiotherapy required for therapy [30].

Use of High-Dose Chemotherapy

Outcomes for patients with recurrent malignant astrocytomas are known to be poor, paving the way for trails with HDCST. With the use of single-agent carmustine, the results were quite disappointing [31]. The use of thiotepa and etoposide within protocols with or without the addition of carmustine in recurrent HGG showed better outcomes [32]. This COG reported their initial cohort of malignant astrocytomas treated with HDCST following disease recurrence and compared their results with historical conventional approach [33]. Twenty-seven patients under the age of 21 years of age entered the trial, and three different preparative regimens were given including thiotepa 900 mg/m^2 over 3 days with etoposide (750 or 1,500 mg/m^2 over 3 days) either alone or in combination with carmustine (600 mg/m^2 over 3 days) or carboplatin (1,500 mg/m^2 over 3 days or using Calvert formula with an AUC of 7 mg/mL/min/day). TRM was high at 19 % while 17 of the 27 subjects developed disease progression. Five of the 27 subjects are long-term survivors of this approach (only one of these needed RT), including 2 with GBM [33]. There were no survivors within the historical cohort, suggesting that dose intensity and HDCST may play a role in the treatment of malignant glioma. Overall patients treated with standard chemotherapy had a 23 % 1-year survival compared to a 41 % 1-year survival for those treated with HDCST. The largest long-term survival difference was when comparing chemotherapy only with those who underwent HDCST transplant where the 4-year estimates of survival were 0 % for chemotherapy alone and 46 % for autologous transplant [33].

The phase 2 Children's Cancer Group CCG-9922 study for centrally reviewed glioblastoma multiforme used myeloablative thiotepa, BCNU, and etoposide followed by focal irradiation for treatment of recurrent disease and had an excellent 2-year PFS of 46 %. The trial however was terminated early due to pulmonary toxicities [4].

Given the positive survival benefit temozolomide, a phase 1 dose escalation study of this agent given with carboplatin and thiotepa resulted in a 30 % survival in a small cohort of 12 subjects at 32–48 months [34].

There have been three recent Italian studies of high-dose chemotherapy that have been recently presented by the Italian Pediatric Hematology/ Oncology Association (AIEOP) at an international conference in Milano [30]. The first study was on eight cases of malignant glioma in children under the age of 3 years at diagnosis treated with either high-dose chemotherapy using high-dose methotrexate, etoposide, cyclophos-phamide, and carboplatin followed by two myeloablative autologous transplants using carboplatin/etoposide for the first and thiotepa/melphalan for the second. Radiation was given to those with progressive disease or those with disease residual at

the completion of chemotherapy. Objective results were seen in five of the six newly diagnosed infants and in one of the two previously treated infants. Three are alive and in remission without having been irradiated at a median follow-up of 64 months. Two subjects died of TRM during the myeloablative cycles and three of progressive disease [35].

Conclusions

Although HDCST is not considered standard therapy for high-grade glioma, presently numerous studies demonstrate survivorship using the HDCST approach. This needs further studies in larger studies. Identification of those likely to benefit from this approach needs assessment.

Hematopoietic Stem Cell Transplant for Brainstem Glioma

Natural History

A description of brainstem gliomas is available in Chaps. 10 and 11. They are hard to treat tumors with dismal long-term outcomes. The mainstay of therapy is radiation with a palliative intent, and numerous trials of radiation techniques and adjuvant chemotherapy have been performed without any survival benefit being demonstrated [36]. Given the very poor outcomes for children with pontine glioma, novel treatments with high-dose chemotherapy have been designed to assess feasibility and efficacy.

Use of High-Dose Chemotherapy

There are limited studies that have investigated the use of HDCST in children with pontine glioma. The majority of studies are small feasibility studies in either recurrent or newly diagnosed pontine glioma utilizing a variety of regimens. Unfortunately as seen in the outcomes of the studies outlined below, this approach has not been found to be very fruitful.

Six newly diagnosed patients with pontine glioma were treated with cyclophosphamide and thiotepa followed by hyperfractionated RT and two of the six were alive seven and 24 months post therapy [8]. However, the one long-term survivor had an atypical contrast-enhancing lesion on imaging raising the possibility that this tumor was different biologically. The median survival in this small series was 12.5 months and one of the six died of toxicity. There were two documented tumor responses before the radiation with one partial response and one minor response.

Seven children with pontine glioma were included in a larger series of 22 subjects enrolled in trial of etoposide and thiotepa. There was one partial response in a child with a recurrent brainstem tumor [37]. Another study of high-risk brain tumors included a long-term survivor of a pontine glioma [10]. Other reports of tumor responses to chemotherapy include a minor response to cyclophosphamide and melphalan [11], and a minor response to busulfan and thiotepa.

There were no long-term survivors in a CCG report describing 16 patients with newly diagnosed (6 patients) and recurrent (10 patients) diffuse intrinsic brainstem glioma. TRM was high (2 of 16 patients), and median survival was 11.4 months for newly diagnosed and 4.7 months for subjects with recurrent tumors [5].

In 1990 Societe Francaise d'Oncologie Pediatrique (SFOP) opened a pilot study of HDCST for children with pontine glioma designed to investigate the feasibility of treating newly diagnosed children [38]. RT was given as per institutional standards. HDSCT was initiated at about 40 to 60 days after the end of RT. The conditioning regimen consisted of oral busulfan × 4 days (150 mg/m^2 per day divided into 4 doses per day) followed by thiotepa 300 mg/m^2 per day for 3 days. Although 35 children were enrolled in the trial, only 24 children proceeded to HDSCT with a median time of 54 days post completion of RT. All 24 children died, with 3 mortalities due to toxicity and the other 21 due to disease progression. The median survival time for the study group was 10±3.6 months. The median time to clinical progression from bone marrow transplantation was 119 days.

The authors conclude that the use of HDCST after radiation therapy is not indicated for children with pontine glioma [38].

Conclusions

HDCST is not indicated for pontine gliomas given the lack of efficacy and significant toxicity associated with its use. Other novel approaches will need to be studied.

High-Dose Chemotherapy for Infants and Rare Brain Malignancies

Long-term effects of radiation are worst when the infant brain is exposed to high doses of radiation. Delays in radiation while preserving outcomes and EFS would be desired by treating neuro-oncologists. The CCG study CCG99703 demonstrated that repetitive cycles of HDCST for children <3 years of age were feasible. The HDSCT backbone consisted of carboplatin and thiotepa. In the 92 children accrued on study, neutropenia, thrombocytopenia, and stomatitis were common, while reports of grade 3 and 4 weight loss or gastrointestinal issues occurred in less than 2 % children. The use of total parenteral and enteral feeding occurred in 42 % and 29 % of children, respectively.

In a recent study, 25 children <3 years of age with malignant brain tumors received tandem HDCST after six cycles of induction therapy. Sixteen patients survived to a median of 52 months (range 18–96) giving a 5-year OS and EFS of 67.8±9.4 % and 55.5±10 %, respectively. Four of 16 patients are long-term survivors without receiving an RT, while 2 received local RT, 3 received craniospinal RT, and 7 received both. Late adverse effects included hypothyroidism (20 %), growth hormone deficiency (30 %), renal tubular damage (40 %), and hearing impairment (50 %). Median value of full scale, verbal, and performance intelligence quotient at a median follow-up of 45 months was 75 (range 67–90), 83 (range 61–112), and 71 (range 69–86), respectively.

The authors conclude that tandem HDCST has the ability to preserve reasonable outcomes in infants with malignant brain tumors with acceptable levels of long-term toxicities [39].

Atypical teratoid rhabdoid tumor is a rare embryonal tumor that occurs mostly in infancy and has a very dismal prognosis. It has a very unique molecular signature that has aided early diagnosis. Although surgery and chemotherapy are considered standard treatment, the use of HDCST has emerged as a treatment approach with reasonable outcomes based on reports in small cohorts of patients. Ginn et al. demonstrated the efficacy of this approach in 33 cases where 14 patients also received RT [40]. Twenty patients were alive at a median follow-up of over 50 months. The conditioning regimen generally used consisted of carboplatin and thiotepa given over a 2-day period followed by a rest of 2 days and subsequent infusion of stem cells. Similarly the report by Lafay-Cousin et al. also shows a significant survival benefit in patients treated with the HDCST approach (OS at 2 years of 47.9 ± 12.1 % versus 27.3 ± 9.5 % for the conventional approach) [41]. The approach however still remains experimental.

Treatment of rare brain malignancies and germ cell tumors of the brains has been attempted with HDCST in resistant and recurrent cases. The treatment remains experimental and needs to be investigated in larger trials. Clearly for responsive tumors, this therapy has proven to have benefit and may help delay or even omit use of radiation treatment and its side effects.

References

1. Finlay JL, et al. Pilot study of high-dose thiotepa and etoposide with autologous bone marrow rescue in children and young adults with recurrent CNS tumors. The Children's Cancer Group. J Clin Oncol. 1996;14(9):2495–503.
2. Heideman RL, et al. Phase I and pharmacokinetic evaluation of thiotepa in the cerebrospinal fluid and plasma of pediatric patients: evidence for dose-dependent plasma clearance of thiotepa. Cancer Res. 1989;49(3):736–41.
3. Calvert AH, et al. Carboplatin dosage: prospective evaluation of a simple formula based on renal function. J Clin Oncol. 1989;7(11):1748–56.
4. Grovas AC, et al. Regimen-related toxicity of myeloablative chemotherapy with BCNU, thiotepa, and etoposide followed by autologous stem cell rescue for children with newly diagnosed glioblastoma multiforme: report from the Children's Cancer Group. Med Pediatr Oncol. 1999;33(2):83–7.
5. Dunkel IJ, et al. High dose chemotherapy with autologous bone marrow rescue for children with diffuse pontine brain stem tumors. Children's Cancer Group. J Neurooncol. 1998;37(1):67–73.
6. Kalifa C, et al. High-dose busulfan and thiotepa with autologous bone marrow transplantation in childhood malignant brain tumors: a phase II study. Bone Marrow Transplant. 1992;9(4):227–33.
7. Dupuis-Girod S, et al. Will high dose chemotherapy followed by autologous bone marrow transplantation supplant cranio-spinal irradiation in young children treated for medulloblastoma? J Neurooncol. 1996;27(1): 87–98.
8. Kedar A, et al. High-dose chemotherapy with marrow reinfusion and hyperfractionated irradiation for children with high-risk brain tumors. Med Pediatr Oncol. 1994;23(5):428–36.
9. Heideman RL, et al. High-dose chemotherapy and autologous bone marrow rescue followed by interstitial and external-beam radiotherapy in newly diagnosed pediatric malignant gliomas. J Clin Oncol. 1993; 11(8):1458–65.
10. Graham ML, et al. High-dose chemotherapy with autologous stem-cell rescue in patients with recurrent and high-risk pediatric brain tumors. J Clin Oncol. 1997;15(5):1814–23.
11. Mahoney Jr DH, et al. High-dose melphalan and cyclophosphamide with autologous bone marrow rescue for recurrent/progressive malignant brain tumors in children: a pilot pediatric oncology group study. J Clin Oncol. 1996;14(2):382–8.
12. Gajjar A, et al. Risk-adapted craniospinal radiotherapy followed by high-dose chemotherapy and stem-cell rescue in children with newly diagnosed medulloblastoma (St Jude Medulloblastoma-96): long-term results from a prospective, multicentre trial. Lancet Oncol. 2006;7(10):813–20.
13. Evans AE, et al. The treatment of medulloblastoma. Results of a prospective randomized trial of radiation therapy with and without CCNU, vincristine, and prednisone. J Neurosurg. 1990;72(4):572–82.
14. Taylor MD, et al. Molecular subgroups of medulloblastoma: the current consensus. Acta Neuropathol. 2012;123(4):465–72.
15. Duffner PK, et al. Postoperative chemotherapy and delayed radiation in children less than three years of age with malignant brain tumors. N Engl J Med. 1993;328(24):1725–31.
16. Sung KW, et al. Reduced-dose craniospinal radiotherapy followed by tandem high-dose chemotherapy and autologous stem cell transplantation in patients with high-risk medulloblastoma. Neuro Oncol. 2013;15(3):352–9.
17. Kim SY, et al. Reduced-dose craniospinal radiotherapy followed by high-dose chemotherapy and autologous

stem cell rescue for children with newly diagnosed high-risk medulloblastoma or supratentorial primitive neuroectodermal tumor. Korean J Hematol. 2010; 45(2):120–6.
18. Gajjar A, Pizer B. Role of high-dose chemotherapy for recurrent medulloblastoma and other CNS primitive neuroectodermal tumors. Pediatr Blood Cancer. 2010;54(4):649–51.
19. Strother D, et al. Feasibility of four consecutive high-dose chemotherapy cycles with stem-cell rescue for patients with newly diagnosed medulloblastoma or supratentorial primitive neuroectodermal tumor after craniospinal radiotherapy: results of a collaborative study. J Clin Oncol. 2001;19(10):2696–704.
20. Foreman NK, Love S, Thorne R. Intracranial ependymomas: analysis of prognostic factors in a population-based series. Pediatr Neurosurg. 1996;24(3):119–25.
21. Merchant TE, et al. Preliminary results from a phase II trial of conformal radiation therapy and evaluation of radiation-related CNS effects for pediatric patients with localized ependymoma. J Clin Oncol. 2004; 22(15):3156–62.
22. Lafay-Cousin L, Strother D. Current treatment approaches for infants with malignant central nervous system tumors. Oncologist. 2009;14(4):433–44.
23. Bouffet E, Foreman N. Chemotherapy for intracranial ependymomas. Childs Nerv Syst. 1999;15(10): 563–70.
24. Grill J, et al. A high-dose busulfan-thiotepa combination followed by autologous bone marrow transplantation in childhood recurrent ependymoma. A phase-II study. Pediatr Neurosurg. 1996;25(1):7–12.
25. Zacharoulis S, et al. Outcome for young children newly diagnosed with ependymoma, treated with intensive induction chemotherapy followed by myeloablative chemotherapy and autologous stem cell rescue. Pediatr Blood Cancer. 2007;49(1):34–40.
26. Venkatramani R, et al. Outcome of infants and young children with newly diagnosed ependymoma treated on the "Head Start" III prospective clinical trial. J Neurooncol. 2013;113(2):285–91.
27. Bandopadhayay P, et al. ANZCCSG BabyBrain99; intensified systemic chemotherapy, second look surgery and involved field radiation in young children with central nervous system malignancy. Pediatr Blood Cancer. 2011;56(7):1055–61.
28. Sung KW, et al. Tandem high-dose chemotherapy and autologous stem cell transplantation for anaplastic ependymoma in children younger than 3 years of age. J Neurooncol. 2012;107(2):335–42.
29. Levin VA, et al. Superiority of post-radiotherapy adjuvant chemotherapy with CCNU, procarbazine, and vincristine (PCV) over BCNU for anaplastic gliomas: NCOG 6G61 final report. Int J Radiat Oncol Biol Phys. 1990;18(2):321–4.
30. Massimino M, Cohen KJ, Finlay JL. Is there a role for myeloablative chemotherapy with autologous hematopoietic cell rescue in the management of childhood high-grade astrocytomas? Pediatr Blood Cancer. 2010;54(4):641–3.
31. Hochberg FH, et al. High-dose BCNU with autologous bone marrow rescue for recurrent glioblastoma multiforme. J Neurosurg. 1981;54(4):455–60.
32. Papadakis V, et al. High-dose carmustine, thiotepa and etoposide followed by autologous bone marrow rescue for the treatment of high risk central nervous system tumors. Bone Marrow Transplant. 2000;26(2):153–60.
33. Finlay J, et al. The management of patients with primary central nervous system (CNS) germinoma: current controversies requiring resolution. Pediatr Blood Cancer. 2008;51(2):313–6.
34. Abrey LE, et al. High-dose chemotherapy with stem cell rescue as initial therapy for anaplastic oligodendroglioma: long-term follow-up. Neuro Oncol. 2006;8(2): 183–8.
35. Ruggiero A, et al. Phase II trial of temozolomide in children with recurrent high-grade glioma. J Neurooncol. 2006;77(1):89–94.
36. Allen JC, Siffert J. Contemporary chemotherapy issues for children with brainstem gliomas. Pediatr Neurosurg. 1996;24(2):98–102.
37. Bouffet E, et al. Etoposide and thiotepa followed by ABMT (autologous bone marrow transplantation) in children and young adults with high-grade gliomas. Eur J Cancer. 1997;33(1):91–5.
38. Bouffet E, et al. Radiotherapy followed by high dose busulfan and thiotepa: a prospective assessment of high dose chemotherapy in children with diffuse pontine gliomas. Cancer. 2000;88(3):685–92.
39. Sung KW, et al. Tandem high-dose chemotherapy and auto-SCT for malignant brain tumors in children under 3 years of age. Bone Marrow Transplant. 2013; 48(7):932–8.
40. Ginn KF, Gajjar A. Atypical teratoid rhabdoid tumor: current therapy and future directions. Front Oncol. 2012;2:114.
41. Lafay-Cousin L, et al. Central nervous system atypical teratoid rhabdoid tumours: the Canadian Paediatric Brain Tumour Consortium experience. Eur J Cancer. 2012;48(3):353–9.

Supportive Care

22

Beverly A. Wilson, Karina L. Black, and Samina Afzal

Despite the many advances in treatments and improvements in survival, the diagnosis and treatment of a pediatric brain or spinal cord malignancy is accompanied by many challenges and stressors which can be overwhelming for the patient, caregivers, and the entire family. Supportive care describes the services and multidisciplinary care required to address the needs of the patient and family in order to meet the physical, informational, psychosocial, emotional, practical, and spiritual needs during all phases of their cancer care [1]. Although some of the supportive care needs are common among families, the diagnosis and treatment of pediatric brain and spinal cord tumors is complex and every family is different, with needs that may be variable throughout treatment. Therefore, it requires a collaborative and multidisciplinary health-care

team to effectively assess and address the supportive care needs in this population [1–4]. The supportive care requirements of these children and families can include the physical (physiotherapy, occupational therapy, speech pathology, dietician, medical, pharmacy), education/informational (often met by nursing and medical team members), as well as psychosocial (social work, psychology, child life, psychiatry). This chapter will discuss the supportive care needs at diagnosis and during the treatment phase as long-term follow-up is addressed in other chapters of this textbook.

Psychosocial and Informational Support

Family Assessment

The diagnosis of a child with a malignancy is a stressful life event, and if the family's patterns of functioning, resources, or coping skills are inadequate, the family can move into a state of crisis making it more difficult to manage the challenges of the new diagnosis [2–5]. Parents experience intense emotional reactions and uncertainty in response to their child's diagnosis including fear, powerlessness, denial, guilt, sadness, anger, and confusion, with many reporting some level of anxiety and depression [1–3]. It is important to reassure families that these intense emotional reactions are normal responses to the child's

B.A. Wilson, B.M.Sc., M.D., F.R.C.P.S.C. (✉)
Department of Pediatrics, Division of Hematology/
Oncology, University of Alberta, Edmonton,
AB, Canada
e-mail: bev.wilson@albertahealthservices.ca

K.L. Black, B.Sc.N., M.N., N.P.
Pediatric Oncology Program, Stollery Children's
Hospital, Edmonton, AB, Canada

S. Afzal, M.B.B.S., F.C.P.S., F.R.C.P.C.H. (UK)
Department of Pediatrics, Division of Oncology,
IWK Health Centre, Halifax, NS, Canada

illness and that the team is there to support and not judge them [3]. During periods of stress, families depend on familiar patterns of family functioning, methods of coping, and problem-solving [5]. It is helpful to complete an assessment of the family, including family composition, history, strengths, vulnerabilities, and preexisting issues. The assessment should include psychosocial and practical resources including employment, socioeconomic status, as well as an assessment of marital–parental and sibling relationships [2–5]. A written summary of the assessment that describes the family and their strengths and vulnerabilities relevant to their child's illness should be shared with the treatment team in order to provide support for the family [3].

Parental–marital relationships are often challenged by the state of uncertainty and stress the diagnosis and treatment of cancer of their child imposed on the relationship [2, 4, 5]. For some parents, who have supported each other through past crisis and have helped each other cope with the significant emotions, they have found their relationship strengthened. For others, this stress exacerbates previous marital problems which can impact the parent's and the whole family's ability to cope [2, 5]. Single-parent households are common in today's society and task overload is common for the single parent of an ill child. When parents are separated or divorced, special efforts are required by the health-care team to ensure both parents are kept informed [4]. The traditional definition of family has changed for many and so we must be respectful of the variations in family structure when performing family assessments. It is also important to learn about any specific beliefs, attitudes, or behaviors related to the families' ethnic background that may influence the families' coping or ideas about care. Misunderstanding often results when the health-care team does not fully consider sociocultural factors that may influence care [4].

Practical Resources

Economic impact adds significantly to the family's distress [4]. Financial and employment security can become compromised as the family

tries to meet the new demands of their child's diagnosis and treatment [1, 6]. Family financial resources are often depleted as mothers typically take responsibility for caring for their child in the hospital, relinquishing employment or household responsibilities. Fathers, even when taking time off in early treatment, ultimately return to work in order to maintain a family income [1, 5, 6]. In a single-parent family, the challenge of caring for the child while maintaining an income is more difficult [5]. There are also added expenses associated with the diagnosis and treatment that add financial burdens on the family (i.e., parking, accommodation, child care) [4, 5]. Early assessment is essential in order to provide support to the family and lessen the economic stress on the family [4]. Additionally, parents may need assistance mobilizing social support for managing daily activities and routine household chores while they are adapting to the diagnosis and treatment demands. Family and household routines are often disrupted, and social workers and members of the health-care team can assist the family in identifying sources of practical support [1, 3, 5].

Informational Needs

Once a child is diagnosed, the families are presented with a great deal of information at a time when they are already feeling overwhelmed [1, 4]. Family members may not be able to absorb and retain any of the initial information presented to them beyond the diagnosis [2]; therefore, good communication by the health-care team, repetition of information, opportunities to ask questions, and written materials are important for assisting families in making sense of the information [1–4]. Gaining information about their child's condition allows parents to feel some control over the situation and regain some peace of mind [1, 6]. The Internet is increasingly being used as a source of information, and families require members of the health-care team to clarify the information they may obtain [6]. Parents are also required to care for their child once discharged home, often responsible for new technical tasks, which can be a source of burden and anxiety [3, 6]. Psychosocial providers can assist families to manage feelings of information overload and problem-solve to meet the treatment demands [3].

Important Patient Considerations: Children and Adolescents

An important yet difficult task for parents is talking to their child about their diagnosis. Parents often require guidance from the team regarding how and when to talk to their children, to do so honestly and at an age-appropriate level, yet in a way that decreases anxiety and increases trust in the treatment team [4]. Even before a diagnosis is made, children may be experiencing distressing symptoms and emotions, having undergone numerous and sometimes painful tests, often in a strange environment and been separated from their peers and family due to illness [2, 3, 5]. Children's reaction to the illness is partly determined by their developmental level, previous experiences, as well as their family's reactions [3, 5]. Older children and adolescents can be variable in the amount of information they want and, while being able to understand more than younger children, may be overwhelmed and less engaged in treatment discussions [3]. Children of all ages can regress when scared. Adolescents may have very personal concerns about how their illness will affect them that may not be apparent to their family or medical team. Children with cancer may display increased sleep, loss of interest in activities, social withdrawal, and other symptoms consistent with depressed mood, although research has not shown greater rates of clinical depression in children with cancer [2]. The psychosocial team plays an important role to support the children and reassure the family that their children's behaviors are not unusual [3].

Normalizing activities as much as possible can be helpful in restoring a sense of safety and normalcy for children following diagnosis [3, 4]. Within the hospital, multidisciplinary team members, particularly child life specialists, can help to normalize daily activities and provide support for required medical procedures [3]. Once discharged from the hospital, parents often need encouragement to allow the child to live life as normal as possible. Parents have to overcome their own fears for their child, to allow them to return to pre-illness activities within the restrictions of the illness. Providing consistent discipline, not overindulging or overprotecting the child, helps to avoid behavioral problems long term and supports the child's sense of self-worth [3, 4]. Although parents may be fearful of injury or exposure to other children, play is important in mental and physical growth, as well as in helping children to cope with anxiety, fear, and frustration [4]. For older children and adolescents, the return to school is an important part on normalizing the child's life in the face of illness [2–5], although today more and more children are also using email and social networking to stay in touch with one another [4]. At any developmental level, relationships with peers provide children with a sense of connection, friendship, and support which is crucial in the development of their identity [3]. The bodily changes and side effects of the disease or treatment can impact the child's sense of self and body image [3, 5] and impact social interaction and independence. Patients at the highest risk for peer difficulties are those with obvious changes in physical appearance and those with central nervous system involvement. Particular attention needs to be paid to assessing and supporting the social relationships and functioning of these children [2, 4].

Important Considerations: Siblings

Siblings of children with cancer are at risk for difficulties from the time their sibling is diagnosed, particularly during the first few months. Family life becomes organized around the hospitalized child and other family roles and responsibilities are disrupted. Siblings can experience feelings of anger, jealously, neglect, worry, anxiety, sleep and eating disturbances, and mood and temperament changes [3–5]. Siblings may attempt to hide these feelings from their parents however, in order to not worry their parents [4, 5]. Older siblings however, may exhibit high levels of empathy and maturity and want to be included in information and care regarding their sibling [3–5]. Psychosocial team members can assist parents in addressing the difficulties as they present and many programs also offer optional sibling support groups.

Nutritional Support

It is well established that children and young adults with cancer experience malnutrition due to their underlying malignancy and treatment-related factors. Diminished nutritional status has been recognized as a contributor in poor wound healing, increased infection risk, and decreased tolerance to chemotherapy [7, 8]. It has also been demonstrated that poor nutrition impacts several outcome measures including quality of life, response to treatment, and overall cost of care [7–9]. Children are particularly sensitive to the effects of malnutrition due to their limited energy stores and increased nutritional requirements needed to attain appropriate growth and neurodevelopment [9].

Along with the numerous factors contributing to poor nutritional status that are commonly seen in many pediatric cancer patients, children diagnosed with CNS tumors often have additional factors resulting from their tumor location and its treatment. For example, patients with diencephalic tumors and medulloblastoma are classified as high risk for development of malnutrition when compared with other types of childhood cancer [7, 9]. Tumors in the posterior fossa, which account for approximately 60–70 % of all pediatric brain tumors, can be associated with suboptimal nutrition due to prolonged nausea and vomiting and neurological impairment prior to diagnosis. Subsequent surgery for these tumors can result in significant swallowing difficulties and aspiration risk [10]. Additionally, a posterior fossa syndrome may develop, which is frequently associated with dysphagia that may not be apparent in the immediate postoperative period [10]. Radiation therapy, whether localized or including

the craniospinal axis, may cause emesis, somnolence, or esophagitis [9, 11]. These factors, along with chemotherapy-associated nausea and vomiting, mucositis, or constipation, may contribute further to a patient's nutritional decline [11].

Nutritional support for patients who are clinically undernourished at diagnosis requires immediate intervention before treatment starts [9]. However, even patients who are nutritional replete at presentation, particularly infants and those with medulloblastoma, require close observation as nutrition may decline rapidly early in the treatment schedule [7, 11]. After tumor resection involving the posterior fossa, postoperative swallowing dysfunction can be anticipated, even in patients without overt clinical signs [10]. Dysphagia may develop if a posterior fossa syndrome occurs. As early recognition and intervention of poor nutritional status may alleviate the need for more aggressive nutritional support later in treatment, involvement of a registered dietician and a speech-language pathologist is critical in the management of this patient population [7, 8, 11].

Strategies for nutritional intervention are numerous. Behavioral and educational techniques, including education of the family and health-care team, are useful for maintaining nutritional status in those patients without preexisting nutritional issues [9]. Modifications to the oral diet, including caloric supplementation by commercial supplemental drinks or caloric additives, are useful in low-risk patient populations [9]. Controlling nausea and vomiting, as well as providing appropriate analgesia for mucositis and esophagitis, is crucial for all patients. Enteral feedings via nasogastric tube or gastrostomy tube should be instituted early in those patients that are unable to maintain their weight by the strategies described [7–9]. Evidence-based recommendations now exist for proactive enteral tube feeding in high-risk patients to avoid the expected nutritional deterioration [11]. For patients with documented abnormalities on swallowing studies, surgically placed feeding tubes are suggested due to the protracted requirement for enteral feeding. The safety of these feeding tubes in this population is well established [8]. Parental nutritional support is occasionally necessary to meet nutritional requirements until the patient is able to tolerate total enteral feeding [9]. Long-term parental nutrition should be avoided where possible however, due to numerous associated complications [9].

The goals of nutritional supportive care in pediatric oncology include the maintenance of body stores, minimization of weight loss, promotion of appropriate growth, and providing quality of life [9]. Well-nourished patients have increased levels of energy which promotes progress during rehabilitation, an important consideration in those with neurological deficits. Nutritional strategies should be integrated as a fundamental feature of supportive care for all children and young adults with CNS tumors including involvement of appropriate healthcare professionals at diagnosis.

Management of Nausea and Vomiting

Despite significant advances in antiemetic management, chemotherapy-induced nausea and vomiting (CINV) remains an important adverse effect of cancer treatment. It has been estimated that as many as 60 % of children with cancer develop nausea or vomiting at some point during chemotherapy treatment [12]. Several types of CINV have been defined, with important implications for both prevention and management:

Acute nausea and vomiting: occurs within 24 h after chemotherapy administration [13]. Most commonly begins within 1–2 h of chemotherapy; the worst most often occurs about 5 or 6 h after chemotherapy administration.

Delayed nausea and vomiting: occurs more than 24 h after chemotherapy administration; may persist for 5–7 days but the duration has not been fully defined. Delayed emesis commonly occurs following the administration of cisplatin, carboplatin, cyclophosphamide, or doxorubicin [13, 14].

Anticipatory nausea and vomiting: occurs prior to administration of chemotherapy. It is a learned or conditioned response linked to visual, gustatory, olfactory, and environmental factors related with previously administered chemotherapy [14].

Breakthrough: refers to nausea, vomiting, and retching that occurs despite antiemetic prophylaxis and/or necessitates the use of rescue medications [14].

Poorly controlled CINV can lead to physical and psychological issues including electrolyte imbalances, dehydration, malnutrition, stress, anxiety, poor functional status, and reduced quality of life as well as financial concerns including additional clinic visits, prolonged hospitalization, and caregivers' loss of time at work [12]. Therefore, good antiemetic therapy is essential for all patients receiving emetogenic chemotherapy.

Antiemetic therapeutic efficacy is influenced by a number of patient characteristics, and each child should be treated according to his or her unique risk factor profile. The risk associated with the presence of multiple risk factors is likely to be cumulative. In an investigation of over 800 chemotherapy-naïve adult patients, the incidence of post-chemotherapy nausea was 20 % in patients having no risk factors and 76 % in those with four risk factors. Factors correlated with a greater risk include being females, prior history of motion sickness, and high anxiety levels; conversely, there was lower incidence in children less than 6 years. Poorly controlled nausea and vomiting in previous cycles increases the likelihood of CINV and anticipatory nausea and vomiting [15].

The proposed pathophysiology of CINV occurs primarily via both the central and peripheral nervous systems. The central mechanism is hypothesized to occur by activation of the chemoreceptor trigger zone (CTZ). The CTZ is located in the area postrema in the floor of the fourth ventricle outside the blood–brain barrier and can be exposed directly to emetogenic substances, such as chemotherapy through the blood system or cerebrospinal fluid (CSF). Once activated, the CTZ releases multiple neurotransmitters, including serotonin and dopamine, which in turn activates the brain stem vomiting center. The vomiting center can be directly stimulated by chemotherapy. The peripheral mechanism is postulated to occur by chemotherapeutic agents causing local gastrointestinal irritation and damage to the gastric mucosa leading to production and release of serotonin and other neuroactive agents by enterochromaffin cells. Serotonin then interacts with 5-HT3 receptors on the vagal afferent terminals in the wall of the bowel and activated receptors send signals to the vomiting center [13]. In both instances, the neurotransmitters may act independently or in combination to induce vomiting. The role of the higher cortical center such as amygdala is less well established but may be involved in anticipatory vomiting. Memory, fear, anticipation, and sensory input, such as smell, are all generated in the higher cortical center and directly stimulate the vomiting center that can result in emesis. Regardless of the source of afferent input, the vomiting center, located in the lateral reticular formation of the medulla oblongata, serves as the final pathway along with efferent impulses to induce emesis [13].

As per the Pediatric Oncology Group of Ontario (POGO), acute chemotherapy-induced nausea and vomiting (CINV) outlines the definition of emetogenicity as the propensity of an agent to cause nausea, vomiting, or retching. Chemotherapy agents are classified into four categories based on their potential to cause nausea and/or vomiting (emetogenic potential) without antiemetic drug treatment: (1) highly emetogenic (HEC), which can cause symptoms in greater than 90 % of patients; (2) moderate risk, which can cause symptoms in 30–90 % of patients; (3) low risk which can cause symptoms in 10–30 % of patients; and (4) minimally emetogenic which can cause symptoms in less than 10 % of patients [16] (Table 22.1) [17]. It is the standard of care that all pediatric patients receiving moderate to highly emetogenic chemotherapy should receive a combination of a 5-HT₃ receptor antagonist plus dexamethasone to prevent acute emesis [18].

Antiemetic Therapy

Role of Dexamethasone in Brain Tumor Patients

Dexamethasone as an antiemetic is either contraindicated or strongly discouraged in children with brain tumors due to the theoretical concern of decreased penetration of chemotherapy agents into the central nervous system. On the other hand, dexamethasone is considered to be the drug of choice to provide temporary relief of symptoms due to an increase in intracranial pressure and edema in children with a brain tumor. It stabilizes the blood–brain barrier (BBB), leading to attenuation of vasogenic brain edema. The mechanism of action of glucocorticoids for control of vasogenic edema is not fully understood. Dexamethasone, most frequently used glucocorticoid, has recently been shown to upregulate Ang-1, which is a strong BBB-stabilizing factor, whereas it downregulates VEGF, a strong permeabilizing factor in astrocytes and pericytes [19]. Dexamethasone may also increase the clearance of peritumoral edema by facilitating the transport of fluid into the ventricular system from which it is cleared by cerebrospinal fluid (CSF). Generally, the dose of dexamethasone required to treat brain edema is much lower than the dexamethasone antiemetic dose.

Treatment of brain tumors is limited by the ability of therapeutic drugs to cross the blood–brain barrier (BBB). The BBB is damaged in patients with a brain tumor, thus facilitating penetration of cytotoxic drugs into tumor tissue. Corticosteroids, by repairing damage to the BBB, may reduce the delivery of chemotherapeutic agents to the brain. This restoration of the BBB may decrease uptake of cytotoxic agents into the brain tissue, reducing the efficacy of chemotherapy in the treatment of a child with a brain tumor [20].

Brain around tumor (BAT) is a transitional zone where the brain tissue is infiltrated with tumor cells. Chemotherapy drugs that are unable to cross the intact BBB show increased penetration into BAT when compared to normal brain

Table 22.1 Emetogenicity of antineoplastics in children. Classification of the acute emetogenic potential of antineoplastic medication in pediatric cancer patients given intravenously (unless stated otherwise) as single agents [17]

High level of emetic risk (>90 % frequency of emesis in absence of prophylaxis)	
Altretamine	Dactinomycin
Carboplatin	Mechlorethamine
Carmustine >250 mg/m²	Methotrexate ≥12 g/m²
Cisplatin	Procarbazine (oral)
Cyclophosphamide ≥1 g/m²	Streptozotocin
Cytarabine 3 g/m²/dose	Thiotepa ≥300 mg/m²
Dacarbazine	
Moderate level of emetic risk (30–90 % frequency of emesis in absence of prophylaxis)	
Aldesleukin >12 to 15 million U/m²	Etoposide (oral)
Amifostine >300 mg/m²	Idarubicin
Arsenic trioxide	Ifosfamide
Azacitidine	Imatinib (oral)
Bendamustine	Intrathecal therapy (methotrexate, hydrocortisone, and cytarabine)
	Irinotecan
Busulfan	Lomustine
Carmustine ≤250 mg/m²	Melphalan >50 mg/m²
Clofarabine	Methotrexate ≥250 mg to <12 g/m²
Cyclophosphamide <1 g/m²	Oxaliplatin >75 mg/m²
Cyclophosphamide (oral)	Temozolomide (oral)
Cytarabine >200 mg to <3 g/m²	Vinorelbine (oral)
Daunorubicin	
Doxorubicin	
Epirubicin	
Low level of emetic risk (10 to <30 % frequency of emesis in absence of prophylaxis)	
Amifostine ≤300 mg/m²	Ixabepilone
Amsacrine	Methotrexate >50 to <250 mg/m²
Bexarotene	Mitomycin
Busulfan (oral)	Mitoxantrone
Capecitabine	Nilotinib
Cytarabine ≤200 mg/m²	Paclitaxel
Docetaxel	Paclitaxel—albumin
Doxorubicin (liposomal)	Pemetrexed
Etoposide	Teniposide
Fludarabine (oral)	Thiotepa <300 mg/m²
5-Fluorouracil	Topotecan
Gemcitabine	Vorinostat
Minimal (<10 % frequency of emesis in absence of prophylaxis)	
Alemtuzumab	Lenalidomide
Alpha interferon	Melphalan (oral low dose)
Asparaginase (IM or IV)	Mercaptopurine (oral)
Bevacizumab	Methotrexate ≤50 mg/m²
Bleomycin	Nelarabine
Bortezomib	Panitumumab
Busulfan (oral)	Pentostatin
Cetuximab	Rituximab
Chlorambucil (oral)	Sorafenib
Cladribine (2-chlorodeoxyadenosine)	Sunitinib

(continued)

Table 22.1 (continued)

Dasatinib	Temsirolimus
Decitabine	Thalidomide
Denileukin diftitox	Thioguanine (oral)
Dexrazoxane	Trastuzumab
Erlotinib	Valrubicin
Fludarabine	Vinblastine
Gefitinib	Vincristine
Gemtuzumab ozogamicin	Vindesine
Hydroxyurea (oral)	Vinorelbine
Lapatinib	

High level of emetic risk (>90 % frequency of emesis in absence of prophylaxis)
Reprinted from Dupuis LL, Boodhan S, Sung L, et al. Guideline for the classification of the acute emetogenic potential of antineoplastic medication in pediatric cancer patients. Pediatr Blood Cancer 2011;57(2):191-8. With permission of John Wiley & Sons, Inc.

tissue though decreased compared to tumor thereby demonstrating a partially damaged BBB in BAT. In a rat model, the concentration of platinum was significantly lower in BAT treated with cisplatin and dexamethasone compared with the rat treated with cisplatin alone, indicating that the efficacy of cisplatin in patients with a brain tumor may be impaired with commitment administration of dexamethasone [21].

Steroids have also shown to decrease the concentration of intravenous contrast media in the tumor and the area around the tumor on imaging studies including computed tomography and MRI, reflecting stabilization of blood tumor and peritumoral BBB [22]. Also, in several carcinoma cell lines, dexamethasone has been shown to enhance resistance to radiotherapy and chemotherapy [13]. This induction of resistance to chemotherapy and radiotherapy by dexamethasone may result in suboptimal clinical responses in children with brain tumors. In view of the above-mentioned evidence, dexamethasone use as an antiemetic should be avoided, if possible, in children being treated for a brain tumor.

The child being treated for a brain tumor will often receive craniospinal radiation, surgery, and chemotherapy. Radiation to the brain often causes nausea and vomiting that can be managed with the use of a 5-HT3 antagonist given prior to radiation. The chemotherapy regimens usually used to treat brain tumors are often platinum based and hence are highly emetogenic. As dexa-

methasone is discouraged, it is very important to maximize alternative antiemetics.

5-Hydroxytryptamine Receptor Antagonists

The development of the 5-hydroxytryptamine (5-HT$_3$) receptor antagonists has greatly improved the control of chemotherapy-induced emesis and these agents are considered the gold standard. However, 5-HT$_3$ receptor antagonist as single agent leads to poor CINV control in patients receiving moderately emetogenic chemotherapy (MEC) and highly emetogenic chemotherapy (HEC) (Table 22.1) [17]. The recently published POGO guidelines recommend 5-HT$_3$ receptor antagonist administered together with nabilone or chlorpromazine in whom corticosteroids are contraindicated [16].

Ondansetron is the most studied 5-HT$_3$ antagonist and is considered an effective first-line antiemetic in children undergoing chemotherapy, radiotherapy, and surgery. Ondansetron is generally well tolerated in children with minimal toxicity. Ondansetron, granisetron, dolasetron, and tropisetron are all 1st-generation 5-HT$_3$ antagonists and have been compared in various studies. First-generation 5-HT$_3$ antagonists (ondansetron, granisetron, or tropisetron) have comparable efficacy in preventing CINV in cisplatin-based chemotherapy when administered with dexamethasone [20]. The efficacy of the intravenous and oral routes of ondansetron is equivalent, and recent studies have demonstrated that the oral formulations are safe, effective, and probably less expensive than the intravenous formulations during non-cisplatin-containing moderately and highly emetogenic chemotherapy [23]. The recommended dose of ondansetron for children receiving moderately or highly emetogenic chemotherapy is 5 mg/m^2/dose (0.15 mg/kg/dose) IV/PO pre-therapy x 1 dose and then q8h for highly emetogenic chemotherapy and every 12 hourly for moderately emetogenic chemotherapy. The ondansetron dose for children receiving chemotherapy with low emetogenicity is 10 mg/m^2/dose (0.3 mg/kg/dose; maximum 16 mg/dose IV or 24 mg/dose PO) pre-therapy × 1 dose [16].

Granisetron is a specific 5-HT$_3$ antagonist, which is well tolerated with the common adverse effects reported being headache, constipation, diarrhea, asymptomatic arrhythmia, and transient elevation of serum transaminase. The intravenous and oral routes are equally efficacious. The usual intravenous dose is 40ug/kg as a single daily dose for chemotherapy of any emetogenicity [24].

A genetic polymorphism has been identified that affects patients' responses to antiemetic therapy following moderate to highly emetogenic chemotherapy. The 5-HT$_3$ receptor antagonists are metabolized by the cytochrome P450 (CYP) enzymes, and patients who have been identified as ultrarapid metabolizers of the isoenzyme CYP2D6 have a significantly higher frequency of vomiting within the first 24 h after chemotherapy with the administration of ondansetron. Alternatively, granisetron is metabolized exclusively by the CYP3A subfamily and so would not be expected to have diminished effect in rapid metabolizers of CYP2D6 and would potentially be an alternative agent in these patients. Conversion to an alternate 5-HT$_3$ antagonist is a simple intervention in patients who do not respond to initial 5-HT$_3$ antagonist and benefit may be observed in 40–50 % of patients; however, genetic polymorphism may not be the only factor responsible [13].

Palonosetron is a newer 2nd-generation 5-HT$_3$ antagonist with a 40-h half-life in adults com-

pared to the 4–8 h for the 1st-generation antagonist. With its longer half-life, this agent shows promise in the control of both acute and delayed nausea and vomiting [20].

Other Antiemetic Medications

Nabilone is a synthetic cannabinoid used in control of CINV. Preliminary animal studies showed that nabilone had significant antiemetic activity against drugs potent in causing emesis, such as cisplatin and carmustine with its primary action on the medulla oblongata and some secondary anxiolytic activity medicated through the forebrain. Nabilone has been reviewed in a meta-analysis concluding that cannabinoids were slightly better at controlling CINV than prochlorperazine, metoclopramide, domperidone, or haloperidol [25]. The antianxiety properties of nabilone may contribute to its antiemetic effect. In a randomized, double-blind, crossover trial, nabilone was compared to prochlorperazine for control of CINV in children aged between 3.5 and 17.8 years. Major side effects commonly experienced during nabilone administration were dizziness, drowsiness, and mood alteration. Dose reduction improved the symptoms without interfering with the efficacy of nabilone. A higher proportion of patients experienced control of CINV during nabilone treatment compared to prochlorperazine and more patients preferred nabilone [26].

Despite the lack of significant supporting evidence, the use of nabilone is recommended in combination with a 5-HT$_3$ antagonist in patients in whom corticosteroids are discouraged. Nabilone is only available in an oral formulation which may restrict its use in the child unable to swallow. The safety and efficacy of nabilone in children less than 4 years has not been established. Generally, nabilone is more effective in adolescent and older children who are refractory to standard prophylaxis [13].

Metoclopramide was one of the first antiemetics used in clinical practice. It was initially thought to be a dopamine antagonist acting centrally in the chemoreceptor trigger zone and peripherally promoting gut motility but was later also found to be a week 5-HT$_3$ receptor antagonist [27]. Prospective trials have evaluated the efficacy and side effects of metoclopramide versus 5-HT$_3$ receptor antagonists administered to control CINV in children receiving antineoplastic therapy. The ability of metoclopramide is marginal in the setting of highly emetogenic antineoplastic therapy. Extrapyramidal reactions (EPR) have been noted in patients treated with metoclopramide. Diphenhydramine is an anticholinergic drug that acts on the cholinergic receptors to prevent or lessen the dystonia caused by metoclopramide [27]. Metoclopramide may have a role in children receiving moderately emetogenic antineoplastic therapy for whom corticosteroids need to be avoided [16].

Chlorpromazine has been evaluated in a single randomized trial and reported to have only moderate success in providing complete vomiting control in children receiving highly emetogenic antineoplastic therapy [16]. There is a limited published experience with chlorpromazine for CINV; however there is extensive general pediatric experience with use of chlorpromazine. As an antiemetic, its efficacy has not been evaluated in combination of 5-HT$_3$ antagonist. Despite lack of evidence, the use of chlorpromazine in combination with a 5-HT$_3$ antagonist may be considered for children who cannot receive dexamethsoane [16]. Sedation and hypotensive effects should be given consideration while using in the outpatient setting.

For the treatment of anticipatory nausea or in children who experience breakthrough nausea and vomiting, benzodiazepines can be prescribed. It should be noted that benzodiazepines, like lorazepam, cause sedation and should be used cautiously with other agents that cause sedation, e.g., chlorpromazine. The antiemetic effect of lorazepam is thought to be independent of its sedative effect and it is believed to act by inhibiting input to the vomiting center [13].

For breakthrough nausea and vomiting, there is a lack of evidence to give specific directions regarding management. The first step will be maximization of the current antiemetic regimen.

For example, if the patient is on low-dose 5-HT$_3$ antagonist prophylaxis, the 5-HT$_3$ antagonist dose should be maximized. If the patient is already on highest antiemetic dose, then addition of other antiemetics should be considered. The choice of other antiemetics will depend on need and circumstances of individual patients [13].

Currently, there is not enough evidence to recommend the routine use of antiemetics to prevent delayed nausea and vomiting. Knowledge about risk factors for delayed emesis is lacking; however, association between delayed emesis and emesis during acute phase strongly suggests rigorous attention to the prevention of acute CINV. Delayed emesis commonly occurs following the administration of cisplatin, carboplatin, cyclophosphamide, or doxorubicin [13, 14].

A novel agent, aprepitant, is an NK-1 receptor antagonist that blocks NK-1 receptors in the brain and gut. Published pediatric experience is limited and of poor quality. It is effective in combination with a 5-HT$_3$ inhibitor and dexamethasone, in the management of acute and delayed onset of vomiting in highly emetogenic protocols especially those containing cisplatinum [19]. Aprepitant is currently only marketed for use in the combination with ondansetron and dexamethasone so it would not be an option in the management of nausea and vomiting in the child with a brain tumor as dexamethasone use is discouraged.

Non-pharmacological Interventions

Various adjunctive non-pharmacological interventions provide control of CINV in children receiving antineoplastic agents of any emetic risk. Nonmedical approaches including acupuncture, acupressure, guided imagery, music therapy, progressive muscle relaxation, and psychoeducational support and information may be effective in children receiving antineoplastic agents [16].

Children may be advised to eat small, frequent meals; to reduce food aromas and avoid stimuli with strong odors as well as avoid spicy, fatty, and highly salty food; and to take antiemetic prior to meals [16].

Endocrinopathy at Diagnosis and During Treatment of Brain Tumor

Midline tumors developing in the hypothalamic–pituitary region account for 15–20 % of all pediatric brain tumors, including craniopharyngioma, optic pathway glioma, hamartoma, germ cell tumor (GCT), suprasellar arachnoid cyst, and hypothalamic pituitary astrocytoma [28]. Intracranial germ cell tumors (icGCT) are classically divided into two main groups called germinoma and non-germinomatous germ cell tumors (NGGCT). Presenting symptoms usually leading to diagnosis of hypothalamic–pituitary lesion include neurological and visual complaints that could be secondary to increased intracranial pressure, ophthalmic compression, or involvement of adjacent structures [28]. Tumors of suprasellar and pineal region show various endocrine abnormalities even before the start of any treatment or surgery [29]. Endocrinal symptoms in midline tumors including diabetes insipidus; changes in weight, height, and growth velocity; precocious puberty; or delayed sexual development less often lead to diagnosis, despite being present long before diagnosis [28].

Growth infiltration or mass effect of the tumor can cause the dysfunction of the pituitary gland manifesting as endocrine abnormalities. Hypothalamic–pituitary axis dysfunction gives rise to endocrinal abnormalities. This influence could be transient and the pituitary gland may regain its ability to secrete hormones after treatment but it could be permanent. Therapeutic modalities, including surgery and radiotherapy, can damage pituitary cells leading to worsening of preexisting hypopituitarism [30].

Precocious Puberty

Precocious puberty (PP) is usually defined as the onset of secondary sexual development before the age of eight years in girls and nine years in boys. Central precocious puberty (CPP) is organic when it is associated with a lesion of

the central nervous system (CNS) and idiopathic when no lesion is detected by the neuroimaging. Etiology of organic CPP is variable and has a direct relationship to the location and type of lesions, indicating that onset of CPP is not resulting from the disruption of putative GnRH pulse generator inhibitory influence but resulting from secretion of stimulatory substances by various lesions. Cerebral imaging is routinely performed in patients with PP to rule out organic lesions. Various lesions have been described as causes of organic CPP, including true tumors such as glioma, germ cell tumor, and pseudotumor including hypothalamic hamartoma [29]. In icGCT, the high testosterone level in males causing the early onset of puberty can be due to an increase in β-hCG. Precocious puberty development in female is more complicated, requiring a rise in LH and FSH in addition to an increase in β-hCG. This could be the reason that PP caused by icGCT is more commonly seen in males than in females [30].

Optic pathway gliomas have been associated with CPP, both with and without NF1; however, PP has not been reported in gliomas located outside the suprasellar area before treatment, indicating that PP in these tumors could be secondary to tumor location and tumor cell type. Neuroactive substances are secreted by hypothalamic astrocytes stimulating the release of GnRH [29].

Diabetes Insipidus

Diabetes insipidus (DI) is often an early clinical manifestation in suprasellar GCT. The mechanism of central DI is considered to be interruption of the transport of the vasopressin neurosecretory granules along the hypothalamic–neurohypophyseal pathway [31]. DI often persists after completion of tumor treatment, indicating continuous need of vasopressin analogue. Sometimes, endocrinal disturbance can manifest long before radiological evidence of tumor in GCT [30]. Unrecognized endocrine symptoms, mainly enuresis, accounted for longest delay in diagnosis of GCT. Delay in seeking medical advice with polyuria and polydipsia could be related to the fact that GCT occurs in older children and adolescents, who may have less parental supervision and who may be less willing to seek medical attention especially for enuresis [28]. Although DI is mostly related to a neurohypophyseal germ cell tumor, there are reports of DI in patients with tumor of the pineal region, even without radiographic evidence of suprasellar/third ventricular disease.

During chemotherapy for GCT, presence of DI is a risk factor for chemotherapy-related complications when cisplatin- and/or ifosfamide-based protocols are used. Despite vigilant monitoring of electrolytes and desmopressin dose adjustment, significant variations in sodium level have been documented leading to adverse clinical manifestations [32].

Since DI is frequent in patient with icGCT, it is strongly recommended to maintain close follow-up in idiopathic DI as a tumor may appear later on imaging. This follow-up should involve test of pituitary functions, neurological examination, and screening for tumor markers [30].

Growth Hormone Abnormality

Growth hormone levels have been found to be reduced in almost 50 % of cases and retarded growth can be an early sign in icGCT located in suprasellar regions [32]. Mass effect or infiltrative lesions exerted by icGCT cause decrease hormone production or secretion leading to either increased or decreased level of cortisol, sexual hormones, TSH, and thyroxin [30]. No endocrine disturbance is pathognomonic of icGCT. If clinical or laboratory evidence of an endocrine abnormality is detected together with neurological symptoms, an icGCT should be considered even if no radiological evidence of tumor is identified. Close follow-up is strongly recommended [30].

Craniopharyngiomas (CRA) are locally aggressive tumors which typically arise in the suprasellar region and can involve the pituitary stalk, the hypothalamus, and the optic pathway. Although most patients have endocrine insufficiency on diagnosis, with growth hormone defi-

ciency being more prevalent, they rarely seek medical attention for endocrine issues. Stunted growth in most pediatric cases is a hallmark of CRA. Abnormal height and weight have been described in more than 50 % of cases with CRA. However, abnormal BMI (body mass index) or BMI progression and abnormal height or growth velocity are rarely the cause of referral despite being present for long [28].

Multimodality treatment for these CRA tumors can be challenging, given the significant risk accompanying any intervention involving the structures in the region. Endocrinopathy is a common iatrogenic complication of treatment of CRA, with either surgical resection or radiosurgery. Hormonal disturbances are markedly increased after gross total resection compared with partial resection, with or without radiation, with over 50 % of patients experiencing at least one endocrinopathy and over 10 % developing panhypopituitarism [33]. Therefore, the effect of aggressive resection on endocrine function should be considered and anticipated when planning surgery for CRA. Obesity is common at diagnosis but is increased posttreatment. Although PP has been found to be associated with CRA, it is mostly reported after either surgery or radiotherapy and it has rarely been described as presenting symptom of CRA [29].

Clinical Implications

There is often significant delay between the onset of symptoms and diagnosis of pediatric brain tumors, including hypothalamic pituitary lesions, compared to the shorter period taken to diagnose other malignancies. Timely diagnosis could provide an opportunity to start treatment possibly avoiding irreversible damage and improving prognosis with minimal side effects [28].

It is important to recognize endocrine symptoms and clinical signs as they can occur long before the diagnosis of hypothalamic pituitary lesions are made. Height, weight, and BMI plotting may be helpful in shortening the time taken to diagnose as in a substantial number of cases changes in these measurements preceded the onset of neuro-ophthalmic-presenting symptoms [28].

Careful history and clinical examination, as well as timely reevaluation needs to be done in patients with abnormal BMI or BMI progression, as the presence of other neurological, ophthalmologic, and endocrine signs and symptoms may be indicative of the presence of an underlying hypothalamic–pituitary lesion.

Posterior Fossa Syndrome

Posterior fossa syndrome (PFS), also known as cerebellar mutism syndrome (CMS), was first described in 1979 by Hirsh after a posterior fossa tumor resection. PFS develops in a subset of patients following resection of posterior fossa tumors including up to 25 % of patients with medulloblastoma [34, 35] . PFS has been described in both pediatric and adult literature but it is more common in children.

PFS typically manifests 1–2 days after resection of a midline posterior fossa tumor and is characterized by diminished speech progressing to mutism as well as other neurological, cognitive, and behavioral impairments [34–36]. After surgery, there is brief interval of 1–2 days of relatively normal speech followed by rapid onset of mutism and emotional lability with high-pitched cry (sole form of vocalization). Most common neurological findings are ataxia and hypotonia. Additional symptoms include striking apathy, lack of initiative, reduced spontaneous movement, inattention or lack of response to visual stimuli, impaired eye opening, oropharyngeal dyspraxia, and urinary retention. Resolution of mutism is often followed by period of dysarthria. The majority of cases of PFS are moderate to severe in intensity [34–36].

Risk Factors

There are no consistent specific demographic, clinical, or radiographic predictors of PFS. Given the absence of symptoms preoperatively, damage from tumor itself is unlikely [36]. Several risk factors for the development of PFS have been proposed. Tumor type has been identified as a risk factor, with high rate of PFS observed with medulloblastoma compared to other posterior fossa tumors. Vermian location has often been related with syndrome; however, a Children's Oncology Group (COG) study found no correlation between vermian location of tumor and PFS. There has been no relationship between PFS and age or gender at diagnosis. Although case studies have cited tumor size as a risk factor, results from the large prospective study are not consistent with this finding. Preoperative brain stem invasion has been linked with risk of PFS in COG prospective study [34–36].

Mechanism of Injury

Splitting of inferior cerebellar vermis was considered as the cause of PFS following identification of correlation between this approach and development of mutism. This theory has been debated because PFS continued to occur despite a change in practice that avoided splitting of vermis. PFS has been observed even without damage to median and paramedian structures [35, 36].

Another theory suggests that vasospasm and subsequent postoperative ischemia may cause PFS, but radiographic findings have not supported this theory. Hydrocephalus was previously hypothesized to be related to PFS but several studies have found no correlation. Previously, PFS has been shown to occur more frequently in patients with radical resection than in patients with residual tumors suggesting that a more aggressive surgical technique is associated with increased incidence of PFS. Recent studies have not supported this. Postsurgical edema resulting from intraoperative manipulation has also been suggested as a leading theory. Some reports have shown increased bilateral edema in cerebellar peduncles in patients with PFS. Recently, it has been documented that left-handedness presurgically, larger tumor size, presence of high-grade tumor, and white matter damage in the right cerebellar regions of the cerebello–thalamo–cerebral pathway are associated with PFS [34, 36, 37].

Neuroradiological Studies

Preoperative and immediate postoperative MR imaging have not reliably differentiated patients with PFS from those without. Neuroimaging studies failed to predict who will develop PFS, but have helped to understand the pathophysiology of the disorder. Damage has been found in the cerebellar vermis, brain stem, dentate nuclei, middle cerebellar peduncle, and superior cerebellar peduncle. Studies demonstrate that the occurrence of PFS is not localizable to a specific neuroanatomical region but rather to disruption of neural circuitry along the dentatothalamocortical outflow tracts [36, 37].

MRI imaging obtained one year after medulloblastoma resection showed increase diffuse cerebellar and brain stem atrophy in patients with PFS compared to patients without PFS, indicating more persistent posttreatment damage to the cerebellum, vermis and brain stem in patients with PFS [37].

Outcome of PFS

Although mutism is transient, speech rarely normalizes and the syndrome is associated with long-term neurological, cognitive, and psychological sequelae. PFS was previously believed to be a transient phenomenon, but recent studies have demonstrated that while some features of PFS may be transient, persistent impairment is common and incomplete recovery of speech and language is frequent [36].

Neurocognitive outcome evaluated at 12 months following PFS in pediatric patients with medulloblastoma has shown significantly lower performance in processing speed, attention, working memory, cognitive efficiency, reading, spelling, and mathematics, indicating that development of PFS places the patient at increased risk of neurocognitive deficit [38].

Supportive Care and Clinical Implications

The role of the multidisciplinary team including family, nurses, physician, speech-language pathologist, occupation therapist, physical therapist, social worker, and child life support is integral to provide care to patient and families with PFS [39]. The emotional impact of PFS on families can be decreased by having a detailed consent prior to surgery including information on the possible alteration in verbal, sensory, and behavioral abilities postsurgically, thus allowing families to better understand the potential postoperative complications thereby reducing fear and anxiety. Postoperatively, patients and families with PFS will require significant education and support to adapt to new situation [39].

The Following Strategies May Help to Alleviate Symptoms of PFS

Mutism and impairment in expressive language and verbal memory result in inability to vocalize routine physical and emotional needs thus interfering with effective coping. Patients need encouragement to express their feelings via age-appropriate therapeutic play activities [39].

Ataxia, hypotonia, and reduced spontaneous movements need continuous support from the nurse, physiotherapist, and occupational therapist to maintain skin integrity and maintenance of full range of motion and muscle tone by minimizing muscle wasting and contractures [39].

Impaired eye opening requires involvement of ophthalmologist in addition to other team members to prevent corneal abrasions [39].

Oropharyngeal dyspraxia demands vigilant support from the dietitian, speech-language pathologist, and occupational therapist to prevent malnutrition and dehydration. Postoperative gag and swallowing reflexes should be assessed prior to starting oral feeds and an alternate feeding route may be necessary until patient regains gag and swallowing reflexes [39].

Impairment of bladder and bowel function necessitates multidisciplinary team support to aid bowel elimination and prevention of renal retention and calculi.

There is no established treatment to facilitate recovery from cerebellar mutism. No known preventive measures can be established without knowing the exact etiology. Previous studies have not definitely identified any specific demographic, clinical, or radiographic features that can predict who is at risk of developing PFS after posterior fossa surgery. Treatment remains supportive.

References

1. Kerr LM, Harrison MB, Medves J, Tranmer J. Supportive care needs of parents of children with cancer: transition from diagnosis to treatment. Oncol Nurs Forum. 2004;31(6):E116–26.
2. Lanskowksy P. Manual of pediatric hematology and oncology: psychosocial aspects of cancer for children and their families. 5th ed. Burlington: Elsevier; 2011.
3. Recklitis C, Casey R, Zeltzer L. Oncology of infancy and childhood. 1st ed. Philadelphia: Saunders; 2009.
4. Wiener L, Hersh S, Alderfer M. Principles and Practice of Pediatric Oncology: Psychiatric and Psychosocial Support for the Child and Family. 6th ed. Philadelphia: Lippincott Williams & Wilkins; 2011.
5. Woodgate R, West C, Wilkins K. Family-centered psychosocial care. In: Baggott C, Fochtman D, Foley G, Kelly K, editors. Nursing care of children and adolescents with cancer and blood disorders. 4th ed. Glenview: Association of Pediatric Hematology/Oncology Nurses; 2011. p. 114–64.
6. Frierdich S. Continuity of care. In: Baggott C, Fochtman D, Foley GV, Petterson Kelly K, editors. Nursing care of children and adolescents with cancer and blood disorders. 4th ed. Glenview: Association of Pediatric Hematology/Oncology Nurses; 2011. p. 165–202.
7. Co-Reyes E, Li R, Huh W, Chandra J. Malnutrition and obesity in pediatric oncology patients: causes, consequences, and interventions. Pediatr Blood Cancer. 2012;59(7):1160–7.
8. Ballal S, Bechard L, Jaksic T, Duggan C. Principles and practices of pediatric oncology: nutritional supportive care. 6th ed. Philadelphia: Lippincott Williams & Wilkins; 2011.
9. Bauer J, Jurgens H, Fruhwald MC. Important aspects of nutrition in children with cancer. Adv Nutr. 2011;2(2):67–77.
10. Newman LA, Boop FA, Sanford RA, Thompson JW, Temple CK, Duntsch CD. Postoperative swallowing function after posterior fossa tumor resection in pediatric patients. Childs Nerv Syst. 2006;22(10):1296–300.
11. Ward E, Hopkins M, Arbuckle L, et al. Nutritional problems in children treated for medulloblastoma: implications for enteral nutrition support. Pediatr Blood Cancer. 2009;53(4):570–5.
12. Rodgers C, Norville R, Taylor O, et al. Children's coping strategies for chemotherapy-induced nausea and vomiting. Oncol Nurs Forum. 2012;39(2):202–9.
13. Dupuis LL, Nathan PC. Options for the prevention and management of acute chemotherapy-induced nausea and vomiting in children. Paediatr Drugs. 2003;5(9):597–613.
14. Schnell FM. Chemotherapy-induced nausea and vomiting: the importance of acute antiemetic control. Oncologist. 2003;8(2):187–98.
15. Doherty KM. Closing the gap in prophylactic antiemetic therapy: patient factors in calculating the emetogenic potential of chemotherapy. Clin J Oncol Nurs. 1999;3(3):113–9.
16. Dupuis LL, Boodhan S, Holdsworth M, et al. Guideline for the prevention of acute nausea and vomiting due to antineoplastic medication in pediatric cancer patients. Pediatr Blood Cancer. 2013;60(7): 1073–82.
17. Dupuis LL, Boodhan S, Sung L, et al. Guideline for the classification of the acute emetogenic potential of antineoplastic medication in pediatric cancer patients. Pediatr Blood Cancer. 2011;57(2):191–8.
18. Jordan K, Roila F, Molassiotis A, Maranzano E, Clark-Snow RA, Feyer P. Antiemetics in children receiving chemotherapy. MASCC/ESMO guideline update 2009. Support Care Cancer. 2011;19 Suppl 1: S37–42.
19. Kim H, Lee JM, Park JS, et al. Dexamethasone coordinately regulates angiopoietin-1 and VEGF: a mechanism of glucocorticoid-induced stabilization of blood-brain barrier. Biochem Biophys Res Commun. 2008;372(1):243–8.
20. Dupuis LL, Nathan PC. Optimizing emetic control in children receiving antineoplastic therapy: beyond the guidelines. Paediatr Drugs. 2010;12(1):51–61.
21. Straathof CS, van den Bent MJ, Ma J, et al. The effect of dexamethasone on the uptake of cisplatin in 9L glioma and the area of brain around tumor. J Neurooncol. 1998;37(1):1–8.
22. Weller M, Schmidt C, Roth W, Dichgans J. Chemotherapy of human malignant glioma: prevention of efficacy by dexamethasone? Neurology. 1997; 48(6):1704–9.
23. Corapcioglu F, Sarper N. A prospective randomized trial of the antiemetic efficacy and cost-effectiveness of intravenous and orally disintegrating tablet of ondansetron in children with cancer. Pediatr Hematol Oncol. 2005;22(2):103–14.
24. Miyajima Y, Numata S, Katayama I, Horibe K. Prevention of chemotherapy-induced emesis with granisetron in children with malignant diseases. Am J Pediatr Hematol Oncol. 1994;16(3):236–41.
25. Tramer MR, Carroll D, Campbell FA, Reynolds DJ, Moore RA, McQuay HJ. Cannabinoids for control of chemotherapy induced nausea and vomiting: quantitative systematic review. BMJ. 2001;323(7303): 16–21.
26. Chan HS, Correia JA, MacLeod SM. Nabilone versus prochlorperazine for control of cancer chemotherapy-induced emesis in children: a double-blind, crossover trial. Pediatrics. 1987;79(6):946–52.

27. Koseoglu V, Kurekci AE, Sarici U, Atay AA, Ozcan O. Comparison of the efficacy and side-effects of ondansetron and metoclopramide-diphenhydramine administered to control nausea and vomiting in children treated with antineoplastic chemotherapy: a prospective randomized study. Eur J Pediatr. 1998;157(10): 806–10.

28. Taylor M, Couto-Silva AC, Adan L, et al. Hypothalamic-pituitary lesions in pediatric patients: endocrine symptoms often precede neuro-ophthalmic presenting symptoms. J Pediatr. 2012;161(5):855–63.

29. Rivarola, Belgorosky A, Mendilaharzu H, Vidal G. Precocious puberty in children with tumours of the suprasellar and pineal areas: organic central precocious puberty. Acta Paediatr. 2001;90(7):751–6.

30. Jorsal T, Rorth M. Intracranial germ cell tumours. A review with special reference to endocrine manifestations. Acta Oncol. 2012;51(1):3–9.

31. Wang Y, Zou L, Gao B. Intracranial germinoma: clinical and MRI findings in 56 patients. Childs Nerv Syst. 2010;26(12):1773–7.

32. Afzal S, Wherrett D, Bartels U, et al. Challenges in management of patients with intracranial germ cell tumor and diabetes insipidus treated with cisplatin and/or ifosfamide based chemotherapy. J Neurooncol. 2010;97(3):393–9.

33. Sughrue ME, Yang I, Kane AJ, et al. Endocrinologic, neurologic, and visual morbidity after treatment for craniopharyngioma. J Neurooncol. 2011;101(3): 463–76.

34. Law N, Greenberg M, Bouffet E, et al. Clinical and neuroanatomical predictors of cerebellar mutism syndrome. Neuro Oncol. 2012;14(10):1294–303.

35. Robertson PL, Muraszko KM, Holmes EJ, et al. Incidence and severity of postoperative cerebellar mutism syndrome in children with medulloblastoma: a prospective study by the Children's Oncology Group. J Neurosurg. 2006;105(6 Suppl):444–51.

36. Wells EM, Walsh KS, Khademian ZP, Keating RF, Packer RJ. The cerebellar mutism syndrome and its relation to cerebellar cognitive function and the cerebellar cognitive affective disorder. Dev Disabil Res Rev. 2008;14(3):221–8.

37. Wells EM, Khademian ZP, Walsh KS, et al. Postoperative cerebellar mutism syndrome following treatment of medulloblastoma: neuroradiographic features and origin. J Neurosurg Pediatr. 2010;5(4): 329–34.

38. Palmer SL, Hassall T, Evankovich K, et al. Neurocognitive outcome 12 months following cerebellar mutism syndrome in pediatric patients with medulloblastoma. Neuro Oncol. 2010;12(12): 1311–7.

39. Parent E, Scott L. Pediatric posterior fossa syndrome (PFS): nursing strategies in the post-operative period. Can J Neurosci Nurs. 2011;33(2):24–31.

Long-Term Sequelae

Sebastien Perreault and Anne-Sophie Carret

Introduction

Over the last decades, the outcome of children with central nervous system (CNS) tumors has significantly improved. Whereas the overall 5-year survival rate was less than 30 % in 1970, the latest data from the Surveillance Epidemiology and End Results (SEER) estimated that 74 % of children with brain tumors survive beyond 5 years. This cure rate is greatly attributable to the inclusion of radiation therapy (RT) as well as chemotherapy in treatment regimen. However as those survivors become young adults, the incidence of late effects is being more apparent. More than two thirds of long-term survivors have at least one chronic medical complication [1]. These sequelae include endocrinopathy, osteoporosis, cerebrovascular disease, neurological and neurosensory dysfunction, secondary neoplasms, as well as psychological complications and neurocognitive impacts.

Medical Long-Term Effects

Endocrinological Effects

Surgery, radiation therapy, and/or chemotherapy like high-dose alkylating agents, platinum analogues, nitrosoureas, and corticosteroid can cause endocrine and metabolic late effects which include gonadal damage, thyroid disorders, and dysfunction of the hypothalamo-pituitary axis. The risk for particular late endocrine effects depends upon the location of the tumor and the treatment modalities that were used [2–4].

Neuroendocrine Dysfunctions

Hypothalamic and pituitary endocrinopathies occur commonly in children following whole-brain or localized cranial radiation therapy (RT) that included these structures in the radiation field. This damage is particularly common in patients with optic pathway/hypothalamic tumors whose tumors may directly compromise this location. Such injury may occur after doses ≥24 Gy. In children treated with RT for non-pituitary-related primary brain tumors, irradiation of the pituitary hypothalamic axis can result

S. Perreault, M.D.
Division of Child Neurology, Lucile Packard Children's Hospital, Stanford University, Palo Alto, CA, USA

Department of Pediatrics, Division of Neurology, CHU Sainte-Justine/Université de Montréal, Montréal, QC, Canada

A.-S. Carret, M.D. (✉)
Department of Pediatrics, Division of Hematology/Oncology, CHU Sainte-Justine/Université de Montréal, Montréal, QC, Canada
e-mail: anne-sophie.carret@umontreal.ca

K. Scheinemann and E. Bouffet (eds.), *Pediatric Neuro-oncology*,
DOI 10.1007/978-1-4939-1541-5_23, © Springer Science+Business Media New York 2015

in delayed growth hormone (GH), adrenocorti-cotropic hormone (ACTH), and thyroid-stimula-tion hormone (TSH) deficiencies. Growth hormone deficiency occurs in nearly 100 % of children who receive ≥36 Gy of RT to the pitu-itary region as seen in the treatment of medullo-blastoma. It is less common with RT doses <24 Gy, but may not become evident until 10 years after treatment. The time course of endo-crine dysfunction is variable, with patients typi-cally having abnormal serum hormone levels long before clinical symptoms develop. If symp-toms occur, the manifestations depend on the specific hormone deficiency [2, 4].

Thyroid Gland

Complications involving the thyroid gland are primarily seen in patients treated with thyroid involved-field radiation and can present as hypo-thyroidism (primary or central) and thyroid tumors (benign or malignant). Risk factors include female gender, young age at treatment, and radiation dose. The risk of developing pri-mary hypothyroidism following craniospinal radiation therapy (CSRT) alone (36 Gy) for medulloblastoma is approximately 20–30 %, while the risk of secondary hypothyroidism is much lower (~3.4 %). Unfortunately, the attempt to decrease the dose of spinal RT (23.4 Gy) with the addition of adjuvant chemotherapy led to an unintended increased incidence of hypothyroid-ism [2]. The theoretical benefit to a radiation reduction dose (23.4 Gy) used more recently was not as important as the adverse effects created by the addition of chemotherapy: 60–80 % hypothy-roidism for RT plus chemotherapy compared to 20 % for RT alone [2, 3]. Hyperfractionated RT, even in the presence of chemotherapy, is associ-ated with a reduction of primary hypothyroidism. Hypothyroidism may contribute to poor growth, lack of energy, and poor school performance, requiring substitutive opotherapy. Since this defi-cit may develop years following treatment, patient must continue to be monitored with T4 and TSH dosages.

Growth

Radiation-induced growth hormone deficiency is due to either damage to hypothalamus or pitu-itary gland, with the hypothalamus identified as the primary site of damage. Cranial irradiation has an immediate suppressive effect on the hypo-thalamic pituitary axis. According to the total cranial dose received, it reduces spontaneous growth hormone (GH) level and alters the normal pubertal rise in spontaneous GH secretions (18 Gy) but also the response to provocative stim-uli (>27 Gy). GH deficiency will develop earlier with doses >30 Gy. In addition, the size and the number of fractions influence growth hormone levels, with a higher incidence of deficiency in patients receiving their cranial RT over 2.5 weeks in 10 fractions compared to same total dose of 24 Gy over 4 weeks in 20 fractions ($p < 0.002$). Duffner et al. showed that GH deficiency could be documented as early as 3 months following completion of cranial RT [2]. In that study, more than 80 % of patients with posterior fossa tumors became GH deficient within the first year post RT completion. Nevertheless, there are reports of GH deficiency identified as late as 6 years follow-ing radiation. Once identified, GH deficiency appears to be permanent. The cause of poor growth in childhood brain tumor survivors can result also from direct inhibition of vertebral growth by spinal irradiation (>35 Gy) leading to short stature. The effects of spinal radiation are both dose and age dependent and are not cor-rected by growth hormone. In contrast to RT effects, chemotherapy given alone can induce temporary growth retardation. Some agents, such as high-dose prednisone and methotrexate, seem to have direct inhibition effects on bone growth. Other factors, which play a role in growth failure, are poor nutrition, undetected hypothyroidism, and precocious puberty.

Yearly measurement of TSH and free T4 and monitoring for growth problems, using standard-ized curves in the setting of endocrine consulta-tion, should be part of the long-term monitoring of childhood brain tumor survivors. Early diag-nosis of mild hypothyroidism and/or GH deficiency permits early intervention to improve growth velocity and quality of life [2–4].

Gonadal Function

Pubertal development can be adversely affected by cranial radiation. Doses >30–40 Gy may result in gonadotropin deficiency, while doses >18 Gy can result in precocious puberty. Spinal radiation generally spares the testes while it can cause ovarian dysfunction in up to 35 % of girls. Chemotherapy may also impair gonadal function, usually more in males than in females. Testicular damage induced by cyclophosphamide is dose dependent. In general, prepubertal patients tend to be more resistant to adverse effects of RT and chemotherapy on gonadal function than postpubertal patients [2, 4, 5].

Osteoporosis

The brain tumor itself and the necessary treatments, especially radiation therapy, poor nutrition, limited weight-bearing exercise, and the development of endocrinopathies interact and all likely affect bone mineral density (BMD) during a crucial period for bone growth and skeletal accretion. Thus, the childhood brain tumor survivors are at increased risk for osteoporotic fractures later in life, depending on the magnitude of the BMD deficit and the potential for recovery. These survivors should be assessed for risk factors for a low BMD and referred to an endocrinologist for a potential bone health assessment and treatment of any hormonal deficiency as well as maximization of nutrition, exercise, and calcium and vitamin D intake [6].

Physical Appearance

Permanent changes to physical appearance and body image are common late effects in childhood brain tumor survivors and can be often overlooked or minimized by clinicians. Visible scars from craniotomies, ventricular derivations, other procedures, and central lines are daily reminders of their experience for almost all of survivors. Additionally, most of them who received cranial irradiation develop variable degree of permanent alopecia. When treated at a young age, many patients have noticeable changes to the bone structure of their skull. Most of the brain tumor survivors are self-conscious about these localized but visible physical changes. Craniospinal irradiation and/or disruption of the pituitary hypothalamic axis can lead to more global changes in physical appearance such as short stature or obesity [4, 7].

Dental and Oral Health

Dental and oral complications are common among head and neck cancer survivors. For these patients, chemotherapy or protocols involving high-dose chemotherapy with stem cell transplantation, radiation therapy to the head and neck region can have a significant impact on normal growth and development of teeth and surrounding structures. Abnormal findings include taste dysfunction, chronic salivary gland dysfunction with increased risk of candidiasis and dental caries, more frequent during the early phase, smaller teeth (microdontia), delayed eruption of teeth, failure of the teeth to develop (hypodontia, tooth agenesis) but also premature loss of teeth, facial disfigurement, and trismus. Risk factors associated with at least one dental problem include: radiation therapy dose to the jaw especially when the total dose exceed 20 Gy (nearly sixfold increase in risk) and total dose of alkylating agents. Cancer survivors prescribed with bone-modifying agents (e.g., bisphosphonates) constitute also a high-risk group for oral and dental complications, especially jaw osteonecrosis. In general, treatment at younger age is associated with a greater potential for such long-term effects. For those reasons, newly diagnosed cancer patients should be referred for a complete oral examination prior to initiation of therapy. The dentist and the oncologist should maintain communication so that each provider is aware of relevant findings and potential complications of treatment. When there are complications affecting growth and development, patients may require the expertise of oral and maxillofacial surgeons, orthodontists, and prosthodontists for comprehensive management [8].

Sleep Disorder

Children treated for a CNS tumor can experience sleep disorders such as disturbed sleep-wake rhythm, increased sleep duration, less flexible in timing of their sleep, and daytime sleepiness, which can significantly impact on their daily performance and their quality of life (QOL). These disturbed sleep patterns are more often described in children with hypothalamic, pituitary, or brain stem lesions as well as in children treated with craniospinal radiotherapy. There is also a strong association of excessive somnolence and psychosocial functioning with fatigue. Routine evaluation of sleep habits during consults at the outpatient clinic may help to better understand the mechanisms behind these disorders and present possible interventions (e.g., melatonin, cognitive therapy, bright light therapy, medications, and/or physical activities) [9].

Cerebrovascular Disease

Stroke

A growing body of literature reports cerebrovascular disease in survivor of childhood CNS tumors. Reported rates of late-occurring stroke and transient ischemic attack (TIA) vary from 267.6 per 100,000 person-years to 548 per 100,000 person-years [10, 11]. In contrast to 2–8/100,000 person-years in a comparable general population, this represents an increase risk of 40- to 100-fold with a cumulative incidence of 6.9 % at 25 years. Strokes usually occur at a mean age of 26 years, 5 to 15 years after completion of therapy. The risk is closely associated to the radiation therapy (RT) dose and targeted field.

The highest risk is observed in patients receiving more than 50 Gy to the cranium and RT involving the circle of Willis [10, 11]. Patients with brain tumors treated with RT and alkylating agents have been identified to be at highest risk of stroke when compared to their siblings with relative risk of 78.3 [10].

The exact mechanism by which RT induces stroke is still under investigation. Radiation has been found to cause excessive production of prostaglandins, prostacyclins, thromboxane, and leukotrienes inducing inflammatory reactions with increased vascular permeability, vasodilatation, vasoconstriction, and microthrombus formation. Changes in medium and large vessels reminiscent of premature atherosclerosis with intima fibrosis and foam cell accumulation with luminal narrowing are observed. Known risks factors such as dyslipidemia and high blood pressure have been reported to accelerate this process both in animal model and in cancer survivors. Since childhood cancer survivors are more likely to develop obesity, lower high-density lipoprotein, insulin resistance, and hypertension, tight control of those risk factors are essential.

Moyamoya

Moyamoya vasculopathy has been characteristically reported in pituitary and chiasmatic tumor patients treated with and without radiation. This vasculopathy is a progressive stenosis of supraclinoid internal carotid arteries resulting in development of collateral blood vessel formation. Radiation to the circle of Willis and neurofibromatosis type I (NF1) have been identified as risk factors [12]. In one large study, 12 patients (3.5 %) out of 345 treated with RT for a primary brain tumor developed moyamoya syndrome at a median time of 38 months in NF1 patients compared to 55 months in those without NF1. Currently there is no standard treatment, but in their cohort, all patients were placed on antiplatelet therapy with daily aspirin and nine underwent revascularization procedures [12].

Vascular Malformations

Children treated with radiotherapy are at an increased risk of vascular malformations. Radiation can weaken the vessel wall and result in cerebral cavernous malformation, telangiectasias of capillaries, and eneurysms. Cavernous malformations consist of closely apposed, dilated vascular channels with no intervening brain parenchyma. Radiation is also believed to stimulate angiogenesis factors eventually leading to these vascular malformations. In patients treated with RT for their primary brain tumors, a large series identified cerebral cavernous malformations in ten of 297 (3.4 %) patients, 6 times higher than in the control population. Cerebral cavernous malformations were found on imaging at a median latency of 37 months (3 to 102 months) after completion of therapy [13]. Most of these lesions are asymptomatic, but a subset may be associated with seizures, headaches, and hemorrhages that may require surgical intervention.

Telangiectasias are commonly found in brain tissue obtained from patients treated with RT. They encompassed vascular malformation consisting of dilated postcapillary vessels, with thin-walled, tortuous, dilated vascular channels, and perivascular leukocyte infiltration. These abnormal vascular structures may become symptomatic after bleeding but are usually consider a benign finding.

Small Vessel Vasculopathy

Small vessel vasculopathy with mineralizing microangiopathy of the basal ganglia and subcortical white matter has also been found to occur from months to years after completion radiation. An autopsy study revealed that 28 of 163 (17 %) patients with leukemia treated with cranial radiation presented mineralizing microangiopathy after RT [14]. Most patients are asymptomatic, but some investigators have correlated their presence with behavioral disorders, neurological deterioration, and dementia.

SMART Syndrome

Stroke-like migraine attacks after radiation therapy (SMART) syndrome has recently been recognized as a specific constellation of signs and symptoms occurring after high-dose RT (usually >50 Gy) to the posterior cerebral lobes or posterior fossa. Patients typically present acute new-onset neurological symptoms including hemiplegia, aphasia, ataxia, and behavior changes associated with migraine-like headache. Symptoms last from hours to several days and the recovery is usually complete. Magnetic resonance imaging (MRI) changes are characteristic with focal leptomeningeal enhancement associated with thickening and T2 signal abnormality on MRI images of subjacent gyri (Fig. 23.1). Cerebrospinal fluid analysis may reveal pleocytosis. Electroencephalography (EEG) can demonstrate diffuse slowing, and hypermetabolism has been observed on [18 F] fluorodeoxyglucose positron-emission tomography imaging. The differential diagnoses range from encephalomeningitis and leptomeningeal dissemination of the primary tumor. Evaluation for bacterial and viral infection as well as leptomeningeal disease with cytology is necessary for full evaluation. Characteristic MRI changes can then be diagnostic. While several patients may have recurrent events, no specific treatment or prophylaxis is clearly effective. Anecdotal treatments including topiramate, carbamazepine, verapamil, propranolol, and warfarin have been reported [15]. The physiopathology remains unknown but may involve dysfunction of the trigeminal vascular system, channelopathy, or vasculopathy.

Secondary Neoplasms

While the overall survival in childhood cancer survivors increases, secondary neoplasms have emerged as a long-term complication of treatment. Two large registries and two population-based studies have estimated a cumulative incidence of subsequent malignant neoplasms

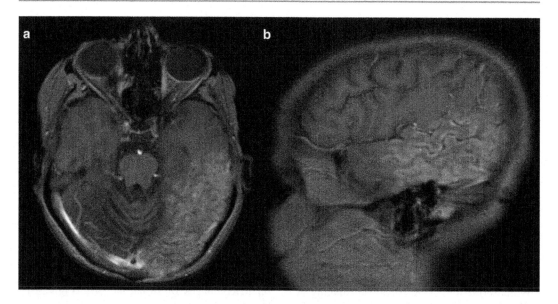

Fig. 23.1 Axial (**a**) and sagittal (**b**) brain MRI T1-weighted images with contrast showing a characteristic SMART syndrome. This 13-year-old female was treated with 39.6 Gy of craniospinal radiation following a diagnosis of medulloblastoma when she was 6 years of age. Seven years later she presented with headache, fever, aphasia, and right hemianopsia. CSF analyses were negative for herpes virus. She recovered completely but presented a total of four similar episodes

(SMNs) in childhood cancer survivors of 3 to 4 % at 20 years posttreatment [16, 17]. Survivors of Hodgkin disease are afflicted with higher rates of breast and thyroid cancers, whereas leukemia and primary CNS tumors have tendency to develop a subsequent CNS tumor. Armstrong et al. reported 76 cases of SMNs in 1877 survivors of CNS malignancies with second CNS tumors (26 %), followed by thyroid (16 %) and sarcoma (11 %). They also observed 171 neoplasms classified as "benign" tumors including 59 meningiomas and 112 nonmelanoma skin cancers. The overall cumulative incidence of a subsequent neoplasm at 25 years was estimated to be 10.7 % (Fig. 23.2) [18]. Most common malignancies are malignant astrocytomas which are overrepresented by glioblastomas, followed by sarcomas and occasionally supratentorial primitive neuroectodermal tumors (sPNET) (Fig. 23.3).

In a study based on an acute lymphoblastic leukemia (ALL) population, the mean time between diagnosis and development of subsequent CNS neoplasm was 11.9 years, with 20.6 years for meningiomas and 8.8 years for all other CNS tumors. In fact, the cumulative inci-

dence of CNS SMNs such as glioblastomas plateaued at 15 years, whereas the cumulative incidence of meningiomas continue to increase beyond 35 years posttreatment [19].

Despite similar histological appearance, secondary malignancies typically behave more aggressively and are resistant to treatment. The overall survival for second glioblastomas is uniformly poor, and second sPNET have an overall survival of 18 % at 18 months compared to 40–50 % at 36 months for a primary sPNET [20]. Subsequent meningiomas have also been found to be more often atypical and prone to relapse.

The development of SMNs is most likely multifactorial, but RT certainly contributes to this process. The vast majority of SMNs develops within the radiation field. At 25 years, the cumulative incidence of SMNs was 7.1 % for patients who received more than 50 Gy to the cranium compared to 1 % for those who did not received RT. A linear dose response is observed with an excess relative risk per Gy of 0.33 for gliomas and 1.06 for meningiomas.

The exact contribution of chemotherapy to the development of SMNs is more difficult to assess

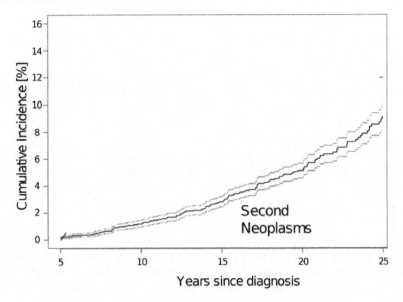

Fig. 23.2 Cumulative incidence of subsequent neoplasms in long-term survivors of childhood central nervous system tumor based on Childhood Cancer Survivors Study. [Reprinted from Armstrong, G.T., Long-term survivors of childhood central nervous system malignancies: the experience of the Childhood Cancer Survivor Study. European journal of paediatric neurology: EJPN: official journal of the European Paediatric Neurology Society, 2010. 14(4): p. 298–303. With permission from Elsevier]

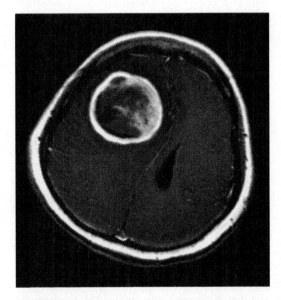

Fig. 23.3 Axial brain MRI T1-weighted image with contrast showing a right frontal subsequent supratentorial primitive neuroectodermal tumor (sPNET). This 17-year-old female patient was treated 7 years earlier with craniospinal radiation for CNS relapse of acute lymphoblastic leukemia. Despite two surgeries, salvage radiation therapy and chemotherapy, she rapidly progressed and died 5 months after diagnosis

partly due to the use of combination chemotherapy regimens. Alkylating drugs, especially cyclophosphamide and epipodophyllotoxins, such as etoposide, have been reported to increase the cumulative incidence of second malignancies up to 4 % compared to 1 % [21]. The majority were acute non-lymphomatous leukemia (ANLL) and acute myeloid leukemia (AML) which tended to occur within the first 3 years after treatment.

Somatic mutations can predispose an individual to develop SMNs. Patients with p53 (Li-Fraumeni syndrome) are more likely to develop sarcoma, primary brain tumor, and ALL after treatment. Therapy may be tailored in order to reduce exposure RT and certain chemotherapy agents, but usually those patients are diagnosed at their subsequent neoplasm. No study has tested systematically all patients with SMNs, but the prevalence of such mutation remains probably low. In six patients with ALL that eventually developed a second CNS tumor, none were carrier of a p53 mutation. Other somatic mutations such as the ataxia telangiectasia mutated gene (ATM) known to be involved in DNA repair possibly play a role. Whereas homozygote patients present a classical phenotype with childhood ataxia, telangiectasia, and immunodeficiency, heterozygotes are at increased risk (odds ratio 5.8) of neoplasm following exposure to radiation. Patients with NF1 are also more likely to develop a secondary malignancy. Sharif et al. reported that 20 % of patients with optic pathway glioma developed SMNs, and half of patients treated with radiotherapy developed an SMN, usually gliomas or malignant nerve sheet tumors [22]. Finally, metabolism and detoxification might also be involved in the development of SMNs especially in those with ANLL and AML. Polymorphisms of NAD (P)H:quinone oxidoreductase (NQO1), glutathione S-transferase (GST), and thiopurine S-methyltransferase (TPMT) have been reported. An ongoing cooperative group study from the Children's Oncology Group aims to address those predisposing factors by enrolling patients with SMNs and assessing their p53, ATM, and polymorphisms status.

The role and benefice of surveillance brain MRI to detect asymptomatic SMNs remains unknown. *Long-Term Follow-Up Program Resource Guide* published in 2008 by the Children's Oncology Group recommends conducting imaging only if the patient presents new-onset symptoms [23]. Experts however suggested surveillance brain MRI every 2 years for patient with NF1 who received RT.

Long-Term Neurological and Neurosensory Sequelae

Long-term survivors of childhood CNS tumors are at high risk of neurologic and neurosensory impairment not only during treatment but also years after completion of their therapy.

Seizures and Epilepsy

Epilepsy may represent a significant problem in a subset of young adult survivors. Studies have reported that between 1 % and 3 % of children with new-onset seizures have a brain tumor and that seizure is the initial presenting symptom at diagnosis in up to 9 % of children with brain

tumor [24]. Patients with slowly growing neoplasms such as dysembryoplastic neuroepithelial tumor (DNET), ganglioglioma, pleomorphic xanthoastrocytoma, and cortically based low-grade astrocytoma are particularly prone to develop epilepsy. The vast majority (81 %) has a supratentorial tumor that generally involves the temporal lobe [25, 26]. Risk factors for poor outcome include having seizures for more than 1 year preoperatively and partial resection. Seizure freedom can be expected in 79 % of patients undergoing a gross total tumor resection versus 43 % for a partial resection. It is still unclear if there is a benefit to perform expanded-field epilepsy surgery with intraoperative electrocorticography in contrast to a brain tumor surgery, where the goal is to remove the tumor and obtain diagnostic tissue. In some instances, chemotherapy and RT have also been reported to improve seizure control.

In a report from the Childhood Cancer Survivor Study (CCSS), the prevalence of epilepsy in long-term survivors of childhood brain tumors was 25 %. Interestingly, 6.5 % had their first seizure more than 5 years after diagnosis of their cancer [27]. Seizures were more frequent in patients treated with RT > 30 Gy to any cortical area (relative risk [RR] 2) and more frequent in children treated at young age. Methotrexate has also been related to late seizure onset, especially in the setting of necrotizing leukoencephalopathy.

Seizure control with antiepileptic drugs appears similar to what can be expected in patients without brain tumor. In a report from Khan et al., 65 % were controlled and 17 % were considered intractable. Uncontrolled seizures were more frequent in children with neurologic deficits, pericavity T2 abnormalities on MRI, and slow waves on EEG [26]. However, another group reported that only 39 % were seizure-free and that 26 % were intractable [25]. For patients who are seizure-free with medication, a slow tapering can be attempted after 2–3 years. In one study, including 62 patients with pediatric brain tumors and epilepsy, 73 % who were weaned off remained seizure-free [26]. Unfavorable risk factors included multiple tumor resections and whole-brain RT.

Motor Dysfunction

Motor impairment is a well-known late-onset sequela, but few studies have specifically been conducted to address this subject. Multiple contributing factors include the tumor itself, hydrocephalus, surgery-associated morbidity, side effects of chemotherapy, and RT. Not surprisingly, it has been reported that compared to their siblings, 49 % of childhood brain tumor survivors had coordination problems and 26 % presented motor difficulties. The onset of those dysfunctions occurred mainly at diagnosis or during treatment. Nonetheless, 4.6 % reported that their impairments appeared more than 5 years posttreatment. Patients who had received at least 50 Gy were found to be at higher risk for motor problems (RR 2.0) compared to those who received less than 30 Gy [27]. Late-onset leukoencephalopathy and cerebral vasculopathy associated with radiation have been hypothesized as possible mechanisms for late-onset motor and coordination impairments.

Primary spinal cord tumors are rare in children and account for 4–8 % of all tumors from the central nervous system. However, due to their location, a significant proportion of patients have long-term sequelae such as weakness, dysesthesia, and sphincter dysfunction. In general, postoperatively 35–70 % will remain stable, 40 to 60 % will improve, and 5 to 40 % will worsen neurologically [28]. Around 40 % of those who deteriorated following surgery will improve within a month, but improvement can be expected up to a year [28]. Postoperative functional outcome is strongly correlated to preoperative neurologic state. The presence of an identifiable tumor plane at surgery, cystic tumor, and improvement in neurological symptoms before discharge has been reported to be associated with overall neurological improvement.

Although initially considered reversible, up to 50 % of patients with postoperative posterior fossa syndrome were found to have permanent neurological dysfunction including cranial nerve neuropathy, hypotonia, and ataxia.

Vincristine and cisplatin commonly used in treatment of patients with brain tumors are known for their neurotoxicity including peripheral neuropathy. Whereas most patients significantly improve following completion of their therapy, young adults continue to present evidence of neuropathy several years later. Long-term follow-up studies have shown that reduction in deep tendon reflexes, raised vibration perception threshold, and abnormal nerve conduction were found in 44 %, 55 %, and 35 %, respectively [29]. Despite the fact that symptoms have been reported to persist in 20–75 % of patients, most had no impact or limitation in their daily activities. The outcome of such peripheral neuropathy 20 to 30 years after treatment is however unknown. As this population is at risk of metabolic syndrome, diabetes-associated neuropathy could add significant morbidity.

Although not extensively studied, pain can also affect daily functioning of long-term survivors of childhood cancer. More than 10 years post diagnosis between 10 and 30 % of patients reported pain or abnormal sensation. 16.7 % were using prescription analgesic drugs and 21 % attributed their pain to cancer and its treatment [30].

Ototoxicity

In targeting the outer hair cells in the organ of Corti and the vascularized epithelium in the lateral wall of the cochlea, high doses of platinum have been reported to cause irreversible early- or delayed-onset hearing loss. These late complications are not only creating functional limitation but also affect speech development, learning, communication, school performance, social interaction, and overall quality of life. Ototoxicity is one of the most common platinum-related neurotoxic effects; it is characterized by a dose-dependent high-frequency sensorineural hearing loss with tinnitus. The variable reported incidence of hearing loss is related to the specific criteria used to define hearing loss, the younger age at start of treatment, the high cumulative doses of platinum compounds (>400 mg/m2 for cisplatin and carboplatin), and the use of concomitant ototoxic treatments including CNS radiation therapy

[31, 32]. Ototoxicity has a general dose dependence, but with considerable interindividual variability. Genetic polymorphisms in enzymes responsible for platinum metabolism (e.g., glutathione S-transferase, thiopurine methyltransferase, catechol O-methyltransferase) may contribute to the substantial interpatient variability in the severity of hearing loss [33, 34]. In addition, higher levels of residual platinum, which can persist for years following treatment, may also contribute to the severity of ototoxicity. Ototoxicity after platinum chemotherapy can present or worsen years after completion of therapy. Radiotherapy (RT) to the normal cochlea or cranial nerve VIII can also cause sensorineural hearing loss. Cranial RT, when used as a single modality, results in ototoxicity when cochlear dosage exceeds 32 Gy. Young age, presence of a brain tumor, and/or hydrocephalus can increase susceptibility to hearing loss. The onset of radiation-associated hearing loss may be gradual, manifesting months to years after exposure. When used concomitantly with platinum, RT can substantially exacerbate the hearing loss associated with chemotherapy. RT to temporal lobe (>30 Gy) and to posterior fossa (≥50 Gy but also ≥30–49.9 Gy) was associated with an increased risk of problems with hearing sounds, tinnitus, and hearing loss requiring an aid [35]. Concurrent administration of platinum and RT results in synergistic ototoxicity, especially in the high-frequency speech range. Care should be taken to distinguish sensorineural hearing loss versus conductive hearing loss due to serous otitis media as seen after RT, which occasionally requires myringotomy. Early detection of ototoxicity in children may minimize the risk for severe impairment in the frequencies required for speech recognition. In children being treated with either cisplatin or carboplatin, extended high-frequency audiometry (i.e., at frequencies above 8 kHz) is more sensitive to early hearing loss than conventional audiometry. This procedure is readily carried out in children more than 5 years old. For younger children, distortion product otoacoustic emissions (DPOAEs) are also more sensitive than conventional audiometry. Various strategies have been considered to minimize platinum ototoxicity. The data were insufficient to support the routine use of otoprotective agents such as amifostine to prevent platinum ototoxicity. A major challenge to the development of otoprotective agents is the lack of consensus on the best ototoxicity assessment criteria, which should include QOL component. Radiation reduction dose to the cochlea has been investigated, including the use of three-dimensional (conformal) RT, intensity-modulated RT (IMRT), and more recently proton therapy [36]. Once treatment is completed, long-term audiometric monitoring should continue according to one of recognized pediatric late effects monitoring guidelines for appropriate management.

Vision

According to a CCSS study, childhood brain tumor survivors are significantly more at risk of developing visual impairment. Legal blindness in one or both eyes was reported in 13 % (RR 17.3), cataracts in 3 % (RR 11.9), and double vision in 17 % (RR 8.8) [27]. Cataracts and late-onset optic neuropathy are a recognized complication of RT. Prolonged uses of corticosteroid such as dexamethasone can also contribute to the development of posterior subcapsular cataracts. Tumors involving the suprasellar area are particularly prone to induce visual field cuts and visual acuity deficits. In patients with craniopharyngioma, 36 % had visual acuity abnormality at presentation without improvement at follow-up, and 44 % had a persistent visual field defect [37]. Studies on ophthalmologic complications of optic pathway glioma have reported visual acuity loss in 20 % to 70 % of patients. Involvement of the posterior chiasmatic area has been reported as a risk factor of poor visual outcome. Finally, long-standing obstructive hydrocephalus from delayed CNS tumor can lead to severe optic atrophy and blindness.

Psychosocial Complications

Cognitive impairment, motor dysfunction, physical appearance, and seizures can contribute to difficulty in several domains such as school, employability, interpersonal relationships, independent living, and emotional functioning. Those challenges and difficulties can translate into poor quality of life for survivors and their families.

Obtaining employment appropriate to one's education and interest can be challenging and constituted an important milestone. Whereas it has been reported that survivors of cancer such as lymphoma and leukemia may expect the same rate of employment than the general population, studies including patients with a history of brain tumor almost uniformly report lower than average employment rate. Survivors from CNS tumors may demonstrate deficits in motor function with limitation in various tasks such as writing, keyboard typing, or driving which can restrict their vocation. After conducting a meta-analysis, De Boer et al. observed that brain tumor survivors are five times more likely to be unemployed (OR 4.74, 95 % CI 1.21–18.65) [1]. The unemployment rate has been estimated to be 26 % in another survey. Risk factors included younger age at diagnosis, lower education or IQ, female gender, epilepsy, and having received RT [1].

While most adult survivors of childhood cancer appear to be doing well in terms of their psychological health and adaptation, a significant proportion (15–30 %) present higher levels of global distress and depression. Fear of secondary neoplasms and health in general is a significant concern and source of stress in this population. Up to 20.5 % of young adults treated for childhood cancer met posttraumatic stress disorder criteria at some point. Threat to life, intensive treatment regimens, painful invasive procedures, and sides effects have been found to lead to stressful experiences.

Social isolation is also a concern in a subgroup of cancer survivors. Some have suggested that missed school and opportunities for social interaction may contribute to this isolation. Physical health problems but also impaired higher executive functions such as initiation, planning, decision making and judgment can affect ones interaction and independency. Mulhern et al. reported that 33 % of long-term survivors of childhood cancer exhibit significant deficiencies in social competence or behavioral problems [38]. It has been observed that only 30 % of young adult survivors of medulloblastoma were able to drive and live independently.

Another assessment of social functioning has been studied through the interpersonal relationship such as marital status. Almost uniformly, studies have shown that survivors of CNS tumors such as medulloblastoma have a lower dating rate. Long-term survivors of childhood and adolescent cancer were less likely to be married than control subjects (rate ratio (RR) for males 0.87, 95 % CI 0.76–0.99), and the rate ratio was even lower for man survivors of CNS tumors (rate ratio 0.48, 95 % CI 0.35–0.66) [39]. The average length of first marriage was in general shorter with higher divorce rates (rate ratio 2.9, 95 % CI 1.7–5.15) compared to control population. Emotional distress, cognitive impairment, chronic fatigue, delayed achieving autonomy from their nuclear families, and physical morbidity certainly contribute to lower rates of marriage for childhood CNS tumor survivors.

Conclusion and Recommendations

As the number of childhood CNS tumor survivors increases, sequelae of therapies are better appreciated. However, very long-term effects 30–40 years after treatment still need to be investigated. Cerebrovascular diseases such as stroke, cognitive dysfunction leading to early dementia, secondary neoplasms, and peripheral neuropathy are likely to constitute an increasing problem in the coming years.

Different resources such as *Long-Term Follow-Up Program Resource Guide* offer valuable guideline and information [23]. To address their specific medical, psychological, and social needs, multidisciplinary and comprehensive clinics are essential. Transition from pediatric neuro-oncology to adult comprehensive care will need to be emphasized and facilitated.

The balance between survival and long-term side effects will certainly be a challenge for decades. Hopefully, tailored therapy to reduce and limit the need for radiation and chemotherapy will lead to improved outcomes with fewer side effects and morbidity.

References

1. de Boer AG, Verbeek JH, van Dijk FJ. Adult survivors of childhood cancer and unemployment: A metaanalysis. Cancer. 2006;107(1):1–11.
2. Duffner PK. Long-term effects of radiation therapy on cognitive and endocrine function in children with leukemia and brain tumors. Neurologist. 2004;10(6): 293–310.
3. Gurney JG, et al. Final height and body mass index among adult survivors of childhood brain cancer: childhood cancer survivor study. J Clin Endocrinol Metab. 2003;88(10):4731–9.
4. Turner CD, et al. Late effects of therapy for pediatric brain tumor survivors. J Child Neurol. 2009;24(11): 1455–63.
5. Armstrong GT, et al. Abnormal timing of menarche in survivors of central nervous system tumors: a report from the Childhood Cancer Survivor Study. Cancer. 2009;115(11):2562–70.
6. Cohen LE, et al. Bone density in post-pubertal adolescent survivors of childhood brain tumors. Pediatr Blood Cancer. 2012;58(6):959–63.
7. Nathan PC, et al. The prevalence of overweight and obesity in pediatric survivors of cancer. J Pediatr. 2006;149(4):518–25.
8. Kaste SC, et al. Impact of radiation and chemotherapy on risk of dental abnormalities: a report from the Childhood Cancer Survivor Study. Cancer. 2009;115(24):5817–27.
9. Verberne LM, et al. Sleep disorders in children after treatment for a CNS tumour. J Sleep Res. 2012;21(4): 461–9.
10. Bowers DC, et al. Late-occurring stroke among long-term survivors of childhood leukemia and brain tumors: a report from the Childhood Cancer Survivor Study. J Clin Oncol. 2006;24(33):5277–82.
11. Campen CJ, et al. Cranial irradiation increases risk of stroke in pediatric brain tumor survivors. Stroke. 2012;43(11):3035–40.
12. Ullrich NJ, et al. Moyamoya following cranial irradiation for primary brain tumors in children. Neurology. 2007;68(12):932–8.
13. Burn S, et al. Incidence of cavernoma development in children after radiotherapy for brain tumors. J Neurosurg. 2007;106(5 Suppl):379–83.
14. Price RA, Birdwell DA. The central nervous system in childhood leukemia. III. Mineralizing microangiopathy and dystrophic calcification. Cancer. 1978; 42(2):717–28.
15. Partap S, et al. Prolonged but reversible migraine-like episodes long after cranial irradiation. Neurology. 2006;66(7):1105–7.
16. Neglia JP, et al. Second malignant neoplasms in five-year survivors of childhood cancer: childhood cancer survivor study. J Natl Cancer Inst. 2001;93(8): 618–29.
17. Inskip PD, Curtis RE. New malignancies following childhood cancer in the United States, 1973–2002. Int J Cancer. 2007;121(10):2233–40.
18. Armstrong GT. Long-term survivors of childhood central nervous system malignancies: the experience of the Childhood Cancer Survivor Study. Eur J Paediatr Neurol. 2010;14(4):298–303.
19. Hijiya N, et al. Cumulative incidence of secondary neoplasms as a first event after childhood acute lymphoblastic leukemia. JAMA. 2007;297(11):1207–15.
20. Sobowale OA, et al. Radiotherapy-induced supratentorial primitive neuroectodermal tumour in a 17-year-old female: a case report and review of the literature. Acta Neurochir. 2011;153(2):413–7.
21. Borgmann A, et al. Secondary malignant neoplasms after intensive treatment of relapsed acute lymphoblastic leukaemia in childhood. Eur J Cancer. 2008; 44(2):257–68.
22. Sharif S, et al. Second primary tumors in neurofibromatosis 1 patients treated for optic glioma: substantial risks after radiotherapy. J Clin Oncol. 2006;24(16): 2570–5.
23. Group CSO, editor. Long-term follw-up guidelines for survivors of childhood, adolescent, and young adult cancers, version 3.0. Arcadia, CA: 2008 www.survivorshipguidelines.org
24. Wells EM, Gaillard WD, Packer RJ. Pediatric brain tumors and epilepsy. Semin Pediatr Neurol. 2012;19(1):3–8.
25. Sogawa Y, et al. The use of antiepileptic drugs in pediatric brain tumor patients. Pediatr Neurol. 2009;41(3):192–4.
26. Khan RB, et al. Seizures in children with primary brain tumors: incidence and long-term outcome. Epilepsy Res. 2005;64(3):85–91.
27. Packer RJ, et al. Long-term neurologic and neurosensory sequelae in adult survivors of a childhood brain tumor: childhood cancer survivor study. J Clin Oncol. 2003;21(17):3255–61.
28. Garces-Ambrossi GL, et al. Factors associated with progression-free survival and long-term neurological outcome after resection of intramedullary spinal cord tumors: analysis of 101 consecutive cases. J Neurosurg Spine. 2009;11(5):591–9.
29. Earl HM, et al. Long-term neurotoxicity of chemotherapy in adolescents and young adults treated for bone and soft tissue sarcomas. Sarcoma. 1998;2(2):97–105.
30. Lu Q, et al. Pain in long-term adult survivors of childhood cancers and their siblings: a report from the Childhood Cancer Survivor Study. Pain. 2011;152(11):2616–24.
31. Whelan K, et al. Auditory complications in childhood cancer survivors: a report from the childhood cancer survivor study. Pediatr Blood Cancer. 2011;57(1): 126–34.
32. Al-Khatib T, et al. Cisplatinum ototoxicity in children, long-term follow up. Int J Pediatr Otorhinolaryngol. 2010;74(8):913–9.

33. Mukherjea D, Rybak LP. Pharmacogenomics of cisplatin-induced ototoxicity. Pharmacogenomics. 2011;12(7):1039–50.

34. Ross CJ, et al. Genetic variants in TPMT and COMT are associated with hearing loss in children receiving cisplatin chemotherapy. Nat Genet. 2009;41(12):1345–9.

35. Hua C, et al. Hearing loss after radiotherapy for pediatric brain tumors: effect of cochlear dose. Int J Radiat Oncol Biol Phys. 2008;72(3):892–9.

36. Paulino AC, et al. Ototoxicity after intensity-modulated radiation therapy and cisplatin-based chemotherapy in children with medulloblastoma. Int J Radiat Oncol Biol Phys. 2010;78(5):1445–50.

37. Chen C, et al. Craniopharyngioma: a review of long-term visual outcome. Clin Experiment Ophthalmol. 2003;31(3):220–8.

38. Mulhern RK, et al. Social competence and behavioral adjustment of children who are long-term survivors of cancer. Pediatrics. 1989;83(1):18–25.

39. Byrne J, et al. Marriage and divorce after childhood and adolescent cancer. JAMA. 1989; 262(19):2693–9.

Neuropsychological Outcomes in Pediatric Brain Tumor Survivors

24

Laura Janzen, Donald Mabbott, and Sharon L. Guger

Introduction

Long-term survival of children with brain tumors has increased over recent decades due to important advances in diagnostics and treatment. Accordingly, attention has turned to the quality of survivorship for the ever-increasing population of pediatric brain tumor survivors (PBTS). Neuropsychological deficits are unfortunately common, with the majority of PBTS showing some form of deficit on formal psychological testing, varying from mild learning difficulties to severe impairment. These difficulties persist over time, and in adulthood, PBTS report the poorest health-related quality of life amongst childhood cancer survivors, secondary to neuropsychological and other treatment-related late effects [1]. Because neuropsychological deficits significantly impact the quality of life, psychosocial functioning, educational attainment, and employment status of PBTS, there is urgent need to identify and minimize these deficits in order to optimize functional outcomes.

Neuropsychological outcomes for individual PBTS are highly variable and depend on multiple, interrelated disease- and treatment-related variables, including characteristics of the tumor (histology, location), required neurosurgical interventions, and adjuvant therapy (chemotherapy and radiation). The manifestation of treatment effects is strongly related to the duration of time since treatment. Neuropsychological effects are moderated by the child's individual characteristics (age at diagnosis, sex, pre-morbid functioning, and genetics) and environmental factors. Targeted interventions may additionally influence long-term neuropsychological outcomes. Further, as the mechanisms of treatment-related neurotoxicity have been elucidated, the potential for risk-adapted treatments, neuroprotective agents, and strategies for neuronal repair has emerged, which could substantially reduce morbidity.

In general, isolating the effect of the myriad predictor variables on neuropsychological outcomes has been difficult. For example, tumor type and location typically dictate the modality and intensity of treatments. Likewise, brain tumors that present in infancy are often very aggressive and require more intensive treatment, making it difficult to disentangle the contribution of age at diagnosis and specific treatments to long-term neuropsychological function.

Despite challenges in attributing the neuropsychological deficits in PBTS to specific causes, a wealth of research has been generated over the past 40 years which has substantially increased our understanding of long-term neuropsychological outcomes. Much of this data has been produced by Canadian researchers, and wherever

L. Janzen, Ph.D. (✉) • D. Mabbott, B.A., M.A., Ph.D.
S.L. Guger, Ph.D.
Department of Psychology, The Hospital for Sick Children, Toronto, ON, Canada
e-mail: Laura.Janzen@sickkids.ca

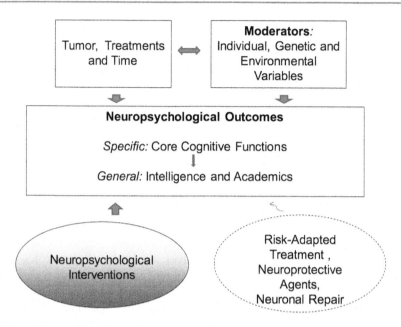

Fig. 24.1 Predictors of neuropsychological outcome in PBTS

possible their contributions are highlighted in this chapter. This accumulated research has led to the development of conceptual models of predictive variables that are related to neuropsychological outcome in PBTS (see Fig. 24.1). The model presented above, adapted from Palmer, 2008 and Askins and Moore, 2008 [2, 3], is used as a framework for this review. The specific and general neuropsychological deficits faced by PBTS are described, along with the predictor and moderating variables which are often interrelated. A review of evidence-based interventions is followed by a discussion of future directions for reducing neuropsychological morbidity and improving research efforts, care, and functional outcomes for survivors.

Neuropsychological Outcomes

There is considerable heterogeneity in individual neuropsychological outcomes for PBTS given the variety of tumor types and/or treatments and associated time and individual factors. As a result, no single neuropsychological phenotype exists. The severity of neuropsychological diffi-

culties experienced by PBTS may range from mild learning or attention difficulties that can be easily accommodated to severe limitations in intelligence and adaptive functioning which restrict independent living. Early research on neuropsychological outcomes of PBTS focused on general measures of intelligence because they were commonly measured in clinical practice, widely understood, and predictive of academic success. Indeed, certain subgroups of PBTS, such as children with medulloblastoma treated with cranial radiation, almost uniformly display intellectual deficits [4]. Likewise, academic achievement is frequently measured because of the significant educational needs of PBTS and the presumed ecological validity of academic performance measures [5].

However, intelligence scores represent a composite of multiple cognitive processes and sole reliance on such broad measures obfuscates more detailed analysis of brain/behavior relations. Similarly, academic performance is multifactorial and may be impacted by behavior, mood, fatigue, and school absences, in addition to cognition [5]. Core cognitive functions, on the other hand, are considered to be "purer" measures of neurocognition in PBTS. These functions, which include attention, processing speed, working memory, psychomotor skills, and new learning, underlie the ability to learn efficiently and retain information [6]. Across all brain tumor patients, core cognitive functions have been shown to be more adversely affected than global intelligence [7, 8], irrespective of treatment. Further, deficits in core cognitive functions have been shown to underlie failure make age-appropriate gains in intelligence and academic achievement [9].

In the largest published meta-analysis of studies of long-term neuropsychological effects in PTBS across all tumor types and locations, Robinson and colleagues [7] analyzed 39 empirical studies and found that relative to normative data, PBTS showed significant and pervasive deficits across a range of specific and general cognitive variables. The largest effect sizes were found for psychomotor skill, attention, visual-spatial skill, verbal memory, and language. Effect sizes for general intelligence and academic achievement were somewhat smaller in magnitude. In terms of their level of performance, PBTS performed almost a full standard deviation below normative level in overall intellectual ability.

Meta-analysis of neuropsychological outcomes in children with tumors of the posterior fossa, collapsing across tumor types and treatments, produced similar findings [8]. Data from 38 individual studies were analyzed and the magnitude of effects across all of the domains ranged from medium to large in size. Again, the largest effect sizes were found for the specific cognitive functions, including attention, psychomotor skill, executive function, and language. Effect sizes for general intelligence and academic achievement were in the moderate range. Age at diagnosis was a significant predictor of outcome; survivors diagnosed younger than 7 years of age showed significantly larger deficits than survivors diagnosed at an older age in the areas of overall cognitive ability, verbal intelligence, and nonverbal intelligence. With respect to their level of performance, children treated for posterior fossa tumors performed near or over a full standard deviation lower than age-matched peers on the specific and general cognitive domains assessed. Thus,

the research to date demonstrates that PBTS, particularly those with posterior fossa tumors who were treated with radiation, show deficits across multiple cognitive domains. Irrespective of the treatment type, core cognitive functions appear to be more vulnerable to disruption in PBTS and, in turn, these specific difficulties lead to declines in general intellectual and academic functioning.

Tumor, Treatments, and Time

Tumor Characteristics

The types and location of brain tumors that arise in childhood differ from those seen in adulthood. Specifically, children are more likely than adults to have primitive neuroectodermal tumors (PNETS), including medulloblastoma and pineoblastoma, choroid plexus tumors, and chiasmatic-hypothalamic gliomas. While supratentorial tumors predominate in adults, children are more likely to have infratentorial tumors. Although there have been conflicting findings, children with supratentorial and infratentorial tumors do not generally differ in overall intelligence, but the pattern of cognitive deficits differs. One study reported that across varying tumor types and with equivalent radiation dose, children with infratentorial tumors performed more poorly on selected measures of core cognitive functions, such as attention and working memory, and were more likely to be diagnosed with a learning disorder relative to survivors of supratentorial tumors, even when controlling for age at diagnosis [10]. As would be predicted based on the functional organization of the brain, tumors in the left hemisphere are associated with greater deficits in verbal and language domains, while midline tumors in the hypothalamic and pineal regions tend to be associated with deficits in declarative memory.

Midline tumors often block cerebrospinal fluid (CSF) flow, resulting in obstructive hydrocephalus which requires neurosurgical intervention. Hydrocephalus has been shown to be a strong predictor of long-term neuropsychological deficits. Specifically, increased severity of hydrocephalus at the time of diagnosis was related to lower intelligence in children with localized infratentorial ependymoma who were assessed prior to or during radiation therapy [11]. While treatment of hydrocephalus by shunting is associated with improved intellectual functioning in the short term, the presence of hydrocephalus severe enough to require shunting (pre- or posttreatment) is associated with poorer long-term intellectual outcomes in patients, regardless of tumor type [12].

Treatments

Surgery and Surgical Complications

While certain tumors, including many low-grade gliomas, require only neurosurgical intervention, this treatment is not necessarily neuropsychologically "benign." Mild intellectual and attention deficits are measurable after neurosurgical intervention but prior to adjuvant therapies [13]. Children with low-grade cerebellar astrocytomas treated only with neurosurgical resection displayed below normative-level performance on measures of general intelligence and academic and adaptive functioning at a mean of 103 days following surgery [14]. Similar results were reported for children who had surgical resections of midline or hemispheric low-grade gliomas; they displayed mild cognitive dysfunction relative to population norms when assessed an average of 111 days after surgery [15]. Cognitive dysfunction was greater in patients with left-hemisphere tumors relative to those with right-hemisphere tumors. Longitudinal studies are needed, however, to determine if there is natural recovery of function for PBTS treated with neurosurgical interventions alone or whether the deficits observed in the initial months following surgery persist.

Perioperative complications confer additional risks to neuropsychological functioning and tend to be more common in very young patients who are already more likely to experience long-term deficits. For example, cerebellar mutism syndrome (CMS) is a postsurgical complication that is seen in approximately 25 % of patients with posterior fossa tumors. The syndrome is characterized by diminished or absent speech, dysarthria, and linguistic difficulties. CMS is often accompanied by ataxia, hypotonia, and emotional lability. Children who develop CMS are more likely to be left handed and have unilateral, localized damage within the cerebello-thalamo-cerebral pathway at the level of the right cerebellum [16]. Disruption of this pathway is thought to interfere with communication between the posterior fossa and left frontal cortical regions that underlie language production [16]. CMS is also associated with increased long-term cognitive deficits compared to those without this complication. Children who develop CMS demonstrate significantly lower performance on measures of processing speed, attention, working memory, executive processes, cognitive efficiency, and academic performance in reading, spelling, and mathematics at one year post diagnosis relative to patients without CMS [17]. Other postoperative complications and infections, difficult-to-control seizures, and antiseizure medication also contribute to neuropsychological morbidity in PBTS.

Radiation

Radiation therapy is generally considered the most significant risk factor for long-term neuropsychological deficits; higher dose and volume of radiation are associated with poorer outcomes, particularly in young children. Children with posterior fossa tumors have been shown to display a 2- to 4-point decline per year in intelligence which is evident at 1 year posttreatment with rapid decline initially following treatment and more gradual decline thereafter [18]. Although there is individual variability in intellectual decline, losses of 25–30 full-scale IQ points are not uncommon and the majority of children treated with cranial radiation prior to 7 years of age require special education. However, much of the research on long-term radiation effects was done with children who received higher doses of radiation than are currently used (5,400 or 3,600 vs. 2,400 cGy craniospinal), and current radiation doses and delivery techniques may be less neurotoxic. Intellectual outcome has been reported to be less impacted in those patients treated with 2,400 cGy dose to the brain and spine [19]; however, this effect has not been observed consistently, leading to questions concerning other patient factors that may influence sensitivity to radiation.

Stereotactic conformal radiotherapy administered directly to the tumor and a margin of surrounding brain protects normal brain tissue and appears to reduce overall cognitive morbidity. Children with low-grade glioma or craniopharyngioma who were treated with conformal radiation therapy showed no decline in learning performance when assessed at a mean of 4–5 years following treatment [20]. Jalali and colleagues showed that conformal radiation administered to pediatric brain tumor patients was associated with clinically significant intelligence declines in one third of the overall sample [13]. In their sample, clinically significant decline in intelligence was associated with younger age at time of treatment and higher radiation dose to the left temporal lobe. Thus, relative to conventional radiation therapy, conformal radiation appears to result in cognitive sparing. However, there continues to be a need for long-term data on specific radiation doses to various brain regions and their associated cognitive outcomes.

Chemotherapy

Understanding the contribution of chemotherapy agents to long-term neuropsychological outcomes in PBTS is complicated as single chemotherapy agents are rarely given in isolation. There is vast literature detailing the neuropsychological effects of methotrexate, much of it in pediatric acute lymphoblastic leukemia (ALL) patients. Methotrexate depletes folate within the central nervous system (CNS) and neuropsychological impairments are related to both individual and cumulative methotrexate doses. For medulloblastoma patients, intrathecal methotrexate, in addition to a standard radiation therapy and chemotherapy protocol, was associated with increased neuropsychological deficits, particularly in those under 10 years of age [21]. Radiation therapy and intrathecal methotrexate seem to have a synergistic effect when combined, and it has been hypothesized that radiation therapy increases the permeability of the blood–brain barrier to neurotoxic chemotherapy.

More recently, methotrexate has been used with brain tumor patients under 3 years of age in an effort to avoid or delay radiation, with positive neuropsychological outcomes. For example, Rutkowski and colleagues reported on intellectual outcomes for 14 children with medulloblastoma diagnosed prior to age 3 years who were treated with chemotherapy-only protocol including intravenous chemotherapy and intraventricular methotrexate [22]. Average IQ at a mean of 5 years post diagnosis was significantly lower than healthy age-matched controls, but higher than historical medulloblastoma controls who received radiation therapy.

The Head Start II protocol utilized postsurgical high-dose chemotherapy followed by autologous hematopoietic cell transplantation to avoid or delay craniospinal radiation, and radiotherapy was required for a minority of patients (33 %). Patients less than 10 years of age at the time of diagnosis demonstrated low average intelligence and visual-motor integration at baseline (following completion of induction therapy, but prior transplant or radiation) [23]. Follow-up testing at a mean of 2.8 years later showed stable cognitive performance with average social-emotional and behavioral functioning. Increased time from diagnosis was associated with lower intelligence, poorer reading, and delayed verbal memory compared to patients more recently diagnosed. Because the full neuropsychological effects of this treatment may not have fully manifested, continued monitoring of this cohort is warranted. Nevertheless, chemotherapy-based protocols that attempt to avoid or delay radiation, particularly in young children, appear to be beneficial to preserving cognitive development.

Glucocorticoid steroids (e.g., prednisone and dexamethasone) are directly associated with acute neurobehavioral difficulties in children and longer-term memory difficulties. Other chemotherapy agents indirectly impact cognitive development and academic performance. Platinum-based chemotherapeutic agents such as cisplatin are ototoxic at higher doses and may induce irreversible, bilateral hearing loss.

Neuropsychological deficits, specifically in the language domains, are thought to be at least partially associated with hearing loss at an early age. Another example is vincristine-related neuropathy which may impact writing and other fine motor functions.

Mechanisms of Treatment-Related Neurotoxicity

Radiation therapy disrupts the protracted process of myelination within the brain, which normally begins prenatally and continues through childhood and adolescence. The resulting white-matter damage is directly related to the nature and severity of neuropsychological impairment. White matter is composed of glial cells that provide structural and physiological support within the CNS and insulate axons (myelin). The functional integrity of white matter is essential for cognitive efficiency as it facilitates the transmission of electrical signals along axons. Thus, glial cells play an important role in neural transmission and are also involved in neurogenesis. These cells are sensitive to treatment-related damage because they are rapidly proliferating.

Observed changes in brain tissue following radiation therapy involve glial atrophy, demyelination, white-matter-specific necrosis, and decline in normal-appearing white-matter volume [24]. Neuroimaging measures of white-matter tissue damage, particularly in prefrontal and frontal regions, predict poor attention [25] and intellectual functioning [26] following cranial radiation. Cranial radiation also has a detrimental impact on the growth of new neurons in the hippocampus [27] with decreased hippocampal volume related to deficits in declarative memory [28].

Time Since Treatment

Regardless of the treatment used, neuropsychological effects appear to be cumulative. The cognitive effects of radiation therapy are measureable as early as one year after treatment and there is continual decline until late adolescence, at which time anticipated age-related gains in cognition begin to plateau. While previously acquired skills and knowledge are retained, there is a slowing in the rate of new skill acquisition, resulting in a steadily increasing gap in performance between PBTS and age-matched peers. Based on a meta-analysis of 29 studies of intellectual and attentional functioning of PBTS across a range of tumor types, locations, and treatments, De Ruiter and colleagues reported that longer time since diagnosis was more highly predictive of overall IQ than either radiation or chemotherapy, accounting for 41 % of the total variance [29].

Moderators: Individual, Genetic, and Environmental Variables

Individual characteristics of the child and the environment may moderate relationships between disease- and treatment-related variables and neuropsychological outcomes. Age at the time of diagnosis is a well-established predictor; children diagnosed at a young age have historically shown poor neuropsychological outcomes. More recently, innovative treatment strategies have been introduced to delay or avoid the use of conventional cranial radiation in very young children (<3 years), resulting in improved neuropsychological outcomes [22]. For reasons not well understood, girls tend to display greater treatment-related neuropsychological impairment than boys, which may be associated with age-related sex differences in brain maturation.

The child's pre-morbid level of functioning is another important moderator of long-term outcomes. Children with above-average cognitive abilities at baseline (e.g., assessment within weeks of diagnosis) tend to show greater declines in standardized scores over time relative to children with lower baseline performance, presumably because they have "more to lose" [30]. Although the IQ point per year decline is typically higher in children with above-average baseline performance than those with lower performance, frank impairment in intellectual functioning in later years is less likely.

On the other end of the spectrum are those brain tumor patients with preexisting neurological or developmental conditions, such as neurofibromatosis type 1 (NF1) who may be at increased risk for developing treatment-related toxicities due to reduced "cognitive reserve" [31]. Identification of this subgroup is particularly important in order to direct early interventions and services.

Genetic variation has also been considered as an additional contributor to individual differences in neurotoxicity following chemotherapy and radiation and neuropsychological outcomes. Sensitivity to radiation-induced neurotoxicity may be mediated by a number of genes related to cellular repair and there is interest in polymorphisms in glutathione S-transferases (GSTs), which have been shown to predict adverse intellectual outcome in medulloblastoma patients [32]. Identifying genetic markers of susceptibility to radiation-induced brain injury may ultimately prove useful in stratifying patients to individualized radiotherapy strategies, brain protection and repair interventions, and targeted rehabilitation programs.

Family functioning interacts with neuropsychological variables to influence long-term outcomes for the survivor and other family members [33]. Neuropsychological difficulties may add to parental burden and general family stress, and in turn, family factors can impact the survivor's adjustment to acquired deficits. Higher socioeconomic status, availability of both parents, and maternal stress level and utilization of supports have been shown to be predictive of higher intelligence in long-term PBTS [34].

Interventions

Comprehensive neuropsychological evaluation is strongly recommended for all PBTS and is essential to characterize the nature and severity of late effects and to provide developmentally appropriate, individualized recommendations for interventions and accommodations. Specific recommendations for classroom-based interventions to support identified areas of need are commonly made following assessment. Supports are often compensatory and may address specific cognitive deficits and/or academic areas (e.g., additional

time to complete tasks or assignments due to slowed processing speed; use of assistive technology and appropriate software such as voice-to-text and/or text-to-voice; direct instruction in subject areas). However, classroom-based interventions (e.g., extra tutoring, audio books, use of a laptop) do not necessarily result in remediation of lagging skills or deficits. Parents of PBTS are often required to advocate for their child's educational and social needs, and parental adjustment, resources, and knowledge of neuropsychological late effects are required for effective advocacy.

Several evidence-based interventions have been examined in PBTS and survivors of other pediatric cancers, with varying degrees of success. Intensive prophylactic academic intervention offered shortly after cranial radiation holds promise for preserving academic skills that are particularly vulnerable (e.g., reading) in young children [35]. These results suggest that there may be a window of opportunity for skills-based intervention in the initial months following radiation before the late effects manifest. For long-term survivors who already display neuropsychological deficits, other approaches have been explored. Butler and Copeland developed a Cognitive Remediation Program (CRP) that incorporated attention training, special education strategies, and aspects of cognitive-behavioral therapy [36]. The results of a multicenter, randomized clinical trial of CRP used with 6–17-year survivors of childhood cancer resulted in modest gains for participants. The treatment was intense (20 two-hour weekly sessions) and lasted 4–5 months. While participants showed statistically significant improvement in academic achievement, used improved coping strategies, and were rated by parents as showing better attention, they did not differ from controls on measures of neuropsychological functioning. Whether these moderate intervention-related benefits were retained over time is unknown.

Because attention deficits are so prevalent in PBTS, pharmacological interventions targeting attention have also been explored. Based on the success of stimulant medication in treating attention and behavioral problems in children with attention-deficit/hyperactivity disorder (ADHD), trials were undertaken to determine the efficacy of stimulants in childhood cancer survivors. In a randomized, double-blind, placebo-controlled trial, methylphenidate (Ritalin) was associated with significantly greater improvement on measures of sustained attention in a group of childhood cancer survivors [37]. Changes in learning and memory, however, were not significant. Mulhern and colleagues reported improvements in parent and teacher ratings of attention and teacher-rated social skills in a sample of childhood cancer survivors who were administered methylphenidate in a randomized, double-blind placebo-controlled trial [38].

Donepezil, an acetylcholinesterase inhibitor, has also been investigated in a pediatric brain tumor sample based on the presumed role of the cholinergic system in neuronal differentiation and synapse formation [39]. In a single-institution open-label pilot study of 11 PBTS who had received radiation therapy, donepezil was associated with improvements in some aspects of executive functioning and memory; however, no differences on other core cognitive domains were found. Tolerability of the drug was problematic and 3 of the 11 patients dropped out of the study prior to completion.

Because pharmacological interventions may not be well tolerated by PBTS and intensive interventions in a clinic setting may not be feasible, other alternatives have been explored. Home-based, computerized cognitive training using the commercially available Cogmed system was found to be feasible and acceptable in a group of school-aged childhood cancer survivors with identified deficits in attention and/or working memory [40]. Using a randomized, controlled design, it was found that participants who complied with the treatment showed significant improvements in visual working memory relative to controls; the gains were maintained over three months following the intervention. It is notable that verbal working memory did not improve and the effect of the intervention on academic achievement and classroom performance were not evaluated. Thus, further work is needed to ascertain whether computer-administered interventions can impact daily functioning in a meaningful way.

Future Directions

With the advent of genomic stratification of tumors, there is potential for patients with genetically lower-risk disease to be treated less intensively, potentially preserving neuropsychological function. While risk-adapted treatments have been applied to medulloblastoma patients, the neuropsychological outcomes and potential for risk-adapted treatment for other tumor types remain to be seen. Another line of research has explored the potential of safe and efficacious neuroprotective agents. When administered prior to radiation or chemotherapy, such agents would guard healthy cerebral tissue from neurotoxicity by enhancing DNA repair and reducing cell death and neuroinflammation. Agents and activities that could be used following neurotoxic treatments to promote neural recovery are also being explored. Cell recovery may be achieved by stimulating the proliferation and/or differentiation of endogenous stem cells or progenitors through voluntary physical exercise, exposure to an enriched environment, and engagement in hippocampal-dependent learning activities. These novel interventions have potential for improving neuropsychological outcomes for PBTS.

Challenges

Despite the promise of novel treatments, interventions, and neural protection/recovery, there have been challenges in accurately identifying patients at highest risk for poor neuropsychological outcomes and providing them with timely, effective interventions. Because of the relatively small number of patients with each tumor type who receive comparable treatment, multicenter collaborative studies are needed to accrue sufficiently large samples to derive meaningful long-term outcome data. Similarly, in order to develop and test the efficacy of neuropsychological interventions, collaborative efforts are required to enroll adequate numbers of patients. Although the Children's Oncology Group (COG) offers a forum to initiate large international trials, there has recently been some success in Canada to carry out collaborative neuropsychological research through the C17, which represents all of the Canadian pediatric hematology, oncology, and stem cell transplant programs [9]. Future collaborative research is necessary to address the acute and ongoing neuropsychological needs of PBTS across the country and ensure equal access to interventions and services.

Longitudinal data which characterize the evolution of neuropsychological deficits from childhood to adulthood have been scarce. Assessment of very long-term neuropsychological outcomes has been challenging due to a loss of contact with patients as they transition from pediatric to adult medical care facilities, which typically occurs at 18 years of age in Canada. Collaborations between pediatric and adult medical and neuropsychology specialists will be necessary in order to follow PBTS into adulthood and identify whether they are at increased risk for pathological aging. Ensuring the continuity of neuropsychological care into adulthood is therefore another important challenge that must be addressed.

Conclusions

Neuropsychological dysfunction is one of the most debilitating potential late effects for PBTS. Children live much longer than adults with the morbidities associated with their disease and treatment. Considerable advances have been made in effectively treating pediatric brain tumors while minimizing neurotoxic effects. At the same time, various interventions offer some promise of reducing or ameliorating neuropsychological sequelae for future PTBS. Knowledge about risk factors and their combined effects helps to identify subgroups of children at highest risk of poor neuropsychological outcomes who require early and intensive interventions.

References

1. Zeltzer LK, Recklitis C, Buchbinder D, Zebrack B, Casillas J, Tsao JC, et al. Psychological status in childhood cancer survivors: a report from the Childhood Cancer Survivor Study. J Clin Oncol. 2009;27(14):2396–404.
2. Palmer SL. Neurodevelopmental impact on children treated for medulloblastoma: a review and proposed conceptual model. Dev Disabil Res Rev. 2008; 14(3):203–10.
3. Askins MA, Moore 3rd BD. Preventing neurocognitive late effects in childhood cancer survivors. J Child Neurol. 2008;23(10):1160–71.
4. Dennis M, Spiegler BJ, Hetherington CR, Greenberg ML. Neuropsychological sequelae of the treatment of children with medulloblastoma. J Neurooncol. 1996;29(1):91–101.
5. Mabbott DJ, Spiegler BJ, Greenberg ML, Rutka JT, Hyder DJ, Bouffet E. Serial evaluation of academic and behavioral outcome after treatment with cranial radiation in childhood. J Clin Oncol. 2005;23(10):2256–63.
6. Mabbott DJ, Rovet J, Noseworthy MD, Smith ML, Rockel C. The relations between white matter and declarative memory in older children and adolescents. Brain Res. 2009;1294:80–90.
7. Robinson KE, Kuttesch JF, Champion JE, Andreotti CF, Hipp DW, Bettis A, et al. A quantitative meta-analysis of neurocognitive sequelae in survivors of pediatric brain tumors. Pediatr Blood Cancer. 2010;55(3):525–31.
8. Robinson KE, Fraley CE, Pearson MM, Kuttesch Jr JF, Compas BE. Neurocognitive late effects of pediatric brain tumors of the posterior fossa: a quantitative review. J Int Neuropsychol Soc. 2013;19(1):44–53.
9. Mabbott DJ, Penkman L, Witol A, Strother D, Bouffet E. Core neurocognitive functions in children treated for posterior fossa tumors. Neuropsychology. 2008; 22(2):159–68.
10. Patel SK, Mullins WA, O'Neil SH, Wilson K. Neuropsychological differences between survivors of supratentorial and infratentorial brain tumours. J Intellect Disabil Res. 2011;55(1):30–40.
11. Merchant TE, Lee H, Zhu J, Xiong X, Wheeler G, Phipps S, et al. The effects of hydrocephalus on intelligence quotient in children with localized infratentorial ependymoma before and after focal radiation therapy. J Neurosurg. 2004;101(2 Suppl):159–68.
12. Reimers TS, Ehrenfels S, Mortensen EL, Schmiegelow M, Sonderkaer S, Carstensen H, et al. Cognitive deficits in long-term survivors of childhood brain tumors: identification of predictive factors. Med Pediatr Oncol. 2003;40(1):26–34.
13. Jalali R, Mallick I, Dutta D, Goswami S, Gupta T, Munshi A, et al. Factors influencing neurocognitive outcomes in young patients with benign and low-grade brain tumors treated with stereotactic conformal radiotherapy. Int J Radiat Oncol Biol Phys. 2010;77(4):974–9.
14. Beebe DW, Ris MD, Armstrong FD, Fontanesi J, Mulhern R, Holmes E, et al. Cognitive and adaptive

outcome in low-grade pediatric cerebellar astrocytomas: evidence of diminished cognitive and adaptive functioning in National Collaborative Research Studies (CCG 9891/POG 9130). J Clin Oncol. 2005;23(22):5198–204.

15. Ris MD, Beebe DW, Armstrong FD, Fontanesi J, Holmes E, Sanford RA, et al. Cognitive and adaptive outcome in extracerebellar low-grade brain tumors in children: a report from the Children's Oncology Group. J Clin Oncol. 2008;26(29):4765–70.

16. Law N, Greenberg M, Bouffet E, Taylor MD, Laughlin S, Strother D, et al. Clinical and neuroanatomical predictors of cerebellar mutism syndrome. Neuro Oncol. 2012;14(10):1294–303.

17. Palmer SL, Hassall T, Evankovich K, Mabbott DJ, Bonner M, Deluca C, et al. Neurocognitive outcome 12 months following cerebellar mutism syndrome in pediatric patients with medulloblastoma. Neuro Oncol. 2010;12(12):1311–7.

18. Spiegler BJ, Bouffet E, Greenberg ML, Rutka JT, Mabbott DJ. Change in neurocognitive functioning after treatment with cranial radiation in childhood. J Clin Oncol. 2004;22(4):706–13.

19. Grill J, Renaux VK, Bulteau C, Viguier D, Levy-Piebois C, Sainte-Rose C, et al. Long-term intellectual outcome in children with posterior fossa tumors according to radiation doses and volumes. Int J Radiat Oncol Biol Phys. 1999;45(1):137–45.

20. Di Pinto M, Conklin HM, Li C, Merchant TE. Learning and memory following conformal radiation therapy for pediatric craniopharyngioma and low-grade glioma. Int J Radiat Oncol Biol Phys. 2012;84(3):e363–9.

21. Riva D, Giorgi C, Nichelli F, Bulgheroni S, Massimino M, Cefalo G, et al. Intrathecal methotrexate affects cognitive function in children with medulloblastoma. Neurology. 2002;59(1):48–53.

22. Rutkowski S, Bode U, Deinlein F, Ottensmeier H, Warmuth-Metz M, Soerensen N, et al. Treatment of early childhood medulloblastoma by postoperative chemotherapy alone. N Engl J Med. 2005;352(10):978–86.

23. Sands SA, Oberg JA, Gardner SL, Whiteley JA, Glade-Bender JL, Finlay JL. Neuropsychological functioning of children treated with intensive chemotherapy followed by myeloablative consolidation chemotherapy and autologous hematopoietic cell rescue for newly diagnosed CNS tumors: an analysis of the Head Start II survivors. Pediatr Blood Cancer. 2010;54(3):429–36.

24. Reddick WE, Glass JO, Palmer SL, Wu S, Gajjar A, Langston JW, et al. Atypical white matter volume development in children following craniospinal irradiation. Neuro Oncol. 2005;7(1):12–9.

25. Mulhern RK, White HA, Glass JO, Kun LE, Leigh L, Thompson SJ, et al. Attentional functioning and white matter integrity among survivors of malignant brain tumors of childhood. J Int Neuropsychol Soc. 2004; 10(2):180–9.

26. Mabbott DJ, Noseworthy MD, Bouffet E, Rockel C, Laughlin S. Diffusion tensor imaging of white matter after cranial radiation in children for medulloblastoma: correlation with IQ. Neuro Oncol. 2006;8(3):244–52.

27. Monje ML, Vogel H, Masek M, Ligon KL, Fisher PG, Palmer TD. Impaired human hippocampal neurogenesis after treatment for central nervous system malignancies. Ann Neurol. 2007;62(5):515–20.

28. Nagel BJ, Delis DC, Palmer SL, Reeves C, Gajjar A, Mulhern RK. Early patterns of verbal memory impairment in children treated for medulloblastoma. Neuropsychology. 2006;20(1):105–12.

29. de Ruiter MA, van Mourik R, Schouten-van Meeteren AY, Grootenhuis MA, Oosterlaan J. Neurocognitive consequences of a paediatric brain tumour and its treatment: a meta-analysis. Dev Med Child Neurol. 2013;55(5):408–17.

30. Palmer SL, Gajjar A, Reddick WE, Glass JO, Kun LE, Wu S, et al. Predicting intellectual outcome among children treated with 35-40 Gy craniospinal irradiation for medulloblastoma. Neuropsychology. 2003; 17(4):548–55.

31. Dennis M, Spiegler BJ, Hetherington R. New survivors for the new millennium: cognitive risk and reserve in adults with childhood brain insults. Brain Cogn. 2000;42(1):102–5.

32. Barahmani N, Carpentieri S, Li XN, Wang T, Cao Y, Howe L, et al. Glutathione S-transferase M1 and T1 polymorphisms may predict adverse effects after therapy in children with medulloblastoma. Neuro Oncol. 2009;11(3):292–300.

33. Peterson CC, Drotar D. Family impact of neurodevelopmental late effects in survivors of pediatric cancer: review of research, clinical evidence, and future directions. Clin Child Psychol Psychiatry. 2006; 11(3):349–66.

34. Carlson-Green B, Morris RD, Krawiecki N. Family and illness predictors of outcome in pediatric brain tumors. J Pediatr Psychol. 1995;20(6):769–84.

35. Penkman L, Scott-Lane L. Prophylactic academic intervention for children treated with cranial radiation therapy. Dev Neurorehabil. 2007;10(1):19–26.

36. Butler RW, Copeland DR, Fairclough DL, Mulhern RK, Katz ER, Kazak AE, et al. A multicenter, randomized clinical trial of a cognitive remediation program for childhood survivors of a pediatric malignancy. J Consult Clin Psychol. 2008;76(3): 367–78.

37. Thompson SJ, Leigh L, Christensen R, Xiong X, Kun LE, Heideman RL, et al. Immediate neurocognitive effects of methylphenidate on learning-impaired survivors of childhood cancer. J Clin Oncol. 2001;19(6): 1802–8.

38. Mulhern RK, Khan RB, Kaplan S, Helton S, Christensen R, Bonner M, et al. Short-term efficacy of methylphenidate: a randomized, double-blind, placebo-controlled trial among survivors of childhood cancer. J Clin Oncol. 2004;22(23):4795–803.

39. Castellino SM, Tooze JA, Flowers L, Hill DF, McMullen KP, Shaw EG, et al. Toxicity and efficacy of the acetylcholinesterase (AChe) inhibitor donepezil in childhood brain tumor survivors: a pilot study. Pediatr Blood Cancer. 2012;59(3):540–7.

40. Hardy KK, Willard VW, Allen TM, Bonner MJ. Working memory training in survivors of pediatric cancer: a randomized pilot study. Psychooncology. 2013;22(8):1856–65.

Quality of Life

25

Annie-Jade Pépin, Anne-Sophie Carret,
and Serge Sultan

Introduction

Quality of life (QoL) is a complex concept. To save life is an essential objective in medicine, but to achieve this goal, we often must make a compromise between prolonging an individual's life and fostering an optimal quality of life. In pediatric oncology and more specifically in neuro-oncology, the morbidity associated to short-term and long-term effects of treatments is a major concern and may affect significantly the QoL. Central questions can also be raised within this field and could include: What are the effects of aggressive treatments which are intensive and prolonged in nature, on the quality of life of these patients? What is the long-term quality of life of these patients and survivors? This chapter is based on research evidence, which comes primarily from reports of the *Childhood Cancer Survivor Studies* [1, 2]. According to Canadian Cancer Statistics, pediatric brain tumors are the second most common type of childhood cancer,

after acute leukemias and the most common solid tumors. Central nervous system tumors are the most common cause of death among all childhood cancers. While some types of brain tumors carry dismal prognosis, others have better prognosis. Over the past decades, the number of childhood brain tumor survivors and life expectancy has increased with the advances in medicine, the new therapeutic approach, the new technologies, and the improvements in supportive care [3]. This phenomenon raises the question of long-term effects of cancer and its treatments on QoL of patients and survivors. Several parameters affect survivors of childhood brain tumors in their daily activities. Alterations within physical, cognitive, and psychological abilities can have consequences on psychological, academic, professional, family, and social levels for the survivors [1, 3, 4]. Studies have reported that 25–93 % of childhood brain tumors survivors suffer from clinically significant distress [3]. Moreover, recent research has shown that about 80 % of these survivors will have long-term sequelae due to the tumor and its treatment. Research reports neurocognitive dysfunction in 90 % of glioma patients, memory problems in 78 %, and attention difficulties in 60 % of cases. These aspects have a pervasive impact with more than 20 % of adult survivors of childhood brain tumors experiencing difficulties in their daily life activities [5]. Physical and cognitive long-term sequelae limit significantly the ability of survivors to find a job [3]: 26 % adults survivors

A.-J. Pépin, Ph.D. • S. Sultan, Ph.D. (✉)
Department of Hematology/Oncology,
CHU Sainte-Justine, Université de Montréal,
Montréal, QC, Canada
e-mail: serge.sultan@umontreal.ca

A.-S. Carret, M.D.
Department of Pediatrics, Division of Hematology/
Oncology, CHU Sainte-Justine/Université de Montréal,
Montréal, QC, Canada

K. Scheinemann and E. Bouffet (eds.), *Pediatric Neuro-oncology*,
DOI 10.1007/978-1-4939-1541-5_25, © Springer Science+Business Media New York 2015

of childhood brain tumor remain unemployed, compared to less than 8 % in a control group of healthy individuals [1]. Similarly, only 26 % of adult survivors of childhood brain tumors complete postsecondary education, and 31 % manage to have full-time employment [3]. Psychological and social disturbances can also make it difficult for survivors to form and take care of a family; 74 % adult survivors of childhood brain tumors were single 5 years after initial diagnosis [1]. All these consequences are significant barriers to an individual's QoL in the long term. The issue of QoL in brain tumor is thus most important during and after treatment. However, despite the importance of the aforementioned effects, the long-term psychosocial of childhood brain tumors still remain poorly known [5].

Factors Related to the Tumor and Treatments

In pediatric oncology, the diagnosis of brain tumor comes with the lowest predictive QoL. For example, Wu et al. (2007) studied the QoL in adolescents with different types of cancer, as well as survivors, using the Minneapolis-Manchester Quality of Life Adolescent Questionnaire (MMQL-AF) [6]. Adolescents who had a brain tumor and adolescents who have leukemia obtained the lowest QoL levels, compared to patients with lymphomas and other solid tumors types. It is very likely that the QoL of these patients is reduced due to developmental and neurocognitive deficits caused by the tumor and its treatment. The localization of the tumor, the type of lesion, and the tumor volume have an impact on the neurocognitive deficits [2]. In the long term, the development of the child may be affected in terms of motor functions, cognition, or social skills. One study has also demonstrated a link between QoL and the health status of this population [7]. However, it is likely that the QoL of these children and survivors is impacted differently depending on the specific type of brain tumor and the type of treatment received. Thus, the number and nature of the physical, cognitive, and developmental deficits caused by the tumor also influ-

ence the long-term QoL of these patients [2]. However, with the current state of knowledge, it is not possible to distinguish the specific effect of cancer or its treatments on QoL dimensions.

As mentioned, the location of the tumor has an impact on the long-term sequelae and the QoL. For example, damage to the right hemisphere may result in visuospatial and visuo-perceptual deficits, while patients with tumors in the left hemisphere may have verbal, memory, language, and intellectual difficulties [8]. Alteration of personality, social judgment, deficits in executive functions (planning, logical reasoning, working memory, abstract thinking, selective attention, etc.), decreased tolerance to frustration, and decreased capacity to work are difficulties encountered by patients with frontal tumors [8]. All these changes in physical, psychological, or social functioning undermine the QoL of the patient and his or her rehabilitation [8]. Tumors located in the fourth ventricle and the posterior fossa were significantly associated with greater fatigue and weakness in the arms and legs, which might interfere with certain activities or social development, contributing to a lower QoL [9]. Similarly, infratentorial tumors were associated with a lower QoL compared to supratentorial tumors [7]. The same authors reported a correlation between the presence of hydrocephalus in children with brain tumors and a lower QoL score. Interestingly, this study did not report a significant difference in QoL between high-grade and low-grade tumors.

The type of treatment received can also have an impact on the QoL, as well as the intensity and the duration of the treatments. Chemotherapy and radiotherapy can have negative effects on the brain development of children with brain tumors and may influence their long-term QoL [7, 10]. For example, one study has shown that radiotherapy is a predictor of poorer QoL, as measured by the physical, emotional, and social dimensions of the Pediatric Quality of Life Scale (PedsQL) (with multiple standardized association coefficient between 4.42 and 9.41) [11]. These results are confirmed when quality of life is measured with the MMQL [9]. In comparison, the standardized coefficients associated with the effect of intensive chemotherapy ranged from 7.65 to

15.06 for the three dimensions of QoL [11]. According to another study, radiotherapy has been identified as a predictor of a poor QoL due to its long-term effects on the intellectual level [9]. A study has shown that childhood brain tumor survivors who were treated solely with radiotherapy had a poorer QoL five years post-treatment, as measured with the PedsQL4.0 self-report, compared to children treated with chemotherapy or a combination of chemotherapy and radiotherapy [10]. Overall, these results demonstrate the significant impact of chemotherapy and radiotherapy on an individual's QoL. It is impossible to ascribe the observed deficits to a specific treatment, due to the diversity of other risk factors, the frequent combination of treatment modalities, and the complexity of some cases. These observed deficits are either cognitive (memory loss, reduced attention, and speed of cognitive processes), emotional (anxiety and depression), or physical (fatigue, pain, decreased physical functions, motor deficits) [7, 10]. Adjuvant treatments can also have effects on the QoL of patients and survivors. For example, glucocorticoids, such as dexamethasone, can cause memory difficulties and emotional disturbances, such as depressive or maniac feelings and emotional lability [2]. Research on the short- and long-term effects of brain tumor treatments needs to better distinguish the individual impact of each treatment (radiotherapy, chemotherapy, adjuvant treatments) on the components of the QoL of patients and survivors.

Definition of QoL

Although sometimes mixed, QoL is distinct from health status. Health status refers to the biological and physiological components of the health of an individual and their functional abilities [8]. In the context of illness, health status is largely defined by the physical and physiological symptoms, as well as functional impairments caused by the illness [8]. The concept of QoL encompasses physical, psychological, and social aspects of an individual. QoL does not only consider the physical and functional impact of the illness but also the impacts on the psychological functioning of the individual, such as one's emotional states and social functioning. While health status is an objective measure, QoL is a subjective measure, because the individual is asked to evaluate the quality of his or her life. This is why it is also referred to as "perceived quality of life" or "subjective quality of life."

According to the World Health Organization (WHO), quality of life is defined as the "individual's perception of their position in life, in the context of the culture and value systems in which they live and in relation to their goals, expectations, standards and concerns" [12]. Niv and Kreitler (2001) identified six major characteristics specific to the concept of QoL in the context of pediatric oncology (see Table 25.1). (1) Quality of life is a subjective concept which is assessed by the person himself or herself, according to their personal standards of what they consider to be a good quality of life [13]. Based on this characteristic, the individual is the most reliable source for measuring his or her own QoL; henceforth, QoL should be primarily measured by self-reported instruments [13]. (2) QoL is phenomenological in nature; the QoL measure is a portrait of the QoL of the individual at the time when it is measured, like a picture of the well-being of that individual at that precise moment [13]. This suggests that the QoL measure cannot assess the causes and history of QoL phenomenon, but only measures the current state of QoL. This characteristic also suggests that QoL changes with time. (3) QoL can be assessed either preferably by the individual himself or herself, as mentioned above, or by a third party, and there are several methods to evaluate it [13]. (4) QoL is a dynamic phenomenon, meaning that it is sensitive to changes in the state of the individual, both psychological (emotional, cognitive) and physical changes [13]. QoL can also change as a function of the individual situation and external changes that the individual is confronted with. (5) QoL consists of several broad areas including subdimensions, such as pain or emotions [13]. (6) QoL is quantifiable; thus, it is possible to assign a score to measure the QoL, and it is possible

Table 25.1 The characteristics of quality of life

Characteristic	Definition
1. Subjective	QoL is an individual perception and the only reliable source for evaluation—it is the person itself
2. Phenomenological	QoL is perceived. It is like a photograph, and it does not permit to obtain clues about causes of the level of QoL
3. Evaluative	QoL can be evaluated
4. Dynamic	QoL is a phenomenon in continuous evolution and is influenced by any changes from the person himself or herself or in his or her environment
5. Multidimensional	QoL is based on several life domains and its measurement calls for several dimensions
6. Quantifiable	QoL can be measured and represented by a score. QoL can be compared across the development of a given individual or between different individuals

Adapted from Kreitler S., Kreitler M.M. Quality of Life in Children with Cancer. In: Kreitler S., Ben-Arush M.W., Martin, A. Pediatric Psycho-oncology: Psychosocial Aspects and Clinical Interventions, 2ed. Oxford, UK: John Willey & Sons, Ltd. 2012. p. 18-31. With permission from John Wiley & Sons, Inc

to compare different QoL scores between different individuals [13]. These characteristics show that QoL is a complex area where there are significant challenges including measurement issues.

Dimensions of QoL

A general consensus has been reached by authors in regard to the three dimensions that include most aspects of QoL: physical functioning, psychological functioning, and social functioning. However, many authors define more specific dimensions. For example, the WHO has identified six respective dimensions for QoL [12].

These dimensions integrate the concepts of health status and subjective QoL:

1. Physical health. This consists of aspects of physical energy, fatigue, pain, and sleep.
2. Psychological aspect. This includes emotions, thoughts, memory, concentration, self-esteem, and the appreciation of physical appearance.
3. Level of independence. This is determined by mobility, ability to perform daily activities, dependence on medical care, and the ability to work.
4. Social relationships. This includes social support and sexual relationships.
5. Environment. This includes financial aspects, security, health care, and other aspects related to the individual's environment.
6. Spirituality, religion, and personal beliefs [12].

Empirical findings in pediatric oncology have shown that the QoL of children is based on (1) the child's symptoms, (2) the level of participation in usual activities, (3) social and family interactions, (4) physical health, as well as (5) emotions and (6) the perception of being ill [14]. These results come from two pilot studies. The first had a cross-sectional design, and the sample included 23 patients who were between 8 and 15 years of age. The second, a longitudinal study with four times of assessment spanning over 2 years, included 13 patients who were 10–18 years old [14]. Both studies were conducted according to a semistructured interview consisting of four questions defined by the researchers ("What makes a good day for you? What makes a bad day for you? Are there some things you like to do that you cannot do now? How has being sick been for you?"), and participants' responses were analyzed using a semantic-content method [14]. This study also showed that the definition of QoL differs depending on whether you ask the children or caregivers, which thereby confirms the need to interview key stakeholders.

Methods: Who Should be the Respondent?

Who is the best person to determine the QoL of an individual? In the context of pediatric neuro-oncology, it is often inevitable that the QoL of the child is rated by a third party, preferably by one of the parents, given the child's suffering and physical and cognitive difficulties related to their illness. Some major questions arise and this raises ethical issues. Is self-reported QoL equivalent to the assessment of QoL by a third party?

To what extent can a parent's assessment of their child's QoL replace the child's own self-reported QoL? Such questions are particularly relevant in neuro-oncology where the ability to respond to verbal material is not always guaranteed. There are two opposing positions on this issue. On the one hand, some researchers attribute a great deal of importance to the individual and subjective nature of QoL and suggest that the child is the best source to evaluate their own QoL, and parental assessments can never replace that of the child [8]. This is why some questionnaires were developed to allow the child to respond in a practical, nonverbal manner (cf. PedsQL preschool version).

On the other hand, other researchers are skeptical about the reliability of self-report measures that are reported by a child, and they perceive the child as being limited in their ability to understand and report their own well-being [8]. Within this framework, the proposed solution is the assessment of the QoL by a third party, preferably the parents or person responsible for the child. This is referred to as a "proxy" [8]. In this way, the point of view of the parent would be perceived as more reliable, valid, and objective than that of the child. However, the assessment of QoL by a third party suggests that the evaluator has the ability to put themselves in the place of the child in order to capture the thoughts and emotions of the child so that they can report the child's perception of QoL and the impact of the illness in their life. This calls on sophisticated skills and a good knowledge of the child's perception of himself or herself. Everyone does not have these abilities, which are necessary in the evaluation of the QoL of the child. This is why, whenever possible, it is recommended to assess the QoL of the child using questionnaires reported by the child himself or herself *and* by the parent. In this way, the two viewpoints are considered, and issues with both methods may be taken into account.

Studies assessing the QoL of children with cancer using self-report and parent-report versions allow for observation of the differences between child and parent reports. Parents generally tend to report higher scores on distress, suffering, and deficits than the child himself or herself [8, 15]. A systematic review measuring the QoL of children with chronic illness, which differentiated between self-reports and parent reports, observed that the areas related to physical functioning, such as physical activity, symptoms, and physical complaints, are evaluated similarly by parents and children, while areas affecting psychological and social dimensions, such as emotions, autonomy, appearance, communication, and mood, give rise to more discrepancies between respondents [15]. Questions regarding physical functioning have correlational effects of $r \geq 0.50$ between self-reports and parent reports, while questions on psychological and social domains result in lower correlations $r < 0.30$ [15]. This suggests that it will be more difficult for parents to accurately assess psychological and social aspects of their child than to assess physical functioning, which is probably more easily observable. Some researchers also speculate that parents tend to project their own distress and symptoms in their assessment of the QoL of their child, reporting a lower perceived QoL for their child than it is in reality. However, this has not been shown systematically yet. A study that assessed psychological functioning of adolescents with brain tumors using self-report, parent-report, and teacher-report versions of the Behavioral Assessment System for Children (BASC) obtained significant differences between QoL scores of different respondents [16]. For the depression dimension, 7 % of adolescents reported a clinically significant score compared to 16 % when considering parent reports and 10 % in teacher reports. For the anxiety measure, 3 % of adolescents report a clinically significant score, while the parents and teachers reports were 12 % and 19 %, respectively [16]. These results demonstrate that there is a substantial difference between the QoL perception of the child assessed by the child himself or herself and that perceived by the parent or a third party, such as a teacher.

Method: What is Response Shift?

The assessment of QoL raises another issue related to adjustment to health status across time. This adaptation is referred to as *response shift*. Response shift is defined as a change in the way in which an individual evaluates his or her own QoL [17]. This change in attitude is the result of a change in the three aspects of the QoL perception of the individual. It can affect (1) the individual's internal standards, (2) personal values, and (3) the conceptualization of QoL over time [17]. In fact, the evaluation of QoL with questionnaires is based on standards, standards of what constitutes a "good" QoL according to the authors of the test, and standards that participants refer to in evaluating their own QoL [17]. An individual who is treated for an illness, refers to his or her life before illness, refers to his or her life before, more or less prescriptively, in order to determine his or her current QoL. The response shift phenomenon is especially present in long-term follow-up in stable conditions, such as remitted cancer. With time, some individuals compare their current QoL to the QoL they had during their treatments, which in turn leads to assess their QoL as better than it was during their treatment. It is a process of reassessing their own personal standards. Response shift may explain the results of some studies in which participants with brain tumors or brain tumor survivors evaluate their QoL as good or sometimes better than the control group of healthy individuals even though their health status has deteriorated [6, 9, 16]. Among these studies, that of Nathan et al., (2007) evaluates the QoL of adult survivors of neuroblastomas and Wilms' tumors in childhood [2]. The results of this study indicate that the QoL of survivors does not differ from that of the normative population. However, these counterintuitive results on the QoL of brain tumors survivors are found in a limited number of studies, compared to the numerous studies demonstrating a poorer QoL in this population. If QoL is used as an important outcome in treatment, it is necessary to take the response shift phenomenon into account. This can be measured with different methods and is grouped into six types of mea-

sures. First, response shift can be measured using an *individualized method*, which integrates the perception and feedback of the patient on his or her definition of QoL, and it includes interviews or paper-and-pencil questionnaires [17]. Second, the *preference-based* method focuses on the importance and the value attributed to the patient's state of health and its various dimensions through the use of questionnaires. Third, the *successive comparison* approach is used to evaluate the patient's judgment on the order of importance of different psychological, physical, and social concepts. These concepts are scored on a continuum, and it must be ordered according to the value the patient attributes to them. Fourth, the *design* approach measures the response shift with questionnaires on the patient's retrospective perception of changes in their standards, ideals, and values perceived after treatment, compared with those before the diagnosis. Fifth, the *statistical* approach evaluates longitudinal data on the QoL of patients in order to observe the evolution of response shift [17]. Finally, the last approach is the *qualitative* method for assessing the response shift, and this involves using semistructured interviews. To our knowledge, this phenomenon has not been systematically studied in pediatric oncology. Future advances in the assessment of response shift will account for this phenomenon in measuring QoL of cancer survivors in order to study the adaptive and nonadaptive long-term implications of response shift. This is a central issue in the use of QoL as a long-term outcome in oncology. In children, the analysis of response shift will also be complicated by developmental changes.

Methods for Quality of Life Measurement

There are different ways to assess QoL in children. Cremeens et al. conducted a literature review of QoL measures in children between 3 and 8 years of age [18]. Some of these measures have been used in pediatric neuro-oncology. Four different formats of QoL instruments were identified and included questionnaires or Likert-based scales, graphical measures, measures based on facial expressions including photographs, cartoons, and visual measures based on a visual, linear scale of QoL [18]. Despite children's difficulties in responding to those questionnaires, the QoL of children is currently primarily evaluated using questionnaires based on Likert-type scales [18]. There are several QoL questionnaires, some of which are generic in nature. Others are specific to pediatric oncology populations. Table 25.2 presents five QoL instruments that have been used in pediatric oncology. References of these five instruments are in Table 25.2. To date, only the PedsQL Brain Tumor Module has been validated specifically with a neuro-oncology population of children. The other instruments have been used in pediatric oncology, but have not been developed for children with cancer.

The Pediatric Quality of Life Inventory Brain Tumor Module is a specific instrument for populations of children with brain tumors. There is a version for parents and one for the patients; both versions have 24 items, respectively. The internal consistency of the different dimensions has ranged from adequate to excellent. The sample used for the validation study of the PedsQL Brain Tumor Module consisted of 51 patients with brain tumors between the ages of 2 and 18. Next, the Pediatric Quality of Life Inventory 3.0 Cancer Module (PedsQL 3.0 Cancer Module) is a 27-item general questionnaire for pediatric cancer patients, with a self-report version and a proxy-report version. The validation study was made with childhood cancer patients, aged between 2 and 18 years (24 of them had brain tumor), compared with healthy children of same range of age. Self-report's internal consistency is adequate and proxy report's internal consistency is good. The third questionnaire is the Minneapolis-Manchester Quality of Life questionnaire (MMQL) which comes in two versions, one for children aged 8–12 (Youth Form; MMQL-YF, 32 items) and one for adolescents aged 13–20 years (Adolescent Form; MMQL-AF, 47 items). The MMQL-YF has adequate internal consistency. The sample for the validation study of the MMQL-YF was children with cancer between 8 and 13 years of age, and of these

children, 12 of them were diagnosed with a brain tumor. The version for adolescents (MMQL-AF) has three additional dimensions: cognitive functioning, self-esteem, and intimate relationships. This version has 47 items. Consistency varied depending on the particular dimension; however, these coefficients ranged from adequate to good. Temporal stability correlation coefficients are adequate over 2 weeks. The validation study of MMQL-AF was conducted with a sample of adolescents with cancer, of which 16 had a brain tumor. The fifth instrument, the Pediatric Oncology Quality of Life Scale (POQOL), was developed specifically for the pediatric oncology population. The 21-item questionnaire must be completed by the parents and has good internal consistency. The validation study was conducted with a sample of children with various types of cancer.

Psychological Aspect of QoL

In the context of cancer, the interaction between the three areas—physical, psychological, and social—is particularly important in enabling the adjustment of the individual faced with the illness and in ensuring their rehabilitation afterwards. Throughout the illness, the psychological state of the patient will vary according to the stages of treatment. In the context of pediatric neuro-oncology, the psychological dimension is also very important, since some personality traits and mood are affected by the tumor and its treatments. Research-based data suggests that psychological distress can persist even after the illness. On average, 25–93 % of children and adults survivors of childhood brain tumors live with significant psychological distress and adjustment difficulties [3]. In children, psychological distress can be expressed in several different ways, by internalized symptoms, such as depression, anxiety, and somatization, and by externalized symptoms, such as antisocial behavior, impulsivity, aggression, and deviance. Among survivors of brain tumors, internalized symptoms are better studied in the literature than externalized symptoms.

Table 25.2 Instrument used to assess QoL in pediatric neuro-oncology

Measure	Domains	Target	Respondents	Number of items	Population used for testing	Psychometric properties	References
PedsQL Brain Tumor Module	1. Cognitive problems 2. Pain and hurt 3. Movement and balance 4. Procedural anxiety 5. Nausea 6. Worry	Brain tumor pediatric patients	Self-report Parent report	24 items	51 pediatric brain tumor patients, aged 2–18 years, and 99 parents of participants	Cronbach's α ranged from 0.76 to 0.92	Palmer S.N., Meeske K.A., Katz E.R., Burwinkle T.M., Varni J.W. The PedsQL™ Brain Tumor Module: Initial Reliability and Validity. Pediatric Blood & Cancer. 2007; 49(3): 287-293
PedsQL 3.0 Cancer Module	1. Pain and hurt 2. Nausea 3. Procedural anxiety 4. Treatment anxiety 5. Worry 6. Cognitive problems 7. Perceived physical appearance 8. Communication	Pediatric cancer specific	Self-report Proxy report	27 items	220 child, aged 2–18 years, with cancer (24 with brain tumor), and 337 of their parents, compared with 105 healthy children aged 2–18 years and 157 of their parents	Cronbach's α = 0.72 (Self-report), 0.87 (parent report)	Varni J.W., Burwinkle T.M., Katz E.R., Meeske K., &Dickinson P. The PedsQL™ in Pediatric Cancer: Reliability and Validity of the Pediatric Quality of Life Inventory™ Generic Core Scales, Multidimensional Fatigue Scale, and Cancer Module. Cancer. 2002;94 (7): 2090-2106
MMQL-YF (8–12 years old)	1. Outlook on life/ family dynamics 2. Physical symptoms 3. Physical functioning 4. Psychological functioning	Pediatric cancer specific	Self-report	32 items	481 healthy children compared with 162 children with cancer (12 with brain tumor), aged between 8 and 13 years old	Cronbach's α ranged from 0.72 to 0.80	Bhatia S., Jenney M.E.M. Wu E., Bogue M.K., Rockwood T.H., Feusner J.H. et al. The Minneapolis-Manchester Quality of Life Instrument: Reliability and Validity of the Youth-Form. Journal of Pediatrics. 2004; 145: 39-46

MMQL-AF (13–20 years old)	1. Physical functioning 2. Cognitive functioning 3. Psychological functioning 4. Body image 5. Social functioning 6. Outlook on life 7. Intimate relations	Pediatric cancer specific	Self-report	47 items	129 healthy adolescents compared with 110 patients with cancer (16 with brain tumor), aged between 13 and 21 years old	Cronbach's α ranged from .67 to 0.89. Test-retest reliability : $r = 0.71$–0.90 ($p < 0.05$), after 2 weeks or more	Bhatia S., Jenney M.E.M., Bogue M.K., Rockwood T.H., Feusner J.H., Friedman D.L. et al. The Minneapolis-Manchester Quality of Life Instrument: Reliability and Validity of the Adolescent Form. Journal of Clinical Oncology. 2002; 20(24): 4692-4698 Wu E., Robison L.L., Jenney M.E.M., Rockwood T.H., Feusner J., Friedman D., et al. Assessment of Health-Related Quality of Life of Adolescent Cancer Patients Using the Minneapolis-Manchester Quality of Life Adolescent Questionnaire. Pediatr Blood Cancer. 2007; 48: 678-686
POQOL	1. Physical functioning 2. Emotional distress 3. Externalizing behavior 4. Response to medical treatment	Pediatric cancer specific	Parent report	21 items	210 parents of children with cancer. Children aged between 6 and 17 years old. Diagnoses was 62 % leukemia, 15 % sarcoma, 6 % Hodgkin's disease, are other dx like Wilm's tumor, neuroblastoma, Burkett's lymphoma, aged between 6 and 17 years old	Cronbach's α = 0.85	Goodwin D.A.J., Boggs S.R., Graham-Pole J. Development and Validation of the Pediatric Oncology Quality of Life Scale. Psychological Assessment. 1994; 6(4): 321-328

Internalized Symptoms

Among internalized symptoms, depression is by far the most commonly studied. Clinical depression has been observed in 38–41 % of adult survivors of childhood brain tumors, in recent studies. However, this proportion could be underestimated, since recent research compared the percentage of clinical depression assessed by professionals and self-reports of depression by patients themselves. Results suggest that 93 % of patients felt depressive symptoms, while professionals identified only 15 % of patients with depression. Studies suggest that depression among childhood brain tumor survivors is underestimated and undertreated. Major depressive symptoms encountered by patients and survivors of brain tumors are dysphoric mood, feelings of hopelessness and helplessness, guilt, low self-esteem, difficulty concentrating, suicidal ideation, and fatigue [19]. Within the empirical literature, it is not yet clear whether fatigue and lack of energy are rather side effects of the cancer and its treatments, or if they are resulting from the depression itself. Depression also may have a negative impact on patients' prognosis. Some studies indicate that among brain tumor survivors, depression is associated with a shorter lifespan. Depression is also associated with a poorer QoL ($r=0.71$ and 0.73) [20]. Risk factors for depression within this population were being a woman, having an individual or family psychiatric history, having cognitive dysfunction, and having physical symptoms and fatigue [19]. A lack of family support or inadequate family support is also a risk factor for depression. Various factors related to the tumor have also been identified, such as the anterior frontal tumor location which is linked with depressive symptoms, apathy and inhibition. Since depressive symptoms in survivors of childhood brain tumors seem quite significant and affect long-term QoL and survival, it means that signs of distress should be taken into consideration and addressed when they are observed in patients and survivors. In fact, early detection of psychological distress would allow for prompt intervention, and this in turn could improve the long-term psychological adjustment of these survivors.

Anxiety symptoms have been the focus of fewer empirical studies. Recent research has reported that 9 % of child and adults survivors of childhood brain tumor who were treated with surgery alone notified anxiety symptoms. A study which looked at the psychological outcomes of childhood brain tumors survivors reported that average scores on the anxiety scale of Brief Symptom Inventory (BSI-18) were $T=45.9$ for the survivors of brain tumors compared with $T=45.4$ for the healthy children comparison group [1]. The results of this study support the fact that childhood brain tumor survivors generally had good psychological health and did not report more symptoms of distress (depression, anxiety, and somatization), compared to healthy children, thus contrasting somewhat with the literature we reviewed on depression alone.

Externalized Symptoms

Compared to internalized symptoms, externalized symptoms have been given less attention within this population. A literature review on emotional, social, and behavioral adjustment childhood brain tumors survivors identified only two studies out of 31 that reported externalized disorders [3]. On average, 7–37 % of child and adult survivors of pediatric brain tumor present with externalized symptomatology, such as aggression, impulsivity, and antisocial and deviant behavior. One hypothesis would be that children with cancer are limited in their adaptive social behavior by their isolation due to multiple hospitalizations and rejection experience from their peers. Therefore, the child has little opportunity to develop adaptive behaviors and social skills, which in turn can influence their social behaviors. However, given the limited number of studies on this topic and the conflicting results, it is difficult to properly assess the importance, implications, and causes of behavioral problems in this population. An alternative hypothesis regards the effects of certain adjuvant treatments, such as glucocorticoids. It has been shown in other type of cancers such as acute lymphoblastic leukemia that the behavioral impact of these treatments can be significant. Glucocorticoids are related to the control of emotions and decline in cognitive functions, like cognitive slowing and memory difficulties that impact the child's ability to adapt to stress and his or her ability of psychosocial adjustment [3, 4]. Recent hypotheses have been proposed on a long-term deregulation of the hypothalamic pituitary adrenal (HPA) axis due to the massive administration of these substances. Such deregulation would result in short- and long-term behavioral and mood difficulties.

Conclusion

The QoL of patients and survivors in pediatric neuro-oncology includes the physical, psychological, and social aspects of the life of the individual. These three aspects are affected by the tumor and its treatment. However, the definition and measurement of QoL poses particular challenges in the long-term follow-up of children with cancer. While traditional research will focus on increased survival, the area of QoL offers two major advantages. First, the routine measurement of QoL in neuro-oncology allows us to assess the areas of functioning where the individual is satisfied or dissatisfied. It therefore helps target more or less precisely the areas that require clinical intervention. Second, the assessment of QoL offers an interesting alternative outcome to be used in trials, and in therapeutic and institutional interventions.

In terms of intervention, early treatment of psychological and social dimensions of QoL could promote better child adjustment at both short and long term. In order to intervene on the perception of difficulties and emotional distress, efforts should focus on early detection of emotional distress in the child and his entourage. A specific approach could target groups that have been identified at greatest risk of deterioration of QoL or emotional distress. To increase the sense of controllability, it is also necessary to focus resources towards the information given to the patient and his or her family. The disclosure of this information helps to educate parents about their child's experience and fosters a resilient, social environment. Thus, a very important area of development in pediatric neuro-oncology is resilience within the child's environment. It is necessary to identify family characteristics that promote long-term resiliency, because optimizing the quality of the social environment is central to the subsequent rehabilitation of the child. Studies report that children with brain tumors are particularly socially isolated and have deficits in social behaviors [3]. Hence, information and psychoeducation on the illness and its consequences would help them combat a feeling of isolation [4]. In the long term, particularly for survivors, professional integration programs may enable survivors to find a job suited to their skills and cognitive deficits. In summary, the assessment of different dimensions of QoL can target the needs of patients and survivors in pediatric neuro-oncology. This can be very helpful in guiding favorable support for better long-term adaptation of patients and survivors and for ensuring optimization of their QoL in the long term.

Acknowledgments The authors would like to thank the Sainte-Justine Foundation for supporting the writing of this chapter and Willow Burns for helping with the English version of the text.

References

1. Zebrack BJ, Gurney JG, Oeffinger K, Whitton J, Packer RJ, Mertens A, Turk N, Castleberry R, Dreyer Z, Robison LL, Zeltzer LK. Psychological outcomes in long-term survivors of childhood brain cancer: a report from the Childhood Cancer Survivor Study. J Clin Oncol. 2004;22(6):999–1006.
2. Nathan PC, Ness KK, Greenberg ML, Hudson M, Wolden S, Davidoff A, Laverdière C, Mertens A, Whitton J, Robison LL, Zeltzer L, Gurney JG. Health-related quality of life in adult survivors of childhood wilms tumor or neuroblastoma: a report from the Childhood Cancer Survivor Study. Pediatr Blood Cancer. 2007;49:704–15.
3. Fuemmeler BF, Elkin TD, Mullins LL. Survivors of childhood brain tumors: behavioral, emotional, and social adjustment. Clin Psychol Rev. 2002;22: 547–85.
4. Meyers CA, Wefel JS. Quality of life. In: Berger MBM, editor. Neuro-oncology: the essentials. 2nd ed. New York: Thieme; 2008. p. 438–46.
5. Dilley KJ, Lockart B. The pediatric brain tumor late effects clinic. In: Goldman S, Turner CD, editors. Late

effects of treatment for brain tumors. New York: Springer; 2009. p. 97–109.

6. Wu E, Robison LL, Jenney MEM, Rockwood TH, Feusner J, Friedman D, Kane RL, Bhatia S. Assessment of health-related quality of life of adolescent cancer patients using the Minneapolis-Manchester quality of life adolescent questionnaire. Pediatr Blood Cancer. 2007;48:678–86.

7. Penn A, Shortman RI, Lowiz AP, Stevens MCG, Hunt LP, McCarter RJ, Curran AL, Sharples PM. Child-related determinants of health-related quality of life in children with brain tumours 1 year after diagnosis. Pediatr Blood Cancer. 2010;55:1377–85.

8. Kreitler S, Kreitler MM. Quality of life in children with cancer. In: Kreitler S, Ben-Arush MW, Martin A, editors. Pediatric psycho-oncology: psychosocial aspects and clinical interventions. Oxford: Wiley; 2012. p. 18–31.

9. Reimers TS, Mortensen EL, Nysom K, Schmiegelow K. Health-related quality of life in long-term survivors of childhood brain tumors. Pediatr Blood Cancer. 2009;53:1086–91.

10. Bhat SR, Goodwin TL, Burwinkle TM, Lansdale MF, Dahl GV, Huhn SL, Gibbs IC, Donaldson SS, Rosenblum RK, Varni JW, Fisher PG. Profile of daily life in children with brain tumors: an assessment of health-related quality of life. J Clin Oncol. 2005; 23(24):5493–500.

11. Sung L, Klaassen RJ, Pritchard S, Yanofsky R, Dzolganovski B, Almeida R, Klassen A. Identification of paediatric cancer patients with poor quality of life. Br J Cancer. 2009;100:82–8.

12. The WHOQOL Group. The world health organization quality of life assessment (WHOQOL): position paper from the world health organization. Soc Sci Med. 1995;41(10):1403–9.

13. Niv D, Kreitler S. Pain and quality of life. Pain Pract. 2001;1(2):150–61.

14. Hinds PS, Gattuso JS, Fletcher A, Baker E, Coleman B, Jackson T, Jacobs-Levine A, June D, Rai SN, Lensing S, Pui C-H. Quality of life as conveyed by pediatric patients with cancer. Qual Life Res. 2004;13:761–72.

15. Eiser C, Morse R. A review of measures of quality of life for children with chronic illness. Arch Dis Child. 2001;84:205–11.

16. Carpentieri SC, Meyer EA, Delaney BL, Victoria ML, Gannon BK, Doyle JM, Kieran MW. Psychosocial and behavioral functioning among pediatric brain tumor survivors. J Neurooncol. 2003;63:279–87.

17. Schwartz CE, Sprangers MAG. Methodological approaches for assessing response shift in longitudinal health-related quality-of-life research. Soc Sci Med. 1999;48:1531–48.

18. Cremeens J, Eiser C, Blades M. Characteristics of health-related self-report measures for children aged three to eight years: a review of the literature. Qual Life Res. 2006;15:739–54.

19. Litofsky NS, Resnick AG. The relationships between depression and brain tumors. J Neurooncol. 2009; 94:153–61.

20. Pelletier G, Verhoef MJ, Khatri N, Hagen N. Quality of life in brain tumor patients: the relative contributions of depression, fatigue, emotional distress, and existential issues. J Neurooncol. 2002;57:41–9.

Palliative Care for Children with Brain Tumors

Lisa Pearlman, Shayna Zelcer, and Donna L. Johnston

Tumors of the CNS are the leading cause of death for all childhood cancers [1]. Children living with incurable brain tumors (BT) follow an expected and progressive trajectory of multiple symptoms and loss of function resulting in a high symptom burden that is distinct from other childhood malignancies. The purpose of palliative care is to optimize quality of life, minimize distress and ease suffering to those children with incurable malignancy and their families throughout the course of illness, and not reserved for the period at EOL. The intent of this chapter is to provide a review of the salient issues of palliative care for children with brain tumors.

L. Pearlman, R.N(EC) N.P.-P, B.A.M.N., A.C.N.P., (✉)
Department of Pediatric Symptom Management &
Supportive Care, Children's Hospital London
Health Sciences Centre, Victoria Hospital,
London, ON, Canada
e-mail: lisa.pearlman@lhsc.on.ca

S. Zelcer, B.Sc., M.D.
Department of Pediatrics, Children's Hospital,
London Health Sciences Center, London,
ON, Canada

D.L. Johnston, M.D., F.R.C.P.C., F.A.A.P.
Department of Pediatrics, Division of Hematology/
Oncology, Children's Hospital of Eastern Ontario,
University of Ottawa, Ottawa, ON, Canada

Every child with an incurable BT has a personal story that is rich in values, culture, and spirituality. An interdisciplinary family-centered and culturally sensitive palliative care approach is vital to comprehensively assess and manage the depth and breadth of needs of this vulnerable population. Incorporating palliative care early in the child's trajectory optimizes symptom management, reduces suffering, and sustains hope and connectedness despite the possibility of death [2]. Certain brain tumors in particular carry a particularly dismal prognosis from the time of diagnosis (e.g., DIPG) and a palliative/supportive care approach may be the only preferred treatment option selected by families.

Principles of Palliative Care

Over the last two decades, palliative care for children has evolved as specialized service delivery which encompasses the total care of children with life-limiting diseases, regardless of outcome [3, 4]. An incurable brain tumor diagnosis affects not only the child but all members of the family. For this reason, events and experiences throughout the child's course of illness and at EOL are remembered and highly relevant to family-centered care. Thus, palliative care is applicable from the time of diagnosis, through active and curative treatment, during the period of EOL, and afterwards in the initial phases of family grief and bereavement [3].

K. Scheinemann and E. Bouffet (eds.), *Pediatric Neuro-oncology*,
DOI 10.1007/978-1-4939-1541-5_26, © Springer Science+Business Media New York 2015

Service deliverables of palliative care include improved communication and continuity of care across different settings; assessment and management of physical, psychosocial, emotional, and spiritual needs; provision of comprehensive specialized pain and symptom management; support with complex and ethical decision-making; enhanced awareness of diverse cultural beliefs about dying and death; specialized care of the dying patient; provision of bereavement care; and staff support and education to improve care delivery and respond to moral distress [2–5]. Palliative care services may or may not be organizationally situated within a pediatric oncology program.

Waldman and Wolfe advocate for a concomitant and holistic care delivery model that includes both palliative care and cancer modifying therapies to afford children with BT and their family opportunities to live to their maximum potential [4]. Without early integration of palliative care, the focus of care then centers on life-prolonging measures, which may result in painful and invasive procedures, additional suffering, and futile resuscitation of a dying child. Opportunities and time to make memories, to create legacies, to enhance meaningful communication about values, and to determine preferences and location for EOL care may be missed if not addressed early in the trajectory of a cancer illness when death is expected.

Uniqueness of Pediatric Neuro-Oncology Palliative Care

Pediatric oncology families have unique relationships with their primary oncologist whom they look to for leadership and direction in all aspects of their child's care, including palliative care. By the very nature of pediatric neuro-oncology, teams caring for children with BT and their families are already well versed with palliative care principles of prognostic uncertainty; high-risk treatment decisions; physical and psychological suffering of the child due to intensive treatment; and the impact of cancer on the entire family [4]. However, in a 2006 survey to the American

Society of Clinical Oncology, a high number of pediatric oncologists reported having no formal pediatric palliative care training and a high level of anxiety in directing complex pain and symptom management [6]. In addition, approximately 40 % of COG institutions did not have access to a specialized pain or palliative care service which is known to foster expertise in palliative care pain/symptom management and ensuring comprehensive care [7].

Timing

Associating palliative care with death and dying creates barriers to meeting the needs of children *living* with brain tumors. Waldman and Wolfe emphasize that prognostic uncertainty and not the likelihood of survival should be the trigger to initiate palliative care. Still, the time to introduce palliative care for children with BT remains unclear, is controversial, and is with little evidence to guide practice [4]. Timing is further complicated by the perceived sharp division between curative cancer therapy and palliative care among pediatric oncologists and parents who view palliative care as giving up hope and representing failure.

Pediatric oncologists often recognize that cure is no longer possible earlier than parents [2]. This is a valuable and critical time to engage parents to focus on a supportive care plan aimed at optimizing comfort and maximizing quality of life. Still, patients are referred late in the child's trajectory, usually after the first relapse or after relapse therapy fails [7, 8].

Cultural beliefs are central to perceptions of illness, end-of-life care, and the dying process. Ethnicity, culture-based values, and language barriers are important patient/family considerations that impact communication about end-of-life care. The location of settings has also been identified as a barrier to implementing palliative care. In an examination of hospice referral patterns among pediatric oncologists, Fowler et al. identified that barriers to referral include inability of hospice settings to administer palliative chemotherapy and blood transfusions [6].

Location of Care

When provided a choice for EOL care, parents prefer for their child to be at home. A home death is linked to improved psychological outcomes for parents and siblings [5]. Home deaths often require the support of hospice/palliative care to provide specialized palliative care nursing, case management, service coordination, availability of 24/7 medical consultation for pain and symptom management, and a home death pronouncement process. Continuity of care with the primary oncology team is important and facilitated by optimizing communication. Studies in location of death in pediatric oncology show that if there is an option of a hospice for the child, then up to one third of families choose that option as location of death [9]. Unfortunately not all children have access to a pediatric hospice, but if available, it is a valued option for children and their families.

Symptom Burden

A landmark paper in pediatric palliative care described the significant presence of symptoms and suffering at the EOL [2]. This study also found that parents were more likely than physicians to report the presence of these physical symptoms. Death from a brain tumor is usually an expected event, yet the multitude of symptoms and care needs can be overwhelming for the patient and family [10]. As end-of-life approaches, suffering becomes more severe and neuro-oncology teams are called upon to manage complex palliative pain and symptoms.

A recent review of symptoms at EOL identified that the mean number of physical symptoms per child was 6.3 and the most frequently reported symptoms were pain, poor appetite, fatigue, lack of mobility, and vomiting [11]. In this study, patients with brain tumors more frequently reported symptoms of incontinence compared to patients with leukemia or solid tumors. In another study that interviewed parents 4–9 years after the death of their child, more than one third of parents felt their child had unrelieved pain near the EOL and more than half of these parents were

still affected by this experience [12]. This further highlights the need for adequate management of physical symptoms.

Jalmsell et al. conducted a retrospective study surveying bereaved parents to determine symptoms at EOL for children with cancer. Thirty-five percent of children in this study died from a brain tumor. Fatigue was reported as being the most debilitating symptom impacting on well-being in the last month of life. Fatigue is multifactorial, unrelieved by rest, and not related to quality of sleep [13]. Children with BT experienced less pain and more difficulties related to bulbar weakness, impaired mobility, and constipation compared to children with leukemia/lymphoma. Loss of appetite and weight loss were not prominent symptoms of children with BT as compared to children with other malignant disease [13]. Pritchard et al. identified in their study that bereaved parents reported changes in the child's behavior and appearance at EOL as being of great concern [14].

Unique Symptom Profile of Children with Brain Tumors

Children with BT describe headache pain to be mild and intermittent, due to increased intracranial pressure. Headaches typically respond to a combination of dexamethasone and non-opioid analgesia. In severe cases, patients may require high doses of dexamethasone and opioid. Neuropathic neck and back pain related to leptomeningeal irritation may require gabapentin, methadone, or ketamine administration.

In the last stage of disease, BT patients may present with severe symptoms as a result of the growing tumor and treatment side effects. This may lead to cognitive decline, impaired level of consciousness, visual and auditory impairment, poor functional status, progressive bulbar weakness, loss of motor function/gait impairment, poor communication, and high need for support for activities of daily living [10, 13, 15].

Bulbar dysfunction leads to difficulties with swallowing, speech, and managing secretions. Augmentative communication can be instituted early in the disease progress to assist with communication at EOL. Dysphagia secondary to posterior fossa and brainstem tumors may affect the child's ability to safely take in fluids and foods by mouth. As the child approaches EOL and becomes more somnolent, the route of medication administration should be changed from the oral route.

As the child with a BT experiences progressive dysphagia, bulbar weakness, cognitive decline, and fatigue, parents may request a nasogastric tube to be inserted for nutrition. Parents of children with BT express deep concern that their child will suffer and starve to death if the child remains hungry yet is unable to eat orally. Parents frequently request the insertion of nasogastric or gastrostomy tubes. Neuro-oncology teams have a key role in guiding and navigating patients and their parents through this ethical struggle ahead of time as part of advance care planning (ACP). Withholding/withdrawing artificial nutrition and hydration is a deeply personal decision for patients and parents, often rooted in religion, country of origin, culture, and tradition. For health care professionals, withholding/withdrawing nutrition is a complex ethical issue. It is important for neuro-oncology teams to facilitate and support this complex decision-making to minimize decisional regret. Parents should be counseled that artificially feeding an unresponsive and dying child will not improve quality of life or change the outcome. Hydration may put the patient at risk for pooling of respiratory secretions, respiratory distress, pleural effusions, and ascites. Parenteral feeding or intravenous hydration may not only jeopardize skin integrity due to frequent voiding and stooling, but the act of changing incontinent patients may trigger incidental or worsening pain.

It is not uncommon for the child with a BT to experience seizures. The goal of seizure management at EOL is distinct from managing chronic epilepsy, particularly in an unresponsive patient. Midazolam is frequently used for its anticonvulsant and sedative properties. It can be administered subcutaneously/intravenously, via the intranasal or buccal route, and as a rapid onset. Seizures that are refractory to midazolam at EOL can be often effectively managed with parenteral phenobarbital (Table 26.1).

Agitation is commonly observed at EOL and presents as restlessness, moaning, and grimacing.

Treatment may include benzodiazepines (lorazepam, midazolam), neuroleptics (methotrimeprazine, haloperidol), reduction of steroid dosage, or administration of opioid if agitation is associated with pain. Agitation can be very distressing for family members necessitating timely and aggressive symptom management.

Declining neurological and cognitive functions predispose patients to choking, aspiration, and falls. Patients with BT are at high risk for skin breakdown related to functional deficits, immobility, and weight gain secondary to steroid use [13]. Patients may present with delayed wound healing and/or wound infection as a result of steroid treatment. With disease progression, leptomeningeal disease, or spinal metastases, patients may develop a neurogenic bowel and bladder and become incontinent of urine and stool.

Corticosteroids are frequently utilized for the relief of progressive neurological symptoms. Initially they provide a marked improvement; however, this efficacy is generally transient [18]. The dilemma often arises whether to further increase the dose of corticosteroids for symptom relief, which often results in a concomitant increase in the side effects of steroids, which are often burdensome in themselves. These adverse effects include hyperphagia, weight gain, body transformation, glucose intolerance, hypertension, mood disturbance, gastrointestinal bleeding and ulcers, and obstructive sleep apnea [18]. Hyperphagia in itself can be of particular concern in those children with swallowing disturbances, as they are permanently hungry and are at risk of choking.

As children approach the final hours of life, respiratory symptoms are greatly impacted by neurological decline and progressive somnolence. Irregular breathing patterns begin to present as hypoventilation, apnea, Cheyne-Stokes respirations, and agonal breathing. These symptoms may be isolated or occur in combination. The loss of gag reflex, inability to swallow, and the buildup of oral and tracheal secretions lead to gurgled respirations referred to as the *death rattle*. This can be particularly difficult for family members to observe [15]. Glycopyrrolate administered SC is used to reduce the production of saliva in unresponsive patients.

Table 26.1 Common medications used in the palliative care of children with brain tumors

Medication	Indication	Route	Initial dosage	Maximum	Frequency
Dexamethasone	Raised intracranial pressure, nausea and vomiting	PO/NG, SC, IV	1–2 mg/kg (initial) 0.25–0.5 mg/kg	4–10 mg/dose	Q6–12 h
Ondansetron	Nausea and vomiting	PO, SC, IV	0.15 mg/kg	8 mg	Q8 h
Morphine	Analgesia, dyspnea	PO/NG SC, IV Continuous Infusion (SC, IV)	0.1–0.3 mg/kg/dose 00.05–0.15 mg/kg/dose 0.01–0.06 mg/kg/h		Q3–4 h Q3–4 h
Hydromorphone	Analgesia, dyspnea	PO/NG SC, IV Continuous Infusion (SC, IV)	0.03–0.1 mg/kg/dose 0.015–0.02 mg/kg/dose 0.001–0.003 mg/kg/h		PO—Q3–4 h SC/IV—Q3–4 h
Fentanyl	Analgesia	IV Continuous IV Transdermal	0.5–2 µg/kg/dose 0.5–2 µg/kg/h Patch: 12.5, 25, 50, 75, 100 µg/kg/h		Q30 min–1h Q72 h
Gabapentin	Analgesia (adjuvant agent for neuropathic pain)	PO/NG	10 mg/kg/day titrate up to 50 mg/kg/day for effect	3,600 mg/day (50–75 mg/kg/day)	Q8 h
Midazolam	Dyspnea, seizures, agitation	Buccal Intranasal SC, IV	0.3 mg/kg 0.1 mg/kg/dose 0.025–0.05 mg/kg/dose		Q 5min (Seizures) to Q4 h
Lorazepam		PO, SC, IV	0.002–0.01 mg/kg/dose		Q4–6–12 h
Methotrimeprazine	Agitation, nausea, vomiting	PO/NG, SC	0.12–0.5 mg/kg/dose		Q4–12 h
Haloperidol	Agitation, delirium	PO, IV SC/IV	PO—0.01–0.2 mg/kg dose SC—0.005–0.06 mg/kg		Q8–12 h
Glycopyrrolate	Increased respiratory secretions or terminal secretions at EOL	PO SC	0–100 µg/kg 4–10 µg/kg		Q6 h Q3–4 h

Based on data from refs [16, 17]

Palliative Sedation

In specific circumstances palliative sedation (PS) may be implemented to alleviate uncontrollable pain, seizures, respiratory distress and existential suffering despite rigorous treatment of refractory symptoms at EOL. There is a paucity of published reports to determine incidence and prevalence of palliative sedation instituted in children with brain tumors. The initiation of PS occurs once the medical team and parents determine that the child has true refractory symptoms causing unbearable suffering. It is imperative that the intent of PS be addressed well before initiation so that parents understand that PS is not intended to hasten death but to support the child through this difficult stage of their dying process. Engaging the parents and the multidisciplinary team early in the process minimizes moral distress and unites the parents and team in shared EOL goals. Such cases require written guidelines and expertise to direct the administration of continuous high-dose opioids and sedation [19].

Psychological Symptoms

Symptom management includes the management of both physical and psychological symptoms. A recent review of symptoms in the palliative phase identified that the mean number of psychological symptoms per child was 3.2, and the main symptoms were sadness, difficulties in talking about their feelings regarding illness and death with parents, fear to be alone, loss of perspective, and loss of independency [11]. Wolfe et al. identified that according to their parents, in the last month of life, children had little or no fun, were more than a little sad, and were not calm or peaceful most of the time [2]. Mood disorders particularly anxiety and depression are not uncommon. Jalmsell et al.'s survey of bereaved parents identified children >9 years old were at higher risk of developing anxiety [13]. These symptoms need to be openly discussed and addressed by psychosocial members of the allied health-care team early on in the trajectory.

Advance Care Planning

ACP is a clinical intervention to facilitate ethical and effective decision-making for children with BT. ACP in a pediatric setting is a process that honors relationships, family-centered care, and cultural values to support decision-making. Open communication is central to good palliative care and is linked to improved decision-making and decreased parental suffering [2, 4].

Pediatric oncologists are called upon to talk openly with patients and parents about aggressive cancer focused treatment, ending life support, and identifying the dying point for patients with incurable BT. Addressing end-of-life decisions including *Do Not Attempt Resuscitation* (DNAR) early on in the trajectory minimizes a potential crisis during a time of acute deterioration or flare-up of refractory pain or symptom. Thus, it is essential to use the time period following the diagnosis of incurable BT to begin the process of identifying goals of care and facilitating the development of EOL care plans. This is highly relevant for children and adolescents whose ability to communicate personal care preferences may be impacted by bulbar dysfunction and cognitive decline.

Decision-Making

End-of-life decision-making is emotionally arduous and intense for parents of children with brain tumors. EOL decisions for children with BT include limiting or ending treatment, withholding/withdrawing artificial hydration and nutrition, determining location of care, and assessing the need for palliative sedation and resuscitation [2, 4, 5, 20]. Parents approach such existential decisions for their child and themselves by weighing decisions regarding their child's suffering, regarding experimental treatment options, and regarding a purely palliative approach to care and recognizing that without treatment their child will die. Parents are further called upon to make decisions related to autopsy, tissue donation, and funeral arrangements. Given the complexity of such decisions, patients and families require guidance and direction from a skilled and supportive multidisciplinary team [10].

Heinze and Nolan performed a qualitative review of published research on parental decision-making for children at EOL over a 10-year period from 2001 to 2011 [21]. In this review of 35 published reports, parental decision-making was positively influenced by the clinical expertise of the treating team, consistent and direct communication about the child's progress, and clear understanding of the prognosis. Other studies rank hope as an important factor in decision-making [10, 22]. The need to have more time with their children has emerged as a prominent theme in parental EOL decision-making studies. Palliative chemotherapy is an intervention that parents value as being important in order to have more time with their child. Studies have demonstrated that clinicians think otherwise and perceive palliative chemotherapy to be invasive with the potential to cause treatment-related side effects, to adversely affect quality of life, and to prolong suffering [11, 22, 23].

Children and chronically ill adolescents themselves often wish to be involved in decisions affecting their future health care, while their parents find this to be a startling fact [20, 24, 25]. Children want to be heard, while their parents have a strong need to protect them from the harsh reality of their disease. Clinicians are reluctant to routinely include children and adolescents in decision-making. In the absence of legal age to consent to treatment, there is consensus that children as young as 14 years old are capable of understanding treatment decisions and consequences of their treatment that could lead to death. Yet, parents and clinicians express worry that adolescents are not developmentally ready to appreciate consequences to treatment/nontreatment options and both groups view discussions as upsetting to children and adolescents. Their ultimate fear is that children and adolescents will lose hope and have adverse outcomes as a result of the knowledge that they have terminal cancer [20, 24].

Hinds et al.'s early research has challenged this perception and contributes new knowledge that dying school-aged children and adolescents were able to articulate their preferences for EOL care [20]. Hinds and her colleagues interviewed 20 patients aged 10–20 years old about their preferences for EOL. Four of these patients had a brain tumor. The mean age was 17 years and 4 months. Results of this study demonstrated that all of the patients in this study were aware of death as a consequence of their decision-making. These 20 patients identified that their EOL preferences were influenced by their concern for others, their wishes to avoid treatment-related adverse events, their choice to end life-prolonging therapy, their readiness to go to an afterlife, and their negative experience of witnessing receive life-sustaining treatment [20].

In a more recent study, Hinds et al. demonstrated that children as young as 5 years old were able to identify cancer-related quality of life issues [24]. She and her colleagues advocate for more opportunities to facilitate younger children to have a voice in treatment-related discussions. End-of-life planning booklets such as *Pediatric My Wishes* and *Voicing My Choices* are easily accessible developmentally appropriate resources that are available in several languages [26]. These booklets are a platform to support school-aged children and adolescents with opportunities to have their needs and preferences explored with a parent or member of the neuro-oncology team.

Autopsy/Organ Donation

When a child dies from a progressive brain tumor, many health-care practitioners or family members may erroneously feel that there is no reason to perform an autopsy. However, postmortem examinations in pediatric oncology are often an important source of new or additional important information for physicians and families alike.

In order for this significant decision to be fully considered, families should be given the opportunity to consider this request ahead of time, before the child approaches EOL. Practitioners should anticipate in advance opportunities to discuss autopsy and when families would be most responsive to the discussion. Guidelines on how to introduce this sensitive topic to parents or guardians of children have been published [27]. In addition, the place of death should not influence the decision.

Postmortem examinations should be offered to families regardless of whether end-of-life care is in the hospital, hospice, or home. A description of the goals of autopsy, including tissue collection for research purposes, and all aspects of the procedure itself should be disclosed. Explanations should describe the different types of autopsies, in particular that the autopsy can be restricted to the whole brain or tumor itself, according to the family's preference. Arrangements should always be made to discuss the autopsy results with the primary care team, and this discussion in itself can be an important step in the family's bereavement process.

Autopsy tissue is an important source for future pediatric brain tumor research. For tumors that can be neither resected nor biopsied, it is the only tissue available. Significant research has been conducted in tissue obtained from autopsy with children with diffuse intrinsic pontine gliomas (DIPG) [28, 29]. As the diagnosis of a DIPG is usually not made by histology but rather by imaging and clinical characteristics, very little is known about the biology of this cancer. Given the dismal prognosis of children with DIPG, a push has been made to advocate for postmortem donation of tissue. Important information has been gathered from these autopsy studies and possible biologic targets for future therapies have been identified [29].

The diagnosis of a primary brain tumor is not considered a contraindication to organ donation, unlike other malignancies, due to the rarity of extra-neural metastases [30]. Tissue donation including cornea, skin, bone, cardiovascular, and connective tissue should be discussed. Failure to disclose eligibility for organ and tissue donation could be a source of grief and bereavement for the family in the future.

Grief and Bereavement

The death of a child has a profound and lasting impact on parents and siblings alike. The loss of a child is described as one of the most stressful life events a parent can experience and the grief is more intense and longer lasting that that of any other type of loss [31, 32]. Parents of children who die from cancer have poor psychosocial outcomes including elevated rates of anxiety, depression, prolonged grief, poor psychological well-being, poor physical health, and poor quality of life. The loss of the ability to communicate by the child with a brain tumor may be particularly difficult for the family and identified as a source of loss and missed opportunity [10, 32, 33].

Bereavement follow-up by the primary neuro-oncology team is an essential component and standard of palliative care. Contact from a team member after a child's death can not only help relieve a family's potential sense of abandonment but also identify families at particular risk and allocate resources to them.

Research

Pediatric palliative care research has concentrated on the EOL care of children with malignant disease with little focus on the multitude of needs that precede EOL. Children with BT have distinct needs, yet they are rarely studied as a separate group [10]. Instead, children with BT are grouped with other childhood malignancies in EOL studies making it difficult to elucidate their unique symptom management burden and palliative care needs.

Current palliative care research is limited by nonrandomized studies, surveys and focus groups of bereaved parents, and retrospective chart analyses [10, 13]. In studies focusing on EOL care, ethics review boards remain conservative in judging harm. Thus, ethics review boards remain reluctant to support prospective studies using dying children and/or their parents despite evidence that neither children nor their parents are negatively impacted or traumatized by the research process [20, 22, 24, 34, 35].

Conclusion

Children with BT experience unique and distressing symptoms that are distinct from other pediatric malignancies. Progressive cognitive impairment and declining overall function are significant quality of life issues impacting on communication, decision-making, and safety.

Children with BT are at high risk of suffering in a cure-focused culture without a palliative care approach initiated early in the trajectory.

In pediatric neuro-oncology, palliative care has always been a part of care delivery and pediatric oncologists have historically been intimately involved in EOL care. Pediatric palliative care is rapidly shifting from a focus of care from dying and death to an emphasis on quality of life and living throughout the course of the child's cancer trajectory regardless of the outcome. Integrating palliative care principles early after diagnosis is particularly relevant to children with brain tumors who may lead a productive and functional life for weeks to months after diagnosis.

References

1. Canadian Cancer Society. Canadian cancer statistics 2008. http://www.cancer.ca/canada-wide/about%20 cancer/cancer%20statistics/~/media/CCS/Canada%20 wide/Files%20List/English%20files%20heading/ pdf%20not%20in%20publications%20section/ Canadian%20Cancer%20Society%20Statistics%20 PDF%202008_614137951.ashx. Accessed 18 March 2013.
2. Wolfe J, Grier HE, Klar N, et al. Symptoms and suffering at the end of life in children with cancer. N Engl J Med. 2000;342(10):326–33.
3. POGO/PCMCH. Report of the Paediatric Palliative Care Work Group; 2011.
4. Waldman E, Wolfe J. Palliative care for children with cancer. Nat Rev Clin Oncol. 2013;10(2):100–7.
5. Epelman CL. End-of-life management in pediatric cancer. Curr Oncol Rep. 2012;14(2):191–6.
6. Fowler K, Poehlin K, Billheimer D, et al. Hospice referral practice for children with cancer: a survey of pediatric oncologists. J Clin Oncol. 2006;24(7):1099–104.
7. Johnston DL, Nagel K, Friedman DL, et al. Availability and use of palliative care and end-of-life-services for pediatric oncology patients. J Clin Oncol. 2008;26(28):4646–50.
8. Johnston DL, Vadeboncoeur C. Palliative care consultation in pediatric oncology. Support Care Cancer. 2012;20(4):799–803.
9. Siden H, Miller M, Straatman L, Omesi L, Tucker T, Collins JJ. A report on location of death in paediatric palliative care between home, hospice and hospital. Palliat Med. 2008;22(7):831–4.
10. Zelcer S, Cataudella D, Cairney AE, Bannister SL. Palliative care of children with brain tumors: a parental perspective. Arch Pediatr Adolesc Med. 2010;164(3):225–30.
11. Theunissen JMJ, Hoogerbrugge PM, van Achterberg T, Prins JB, Vernooij-Dassen MJFJ, van den Ende

CHM. Symptoms in the palliative phase of children with cancer. Pediatr Blood Cancer. 2007;49(2):160–5.
12. Kreicbergs U, Valdimarsdottir U, Onelov E, Bjork O, Steinek G, Henter JI. Care-related distress: a nationwide survey of parents having lost their child to cancer. J Clin Oncol. 2005;23(36):9162–71.
13. Jalmsell L, Kreicbergs U, Onelov E, et al. Symptoms affecting children with malignancies during the last month of life: a nationwide follow-up. Pediatrics. 2006;117(4):1314–20.
14. Pritchard M, Burghen E, Srivastava DK, et al. Cancer related symptoms most concerning to parents during the last week and last day of their child's life. Pediatrics. 2008;121(5):1301–9.
15. Hendricks-Ferguson V. Physical symptoms of children receiving pediatric hospice care at home during the last week of life. Oncol Nurs Forum. 2008; 35(6):108–15.
16. Hauer J, Duncan J, Scullion BF. Pediatric pain and symptom management guidelines. Boston: Dana Farber Cancer Institute/Children's Hospital; 2011.
17. Harlos M. Paediatric symptom management and palliative care pediatric drug doses. Winnipeg: Winnipeg Regional Health Authority. Unpublished data (with permission MH), 2008.
18. Dietrick J, Rao K, Pastorino K, et al. Corticosteroids in brain cancer patients: benefits and pitfalls. Expert Rev Clin Pharmacol. 2011;4(2):233–42.
19. Postovsky S, Moaed B, Krivoy E, et al. Practice and palliative sedation in children with brain tumours and sarcomas at end of life. Pediatr Hematol Oncol. 2007;24(6):409–15.
20. Hinds P, Drew D, Oakes LL, et al. End-of-life preferences of pediatric patients with cancer. J Clin Oncol. 2005;23(36):9146–54.
21. Heinze KE, Nolan MT. Parental decision making for children with cancer at the end of life: a meta ethnography. J Pediatr Oncol Nurs. 2012;29(6):337–45.
22. Tomlinson D, Bartels U, Gammon J, et al. Chemotherapy versus supportive care alone in pediatric palliative care for cancer: comparing the preferences of parents and health care professionals. CMAJ. 2011;183(17):1252–8.
23. Kassam A, Skiadaresis J, Habib S, Alexander S, Wolfe J. Moving toward quality palliative cancer care: parent and clinician perspectives on gaps between what matters and what is accessible. J Clin Oncol. 2012;31(7):910–5.
24. Hinds PS, Menard JC, Jacobs SS. The child's voice in pediatric palliative and end-of-life care. Prog Palliat Care. 2012;20(6):337–42.
25. Knapp C, Komatz K. Preferences for end-of-life care for children with cancer. CMAJ. 2011;183(17):1250–1.
26. Aging with dignity. My Wishes 2012. http://www.agingwithdignity.org/index.php. Accessed 18 March 2013.
27. Broniscer A. Autopsy. In: Wolfe J, Hinds PS, Sourkes BM, editors. Textbook of interdisciplinary pediatric palliative care. Philadelphia: Saunders; 2011. p. 221–6.
28. Broniscer A, Baker JN, Baker SJ, et al. Prospective collection of tissue samples at autopsy in children

with diffuse intrinsic pontine glioma. Cancer. 2010;116(19):4632–7.

29. Angelini P, Hawkins C, Laperrierre N, Bouffet E, Bartels U. Post mortem examinations in diffuse intrinsic pontine glioma: challenges and chances. J Neuroncol. 2001;101(1):75–81.

30. Punnett AS, McCarthy LJ, Dirks PB, et al. Patients with primary brain tumors as organ donors: case report and review of the literature. Pediatr Blood Cancer. 2004;43(1):73–7.

31. Wheeler I. Parental bereavement: the crisis of meaning. Death Stud. 2001;25(1):51–66.

32. Whittam EH. Terminal care of the dying child: psychosocial implications of care. Cancer. 1993; 71(10):3450–62.

33. Cataudella DA, Zelcer S. Psychological experiences of children with brain tumors at end of life: parental perspectives. Palliat Med. 2012;15(11):1191–7.

34. Olcese ME, Mack JW. Research participation experiences of parents of children with cancer who were asked about their child's prognosis. J Palliat Med. 2012;15(3):269–73.

35. Wolfe J. Parents of children with serious illness are more resilient than credited. J Palliat Med. 2012;15(3):258–9.

Eric Bouffet, Nisreen Amayiri, Adriana Fonseca, and Katrin Scheinemann

Introduction

Great disparities exist in the care of children with cancer around the world. It is estimated that more than 80 % of all pediatric cancers occur in countries with limited resources and most disparities are related to differences in healthcare resources and organization of healthcare systems. However, in addition to economic barriers, other issues may limit the quality of care delivered to this vulnerable population. In this chapter, we will review the challenges associated with the management of central nervous system tumors in the pediatric population in countries with limited resources and will provide some suggestions and recommendations based on recent successful experiences [1].

Incidence of CNS Tumors in Countries with Limited Resources

There are only few reports on childhood brain tumors in countries with limited resources. Most publications represent single institution experiences rather than collaborative studies [2]. The incidence of childhood brain tumors is difficult to estimate in these countries due to the lack of population-based cancer registries [3]. There are indeed numerous obstacles for the implementation of cancer registries in developing countries. Many of these countries face general problems of poverty, which make cancer diagnosis, treatment, and compliance a low priority. In addition, some low-income countries have large shifts in population due to wars, migration, or rapid changes in incidence of birth or death, which result in inaccurate age-specific population estimates. Infection and malnutrition are major causes of death in children from developing countries; thus, cancer treatment gets little attention from healthcare authorities. Due to the complexity of the care of pediatric brain tumor patients, even when epidemiologic studies are available, these patients are often not included [4]. However, proper cancer registries would be the first step to appreciate the extent of the problem in order to implement cancer programs (Table 27.1).

E. Bouffet, M.D.
Department of Hematology/Oncology,
The Hospital for Sick Children,
University of Toronto, Toronto, ON, Canada

N. Amayiri, M.D.
Department of Pediatrics, King Hussein Cancer Center,
Amman, Jordan

A. Fonseca, M.D.
Department of Pediatrics, McMaster Children's Hospital,
Hamilton, ON, Canada

K. Scheinemann, M.D. (⊠)
Department of Pediatrics, Division of Hematology/
Oncology, McMaster Children's Hospital,
McMaster University, Hamilton, ON, Canada
e-mail: kschein@mcmaster.ca

Table 27.1 Pediatric brain cancer registration data included in the C15-1X for the period of 1998–2002 by continent

Continent	Countries included/ submitted data	PBCR included/ submitted data	Geographic coverage by continent (%)	Population coverage in millions (%)
Africa	5/14	5/16	31	8.8 (1 %)
Asia	15/18	44/77	57	152.3 (4 %)
Europe	29/30	100/120	83	238.8 (33 %)
North America	2/2	54/58	93	258.5 (80 %)
Oceania	4/6	11/13	85	23 (73 %)
South and Central America	8/11	11/29	38	22.7 (4.3 %)

Reprinted from Curada MP, Voti L, Sortino-Rachou AM. Cancer registration data and quality indicators in low- and middle-income countries: their interpretation and potential use for the improvement of cancer care. Cancer Causes Control 2009; 20(5):751-756. With permission from Springer Verlag
PBCR Population based Cancer Registry

Registries may also help to identify unique genetic or environmental risks and allow proper and timely intervention to improve detection and outcome.

Available data suggest a low incidence of CNS tumor in countries with limited resources. While the incidence of pediatric brain tumor in the CBTRUS (Central Brain Tumor Registry of the United States) was 4.92/100,000 person-years for children less than 15 years during the period 2004–2008 [5], Manoharan et al. reported an incidence of 0.9/100,000 in the Delhi Population Based Cancer Registry (PBCR) for the period 2003–2007 [6]. In Colombia, a country with a population of 47,000,000, there is a rough estimate of 400 new pediatric brain tumors per year. Whether this lower incidence is real or related to other factors is unknown. One common proposed cause of lower reported incidence of childhood cancer in general in low-income countries is the high mortality rate in young children (under the age of 5 years) that may lead to early death before the child develops cancer. However, there is no statistical reason that this high rate of premature death should influence the overall incidence of childhood cancer. Using data from the International Agency for Cancer Research (IARC), Howard et al. reported a close correlation between the reported incidence of childhood leukemia and the mean annual per capita gross national income [7]. There is no similar study for childhood brain tumors. However, it is very likely that in many low-income countries, children with brain tumor die before diagnosis.

Delay in the Diagnosis of CNS Tumors

Despite advances in neuroimaging, timely diagnosis of CNS tumors remains a problem in high-income countries. There are no specific studies that have analyzed differences in the delay to diagnosis of CNS tumors between high- and low-income countries. However, the issue of late diagnosis of CNS tumors is obvious for neurosurgeons and oncologists who practice in these countries. Beyond the usual challenges of nonspecific symptoms such as vomiting, failure to thrive, hypoactivity, headaches, or visual disturbance that are usual factors involved in delayed diagnosis [8], access to neuroimaging facilities is the main obstacle that patients and families face. The limited number of CT or MRI scans; long waiting lists, particularly when sedation is needed; and in many places the prohibitive cost of these tests are among the many reasons that delay or prevent the diagnosis of brain tumor in children in these countries. In most places, the imaging study will be limited to the brain and it is exceptional to have preoperative imaging of the spine when a malignant brain tumor such as medulloblastoma is suspected. Once a brain tumor is diagnosed on imaging, then confirmation of the correct diagnosis would mean a referral to a specialized center able to take care of these children.

Most developing countries lack specialized centers whether due to unavailability of experienced staff or shortage of equipment [9], and even when they have one, families from rural areas often face difficulties to access these specialized centers due to financial costs and difficulties in transportation, which will also complicate future compliance during treatment and follow-up.

In some countries like Panama, programs have been developed to increase awareness of early signs and symptoms of pediatric brain tumors for primary care physicians. The primary objective is to increase early diagnosis and referral of these patients. Programs like this one are being currently developed in other countries like Colombia, addressing the most common malignancies in childhood.

Cultural Barriers

Cancer is a condition that relates to fate, myths, and beliefs. The diagnosis of brain tumor is a devastating event for the families; often they tend to seek help from local "healers" or use complementary and alternative medicine. As a result, this may affect the natural history of the disease and delay the diagnosis of cancer even more [10]. A classical example is the increased incidence of blindness associated with optic pathway gliomas seen in countries with limited resources.

Brain tumor diagnosis has in some cultures a negative perception and stigmatization. Families may refuse to be referred to a cancer center, trying to avoid the risk of marginalization associated with this condition. Stigma like the belief that cancer equates death or mental and physical disability and cultural myths might also influence parental or family decisions including treatment abandonment. Because the social stigmata of cancer can be so powerful, social barriers must be fully understood before any strategy is implemented in low-income countries.

Some cultural choices, like treating boys over girls, may affect incidence, survival, and mortality data of cancer in some cultural contexts [11]. Other social factors are critical, such as financial and transportation difficulties that have been identified as major sources of abandonment of treatment [12].

Management of Pediatric Brain Tumors in Countries with Limited Resources

Neurosurgery

With a few exceptions, neurosurgical management is generally the first step in the treatment of pediatric brain tumors. Neurosurgeons in low-income countries are overloaded with work and neurosurgical units are generally understaffed. Neurosurgery in these countries faces two main challenges, i.e., quality and quantity in both resources and qualified personnel [9]. The World Health Organization African Subcommittee conducted a survey on African neurosurgical services in the late 1990s. This survey reported a ratio of one African neurosurgeon per 1,352,000 individuals compared to 1/121,000 in Europe and 1/81,000 in North America [13]. Similar figures are described in the South Asian continent.

In addition, there are a limited number of neurosurgeons with a pediatric expertise in low-income countries, and thus, general neurosurgeons, when available, are expected to operate on children. In such conditions, specific knowledge of the principles of pediatric neuro-oncology is important and unfortunately many general neurosurgeons are not familiar with this specialty. As a result, in most places, surgical intervention is limited to the insertion of ventriculoperitoneal shunts for the management of hydrocephalus. Attempt to complete or near complete surgical resection is not a common practice, and surgery is usually limited to a biopsy to allow histological diagnosis. Unfortunately, less than gross total resection greatly impact survival of children with brain tumor like ependymoma or/and would upgrade risk status for some other tumors like medulloblastoma.

Neuronavigation and the use of intraoperative microscope are known to facilitate surgery and to improve tumor resection; however, these equipments are scarce in low-income countries or are only available in selected private practices; trained neurosurgeons with the expertise to use these techniques are limited. A recurrent challenge in this context is the management of children who underwent incomplete tumor resection. Most often, neurosurgeons consider that there is no role for further surgery and they refer the child to radiation oncologists or pediatric oncologists for adjuvant treatment. While local oncologists are often unsuccessful in trying to convince referring neurosurgeons to proceed to second look surgery in the context of an incomplete resection, telemedicine experiences that involve a contact between neurosurgeons appear to offer a unique opportunity to discuss such technical issues and to optimize the quality of surgical management [14].

Postoperative intensive care with good monitoring of intracranial pressure, fluids, and electrolyte balance is crucial when caring with brain tumor patients especially when hormonal problems are expected like in craniopharyngioma surgery. The lack of such specialized multidisciplinary care will increase perioperative morbidity and mortality.

Another issue identified in some of the twinning programs is the lack of communication between neurosurgeons and pediatric oncologist. Often, these patients are not referred for further adjuvant therapy and frequently a suboptimal surgical resection is the only treatment modality. This seems to be a more prevalent issue, if the surgical management is performed by a non-pediatric neurosurgeon and at an institution where appropriate pediatric oncology or radiation therapy is not available.

Neuropathology

Experienced pathologists able to differentiate subtypes of pediatric neurological tumors are absent in many developing countries. The lack of trained personnel and inadequate technical equipment are therefore limiting the possibility to achieve a timely and accurate diagnosis in many places. Often, clinicians are faced with long turnover times—sometimes exceeding 1 month—before a diagnosis is proposed [15]. Availability of some important staining techniques may also compromise the possibility to accurately identify

tumor types. A classical example is the availability of the BAF47 staining. This staining that has now become part of the standard battery of immunohistochemical staining performed in the context of embryonal tumors of the central nervous system.

In a report on a telemedicine twinning experience between Canada and Jordan in pediatric neuro-oncology between two multidisciplinary programs, the most common recommendation was a review of the neuropathology, resulted in several cases in a change in the initial diagnosis or in the grading of the tumor with significant consequences in term of subsequent management [14]. Those results have been replicated in the ongoing twining program between Canada and Colombia. However, a number of factors are limiting this practice that would greatly benefit pediatric neuro-oncology programs in countries with limited resources. In this context, it is likely that a significant number of children are treated without an adequate diagnosis.

Radiation and Radiotherapy Services

Radiation therapy is a critical component of treatment of many central nervous system tumors in children; however, limited radiotherapy machines and personnel make them available only at large centers with long waiting lists. There is evidence that delay in starting radiotherapy has a negative impact on survival in medulloblastoma and there is no doubt that the extent of neurological recovery will be closely dependent on the time to initiate radiation in patients with diffuse intrinsic pontine glioma (DIPG).

Radiation indications, treatment volumes, and doses are determined by tumor histology, extent of disease, anticipated pattern of spread, and expected pattern of failure. In malignant CNS tumors such as medulloblastoma and ependymoma, excellent survival rates have been reported, particularly in patients with average risk features (complete resection and absence of metastatic disease and no anaplastic features). Survival rates are above 90 % in patients with pure germinoma, regardless of metastatic stage, with a combination of chemotherapy and radiation. However, access to radiation oncology services is a prerequisite for successful outcome and the number of functioning radiotherapy machines available in most countries with limited resources is the main barrier to optimal patient care. It is clear that pediatric neuro-oncology programs cannot be developed or implemented in countries, which have no radiation oncology services. A survey of radiotherapy equipments in Africa conducted in 1998 reported that 9/56 countries had no radiotherapy at all, 24 had orthovoltage facilities only, and 2/3 of the megavoltage equipments available in the continent were located in two countries (Egypt and South Africa) [16]. The supply of radiation equipments available in the continent represented at that time 18 % of the estimated needs. Appropriate maintenance of the radiation equipment is also an issue in countries where there is only one radiotherapy machine; the treatment could get interrupted for an undetermined period of time or waiting times can increase considerably if the machine goes out of service.

As a consequence, access to radiation is a major issue in most countries with limited resources, and delay in initiation and/or continuation of radiation treatment is a common problem.

In several places, pediatric oncologists are trying to overcome this problem by designing protocols that offer postoperative chemotherapy prior to radiation, in particular for medulloblastoma patients. Although this is not an ideal option, this approach may help prevent early recurrence or dissemination following initial surgery. Another limiting factor in the management is the number of well-qualified personnel with an expertise in CNS radiation techniques and more specifically in pediatrics. Craniospinal radiotherapy (CSI), which is commonly used in the management of medulloblastoma patients, is one of the most complex radiotherapy techniques, and evidence from several medulloblastoma trials has suggested that the quality of CSI impacts outcome. Some groups have started to

address specific issues related to the availability of radiation machines. In particular, a group in Cairo has run a randomized trial that has shown similar survival between patients with DIPG treated with normal fractionation (30 sessions at 1.8 Gy each) and hypofractionation (13 sessions of 3 Gy each) [17]. The results of this trial may benefit DIPG patients in countries that face limitations in the access to radiation services.

Ideally, the radiotherapeutic management of children with CNS tumor in countries with limited resources would benefit from a central referral system that would review and validate indications and facilitate timely access to the most appropriate equipment. Hopefully, cooperative groups and support groups will be able to advocate for the development of such process.

Pediatric Neuro-Oncologists

Dedicated pediatric oncologists interested in neuro-oncology are rare. In most of the countries with limited resources, pediatric oncologists are few and usually overworked. Their time is committed to clinical responsibilities and continuous medical education might not be a priority. In the absence of oncologists with specific training in pediatric neuro-oncology, treatment may lean more toward use of radiation rather than chemotherapy. This is particularly the case in the management of low-grade tumors such as low-grade gliomas of the optic pathways, of the brainstem, or of the spinal cord that can be managed with low-dose chemotherapy in most situations.

Absence of properly designed chemotherapy protocols suitable for developing countries, the intermittent supply of chemotherapeutic drugs, and absence of well-trained nurses would also affect the medical management of childhood brain tumors in these conditions. Some of the twinning programs and teleconference tumor boards have attempted to provide modified protocols that can be used in countries with limited resources (Table 27.2).

Table 27.2 Comparison of available resources in high-, middle-, and low-income countries

	DCs ($n=103$) vs. COG ($n=145$)	DCs ($n=103$) vs. HIC ($n=37$)
Centers seeing ≥150 newly diagnosed pediatric oncology patients per year	34 (33 %) vs. 24 (16.5 %) $p=0.004$	34 (33 %) vs. 10 (27 %) $p=0.6$
Centers seeing ≥15 newly diagnosed brain tumor patients per year	42 (40.7 %) vs. 60 (58.2 %) $p=0.9$	42 (40.7 %) vs. 22 (32 %) $p=0.07$
Centers with dedicated NO	NA	48 (46.6 %) vs. 27 (73 %) $p=0.004$
Availability of a general LTFU team	NA	69 (67 %) vs. 33 (89.2 %) $p=0.006$
Dedicated NO LTFU team for children	8 (7.7 %) vs. 43 (29.6 %) $p≤0.001$	8 (7.7 %) vs. 7 (21.1 %) $p=0.03$
Availability of disease-specific guidelines for the treatment of children with brain tumors	NA	71 (68.9 %) vs. 36 (97.3 %) $p<0.001$
Dedicated NO LTFU team for >21 years	14 (13.6 %) vs. 42 (30 %) $p≤0.001$	14 (13.6 %) vs. 12 (31.6 %) $p=0.02$
Formal NS evaluation in >50 % of irradiated children	9 (8.7 % vs. 78 (53.7 %) $p<0.001$	9 (8.7 %) vs. 17 (45.9 %) $p<0.001$
Availability of GH	NA	63 (61.2 %) vs. 35 (94.6 %) $p<0.001$

Reprinted from Qaddoumi I, Unal E, Diez B, et al. Web-based survey of resources for treatment and long-term follow-up for children with brain tumors in developing countries. Childs Nerv Syst 2011; 27(11):1957-1961. With permission from Springer Verlag
DC low income country, *COG* Children's Oncology Group, *HIC* high-income countries, *NO* neuro-oncology, *LTFU* long-term follow-up, *NS* neuropsychological, *GH* growth hormone, *NA* not assessed

Multidisciplinary Meetings

In pediatric neuro-oncology, there is a critical need for interaction between disciplines such as neurosurgery, neuroradiology, neuropathology, radiation oncology, and oncology. Optimization of cancer treatment depends on careful orchestration of the different treatment modalities in order to provide patients with maximal benefit. Discussions among team members will allow organizing the treatment plan for each specific patient.

Multidisciplinary meetings are part of the standard of care in many institutions in high-income countries. France and the UK have required for each newly diagnosed pediatric neuro-oncology patient review of the case and the agreement on a treatment plan by a multidisciplinary team of experts. High-income countries have also formed national wide neuro-oncology multidisciplinary groups like the Pediatric Canadian Brain Tumor Consortium, where neurosurgeons, neuro-oncologist, neuroradiologist, and allied healthcare member can share their

concerns and experiences and develop a national standard of care treatment approach.

Implementation of multidisciplinary neuro-oncology programs in countries with limited resources is slow. Most physicians in low-income countries still work in silo and are not convinced of the benefit of a dialog between team members, particularly with physicians outside their area of expertise. The role of the pediatric oncologist in this context is critical, even when patients may not require chemotherapy. Multidisciplinary meeting should involve all team members with no exception, in order to discuss every aspect of the care of the patient. In this context, the presence of radiologists, pathologists, neurosurgeons, oncologists, and radiation oncologists at these meetings is critical.

Treatment Side Effects

During the course of treatment, children with brain tumors are prone to many challenges whether related to their original disease or to the applied

Table 27.3 Comparison of centers from low- and upper middle-income countries regarding center characteristics, availability of resources and follow-up resources

	L-LMIC (n=45)	UMIC (n=58)	p Value
# of pediatric oncology patients per year			(≥150 cases/year)
<49	11	17	
50–99	5	22	
100–149	4	10	
150–199	4	3	
>200	21	6	
# of brain tumor patients per year			(≥30 cases/year) 0.34
<4	10	9	
5–14	15	27	
15–29	7	11	
30–49	5	7	
>50	8	4	
Dedicated brain tumor team	Yes, 17 (37.8 %)	Yes, 31 (53.4 %)	0.08
Dedicated LTFU clinic for pediatric oncology patients in general	Yes, 28 (62.2 %)	Yes, 41 (70.7 %)	0.2
Availability of follow-up programs for survivors >21 years in the setting	Yes, 18 (40 %)	Yes, 30 (51.7 %)	0.16
Availability of institutional treatment guidelines for the different brain tumors	Yes, 24 (33.8 %)	Yes, 47 (66.2 %)	0.002
Availability of GH	Yes, 22 (48.9 %)	Yes, 41 (70.7 %)	0.02

Reprinted from Qaddoumi I, Unal E, Diez B, et al. Web-based survey of resources for treatment and long-term follow-up for children with brain tumors in developing countries. Childs Nerv Syst 2011; 27(11):1957-1961. With permission from Springer Verlag

L-LMC low- and middle-income countries, *UMIC* upper middle-income countries, *HIC* high-income countries, *LTFU* long-term follow-up, *NS* neuropsychological, *GH* growth hormone

treatment protocols. They may require physical and occupational rehabilitation, mental and psychosocial support, and reintegration programs. When present, visual and hearing deficits need to be assessed, and patients should be directed to specific facilities that will help them to deal with these difficulties. These are generally not a priority in low-income countries, and physicians should be aware that the use of, for example, ototoxic medications can lead to irreversible hearing loss and usually correcting devices are unaffordable.

Supportive therapy during treatment is also a concern in developing countries; appropriate nutritional support during chemotherapy and radiotherapy can be a challenge, and dietitians dedicated to pediatric oncology are not a reality in most of these countries; prophylactic antibiotics and antifungal are part of the practice in some of these countries, but their use is inconsistent due to the lack of treatment protocols.

Many children will also need hormonal supplementation after brain irradiation. Availability of regular endocrine testing and daily administration of hormone replacement, like growth hormone, may be challenging in countries with limited resources. In reality, most children with CNS tumors are very early lost to follow-up in countries with limited resources. A recent international survey showed that the number of aftercare program in countries with limited resources was limited [18]. It is clear that well-designed programs for assessment of aftercare morbidities are difficult to implement in this context (Table 27.3).

Palliative Care

Owing to the delayed diagnosis, many children with brain tumor diagnosed in countries with limited resources present with advanced disease, and very often in this context, supportive care and palliative treatment would be the most appropriate option. In addition, a number of pediatric brain tumors have a poor prognosis, such as high-grade glioma, DIPG, or atypical teratoid rhabdoid tumors. It is expected that in such context, a majority of patients will eventually succumb to their disease. Pain control and proper palliative care interventions would be important at this stage. Low-income countries are particularly lacking such services [19] and families often perceive palliative care as an abandonment of treatment. Other issues are critical such as access to appropriate pain medications. There is an obvious need to develop palliative care guidelines that address the need of the pediatric brain tumor population in these countries and that also take into account local or regional specificities, either social or cultural or religious. A recent work conducted in families of children diagnosed with DIPG in Jordan suggested that it is possible to address palliative care issues at an early stage and this approach can facilitate the implementation of end of life decisions [20].

Twinning Programs

In the face of the many challenges associated with the management of childhood brain tumor in countries with limited resources, efforts have been developed to implement neuro-oncology programs through twinning initiatives. Support from high-income countries to pediatric oncologists in countries with limited resources provides scientific expertise and can improve management of CNS tumors in these countries. Such initiatives have shown success in the management of childhood leukemia [6], demonstrating that proven treatment regimens can be adapted for use in countries with limited resources.

Previous experience with neuro-oncology twinning programs and teleconference tumor boards [14] have shown that with very little resources, a difference can be made in the diagnosis and therapeutic approaches of these unprivileged children. Although the multidisciplinary care in neuro-oncology requires specific

attention, successful twinning initiatives have been described with significant impact on management and outcomes [21, 22].

Conclusion

The concept of pediatric neuro-oncology is still at its infancy in countries with limited resources. Appropriate neuroimaging facilities, neurosurgical units, radiation equipment, and pediatric oncology services are prerequisites for the implementation of such programs. A number of programs have been recently implemented, often in the context of twinning initiatives and teleconferenced tumor boards, attempting to provide expertise and therapeutic approaches adapted to the needs of these countries.

References

1. Ribeiro RC, Steliarova-Foucher E, Magrath I, Lemerle J, Eden T, Forget C, Mortara I, Tabah-Fisch I, Divino JJ, Miklavec T, Howard SC, Cavalli F. Baseline status of paediatric oncology care in ten low-income or mid-income countries receiving My Child Matters support: a descriptive study. Lancet Oncol. 2008;9(8):721–9.
2. Asirvatham JR, Deepti AN, Chyne R, Prasad MS, Chacko AG, Rajshekhar V, Chacko G. Pediatric tumors of the central nervous system: a retrospective study of 1,043 cases from a tertiary care center in South India. Childs Nerv Syst. 2011;27(8):1257–63.
3. Curado MP, Voti L, Sortino-Rachou AM. Cancer registration data and quality indicators in low and middle income countries: their interpretation and potential use for the improvement of cancer care. Cancer Causes Control. 2009;20(5):751–6.
4. Usmani GN. Pediatric oncology in the third world. Curr Opin Pediatr. 2001;13(1):1–9.
5. Dolecek TA, Propp JM, Stroup NE, Kruchko C. CBTRUS statistical report: primary brain and central nervous system tumors diagnosed in the United States in 2005-2009. Neuro Oncol. 2012;14(5):v1–49.
6. Howard SC, Metzger ML, Wilimas JA, Quintana Y, Pui CH, Robison LL, Ribeiro RC. Childhood cancer epidemiology in low-income countries. Cancer. 2008; 112(3):461–72.
7. Manoharan N, Julka PK, Rath GK. Descriptive epidemiology of primary brain and CNS tumors in Delhi, 2003-2007. Asian Pac J Cancer Prev. 2012;13(2):637–40.
8. Dang-Tan T, Franco EL. Diagnosis delays in childhood cancer: a review. Cancer. 2007;110(4):703–13.
9. El-Fiki M. African neurosurgery, the 21st-century challenge. World Neurosurg. 2010;73(4):254–8.

10. Hamidah A, Rustam ZA, Tamil AM, Zarina LA, Zulkifli ZS, Jamal R. Prevalence and parental perceptions of complementary and alternative medicine use by children with cancer in a multi-ethnic Southeast Asian population. Pediatr Blood Cancer. 2009;52(1):70–4.
11. Bhopal SS, Mann KD, Pearce MS. Registration of cancer in girls remains lower than expected in countries with low/middle incomes and low female education rates. Br J Cancer. 2012;107(1):183–8.
12. Mostert S, Arora RS, Arreola M, Bagai P, Friedrich P, Gupta S, Kaur G, Koodiyedath B, Kulkarni K, Lam CG, Luna-Fineman S, Pizer B, Rivas S, Rossell N, Sitaresmi MN, Tsimicalis A, Weaver M, Ribeiro RC. Abandonment of treatment for childhood cancer: position statement of a SIOP PODC Working Group. Lancet Oncol. 2011;12(8):719–20.
13. El Khamlichi A. African neurosurgery: current situation, priorities, and needs. Neurosurgery. 2001;48(6):1344–7.
14. Qaddoumi I, Mansour A, Musharbash A, Drake J, Swaidan M, Tihan T, Bouffet E. Impact of telemedicine on pediatric neuro-oncology in a developing country: the Jordanian-Canadian experience. Pediatr Blood Cancer. 2007;48(1):39–43.
15. Berezowska S, Tomoka T, Kamiza S, Milner Jr DA, Langer R. Surgical pathology in sub-Saharan Africa–volunteering in Malawi. Virchows Arch. 2012;460(4):363–70.
16. Levin CV, El Gueddari B, Meghzifene A. Radiation therapy in Africa: distribution and equipment. Radiother Oncol. 1999;52(1):79–84.
17. Zaghloul M, Ahmed S, Eldebaway E, Mousa A, Amin A, Elkhateeb N, Sabry M. Hypofractionated radiotherapy for pediatric diffuse intrinsic pontine glioma (DIPG): a prospective controlled randomized trial. Neuro Oncol. 2012;14:i26–32.
18. Qaddoumi I, Unal E, Diez B, Kebudi R, Quintana Y, Bouffet E, Chantada G. Web-based survey of resources for treatment and long-term follow-up for children with brain tumors in developing countries. Childs Nerv Syst. 2011;27(11):1957–61.
19. Delgado E, Barfield RC, Baker JN, Hinds PS, Yang J, Nambayan A, Quintana Y, Kane JR. Availability of palliative care services for children with cancer in economically diverse regions of the world. Eur J Cancer. 2010;46(12):2260–6.
20. Qaddoumi I, Ezam N, Swaidan M, Jaradat I, Mansour A, Abuirmeileh N, Bouffet E, Al-Hussaini M. Diffuse pontine glioma in Jordan and impact of up-front prognosis disclosure with parents and families. J Child Neurol. 2009;24(4):460–5.
21. Qaddoumi I, Musharbash A, Elayyan M, Mansour A, Al-Hussaini M, Drake J, Swaidan M, Bartels U, Bouffet E. Closing the survival gap: implementation of medulloblastoma protocols in a low-income country through a twinning program. Int J Cancer. 2008;122(6):1203–6.
22. Baskin JL, Lezcano E, Kim BS, Figueredo D, Lassaletta A, Perez-Martinez A, Madero L, Caniza MA, Howard SC, Samudio A, Finlay JL. Management of children with brain tumors in Paraguay. Neuro Oncol. 2013;15(2):235–41.

Index

K. Scheinemann and E. Bouffet (eds.), *Pediatric Neuro-oncology*,
DOI 10.1007/978-1-4939-1541-5, © Springer Science+Business Media New York 2015

CPSIA information can be obtained at www.ICGtesting.com
Printed in the USA
LVOW05*1759290315

432474LV00004B/7/P

9 781493 915408